The Art of the Shoe

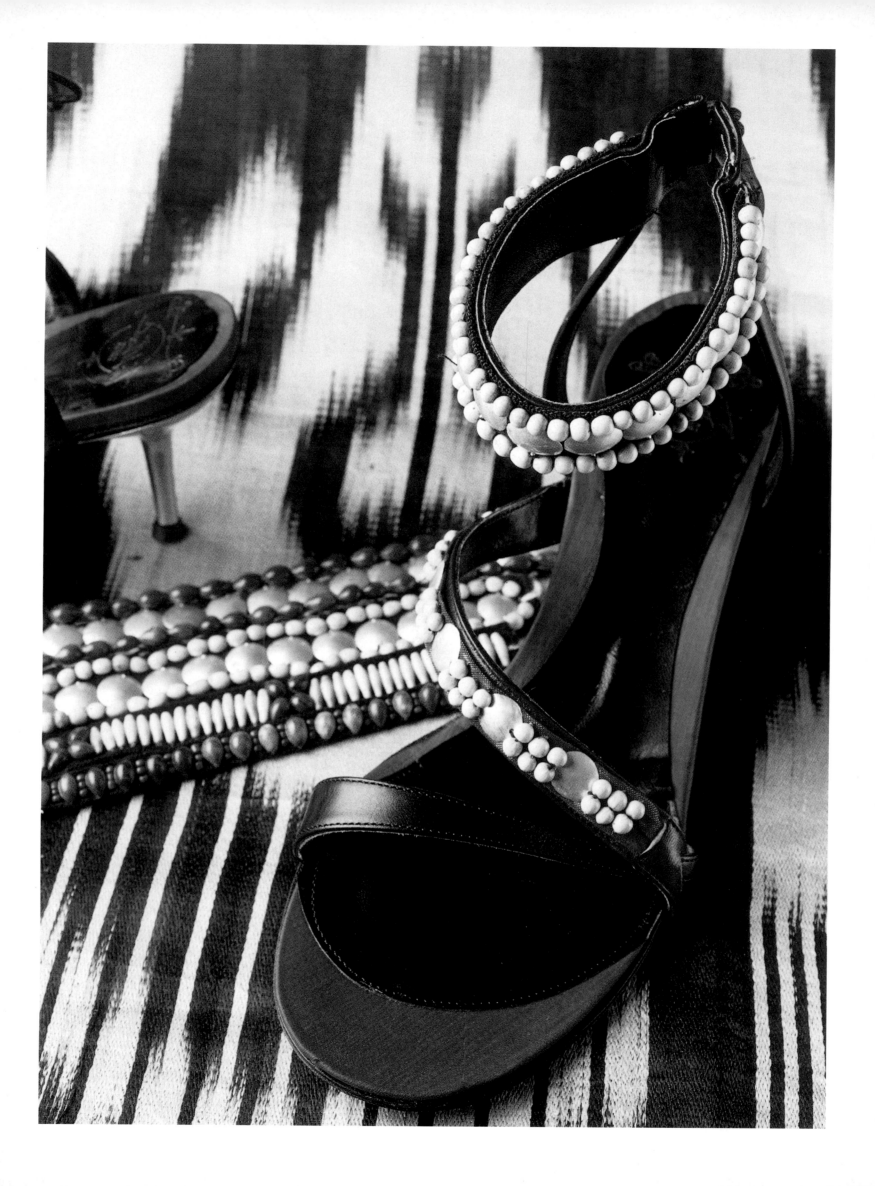

The Art of the Shoe

Marie-Josèphe Bossan

Author: Marie-Josèphe Bossan

Translator: Rebecca Brimacombe

ISBN 1-85995-803-6

Printed in France

Special thanks to the city of Romans, France, and Joël Garnier for his photographs.

Contents

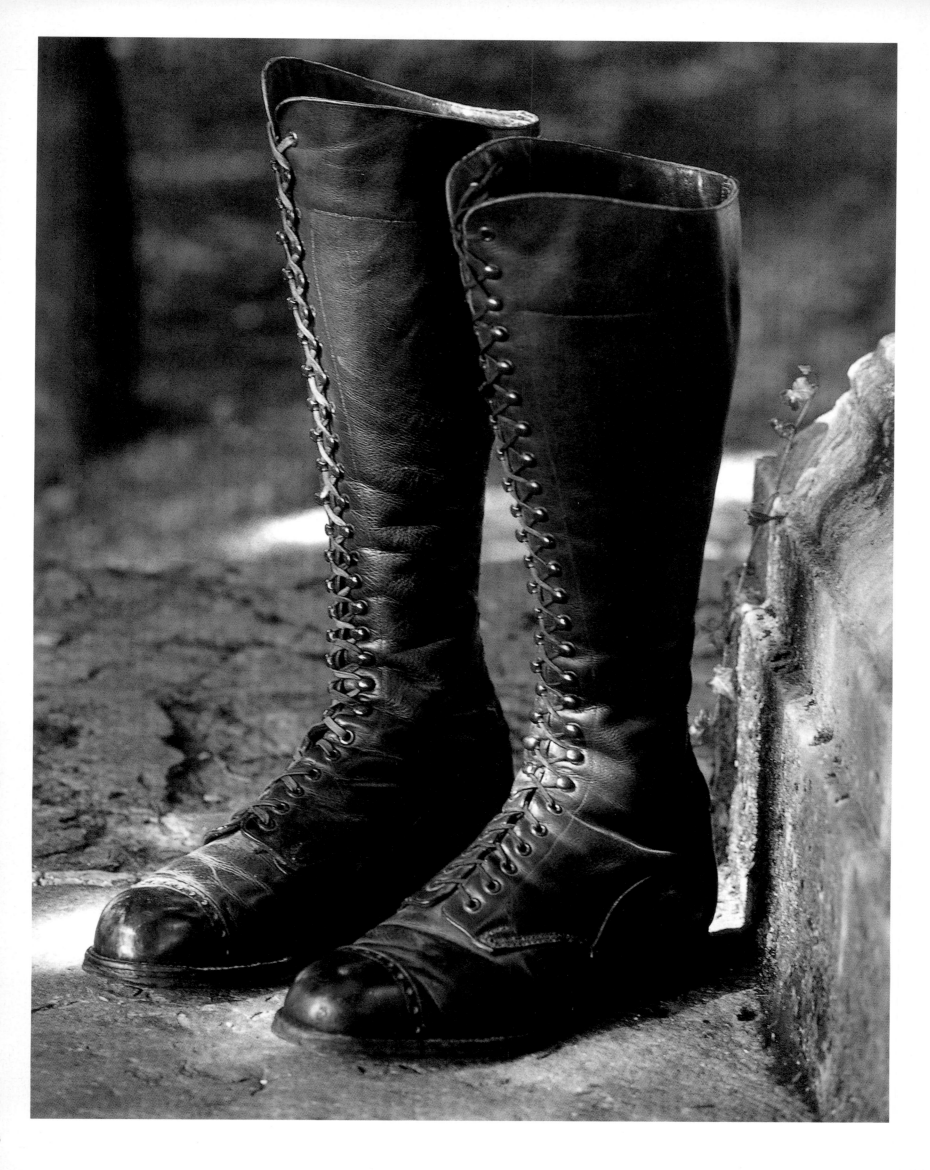

Introduction

The Shoe: Object of Civilization and Object of Art

Aside from noticing a shoe for its comfort or elegance, contemporaries rarely take interest in this necessary object of daily life. However, the shoe is considerable in the history of civilization and art.

In losing contact with nature, we have lost sight of the shoe's profound significance. In recapturing this contact, in particular through sports, we begin its rediscovery. Shoes for skiing, hiking, hunting, football, tennis or horseriding are carefully chosen, indispensable tools as well as revealing signs of occupation or taste.

In previous centuries, when people depended more on the climate, vegetation and condition of the soil, while most jobs involved physical labour, the shoe held an importance for everyone which today it holds for very few. We do not wear the same shoes in snow as in the tropics, in the forest as in the steppe, in the swamps as in the mountains or when working, hunting or fishing. For this reason, shoes give precious indications of habitats and modes of life.

In strongly hierarchical societies, organized by castes or orders, clothing was determinant. Princes, bourgeoisie, soldiers, clergy and servers were differentiated by what they wore. The shoe revealed, less spectacularly than the hat, but in a more demanding way, the respective brilliance of civilizations, unveiling the social classes and the subtlety of the race; a sign of recognition, just as the ring slips only onto the slenderest finger, the "glass slipper" will not fit but the most delicate of beauties.

The shoe transmits its message to us by the customs which impose and condition it. It teaches us of the deformations that were forced on the feet of Chinese women and shows us how in India, by conserving the unusual boots, the nomadic horsemen of the North attained their sovereignty over the Indian continent; we learn that ice-skates evoke the Hammans while babouches suggest the Islamic interdiction to enter holy places with covered feet.

Sometimes the shoe is symbolic, evoked in ritual or tied to a crucial moment of existence. One tells of the purpose high-heels served: to make the woman taller on her wedding night in order to remind her that it is the only moment when she will dominate her husband.

The boots of the Shaman were decorated with animal skins and bones in order to emulate the stag; as the stag, he could run in the world of spirits. We are what we wear, so if to ascend to a higher life it is necessary to ornate the head, if it becomes an issue of ease of movement, it is the feet that are suited for adornment. Athena had shoes of gold, for Hermes, it was heels. Perseus, in search of flight, went to the nymphs to find winged sandals.

Tales respond to mythology. The seven-league boots, which enlarged or shrunk to fit the ogre or Little Thumb, allowed them both to run across the universe. "You have only to make me a pair of boots," said Puss in Boots to his master, "and you will see that you are not so badly dealt as you believe."

Does the shoe therefore serve to transcend the foot, often considered as the most modest and least favored part of the human body? Occasionally, without a doubt, but not always. The barefoot is not always deprived of the sacred and, thus, can communicate this to the shoe. Those who supplicate or venerate are constantly throwing themselves at the feet of men; it is the feet of men who leave a trace on humid or dusty ground, often the only witness to their passage. A specific accessory, the shoe can sometimes serve to represent he who has worn it, who has disappeared, of whom we do not dare to retrace the traits; the most characteristic example is offered by primitive Buddhism evoking the image of its founder by a seat or by a footprint.

Made of the most diverse materials, from leather to wood, from fabric to straw, or whether plain or ornamented, the shoe, by its form and decoration, becomes an object of art. If the form is sometimes more functional than esthetic – but not always, and there will be a place to explain many aberrant forms – the design of the cloth, the broidery, the incrustations, the choice of colours, always closely reveal the artistic characteristics of their native country.

The essential interest comes from that which it is not; weapons or musical instruments are reserved for a caste or a determined social group, carpets are the products of only one or two civilizations, it does not stand up as a "sumptuous" object of the rich classes or a folkloric object of the poor. The shoe has been used from the bottom to the top of the social ladder, by all the individuals of any given group, from group to group, by the entire world.

Jean-Paul Roux,
Honorary Director of Research at the C.N.R.S.
Honorary Tenured Professor of the Islamic Arts
at the School of the Louvre

1. "Akha" sandal, dress of the Akha tribes of the Golden Triangle
   (box of recycled coca and jungle seed, 6 cm steel heel, leather). Trikitrixa, Paris.
2. Aviator Boots, c. 1914, France.

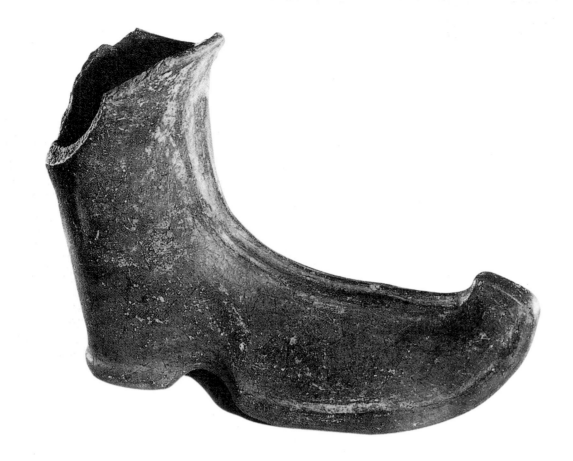

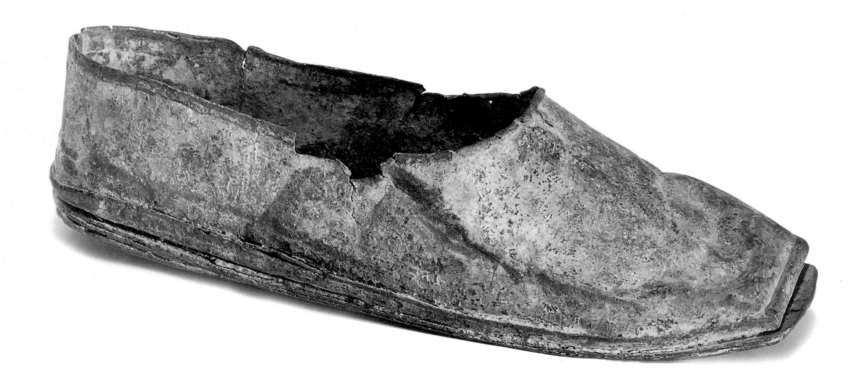

3. Clay model of shoe with upturned toe from an Azerbaijanian tomb,
13th-12th century BC. Bally Museum, Schönenwerd, Switzerland.
4. Iron shoe. Syria, 800 BC. Bally Museum, Schönenwerd, Switzerland.

From Antiquity up to our days

Prehistory

Prehistoric man evidently was unfamiliar with shoes: the Stone Age markings that are known to us all indicate bare feet. But the cave paintings discovered in Spain dating from the Upper Paleolithic period (around 14,000 BC) show Magdalenian man dressed in fur boots. According to the French paleontologist and prehistorian Father Breuil (1877-1961), Neolithic man covered his feet with animal skins as protection in a harsh environment. It seems that man has always instinctively covered his feet to get about, although there remains no concrete evidence of the shoes themselves. Prehistoric shoes would have been rough in design and certainly utilitarian in function. The well-preserved boots worn by Ötzi the Iceman discovered in an Alpine glacier are an excellent example. Their deerskin uppers and bearskin soles enabled him to travel long distances to trade. These materials were chosen primarily for their ability to shield the feet from severe conditions. It was only in Antiquity that the shoe would acquire an aesthetic and decorative dimension, becoming a true indicator of social status.

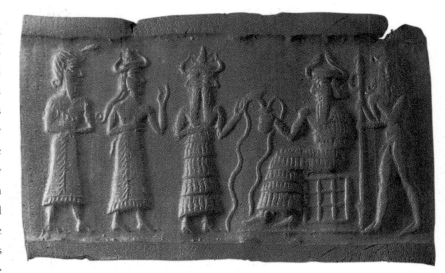

Antiquity
The Shoe in Ancient Eastern Civilizations

From the first great civilizations flourishing in Mesopotamia and Egypt in the 4th millennium BC arose the three basic types of footwear: the shoe, the boot, and the sandal. An archeological team excavating a temple in the city of Brak (Syria) in 1938 unearthed a clay shoe with a raised toe. Dating over 3,000 years before the birth of Christ, it proves that this city shared features with the Sumerian civilization of Ur in Mesopotamia: raised-tipped shoes are depicted on Mesopotamian seals of the Akkadian era around 2600 BC. Distinguished from Syrian models by a much higher tip and embellished with a pompom, in Mesopotamia this type of shoe became the royal footwear of the king. The raised-toe form is attributable to the rugged terrain of the mountain conquerors that introduced it. After its adoption by the Akkadian kingdom, the form spread to Asia Minor where the Hittites made it a part of their national costume. It is frequently depicted in low-reliefs, such as the Yazilikaya sanctuary carvings dating to 1275 BC. Seafaring Phoenicians helped spread the pointed shoe to Cyprus, Mycenae, and Crete, where it appears on palace frescoes depicting royal games and ceremonies. Cretans are also depicted wearing raised-tipped ankle boots in the painted decorations of Rekhmire's tomb (Egypt 18th dynasty, 1580-1558 BC), indicating contact between Crete and Egypt during this era. The Mesopotamian empire of Assyria dominated the ancient east from the 9th to the 7th century BC and erected monuments whose sculptures depict the sandal and the boot. Their sandal is a simplified shoe composed of a sole and straps. Their boot is tall, covering the leg; a type of footwear associated with horsemen. From the middle of the 6th century to the end of the 4th century BC, the Persian dynasty, founded by Cyrus the Great II around 550 BC, gradually established a homogeneous culture in the ancient east. Processional bas-reliefs carved by sculptors of the Achaemenidian kings offer a documentary record of the period's costume and footwear.

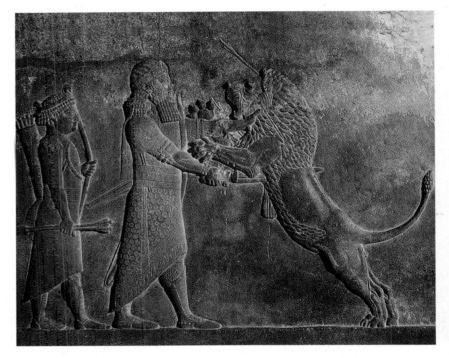

In addition to images of boots, there are shoes made of supple materials and of leather shown completely covering the foot and closing at the ankle with laces. For a deeper understanding of how the shoe evolved from its origins to the present day, it is important to look at ancient civilizations in their historical context. Additionally, an analysis of the primary biblical texts will shed new light on the subject and give greater relevance to the history of the shoe.

5. Cylindrical seal and its stamp. Akkad Dynasty, Mesopotamia, around 2340-2200 BC. Height: 3.6 cm. Louvre Museum, Paris.

6. "Lion put to death by the King," low-relief from the Palace of Assurbanipal at Nineveh, 638-630 BC, British Museum, London.

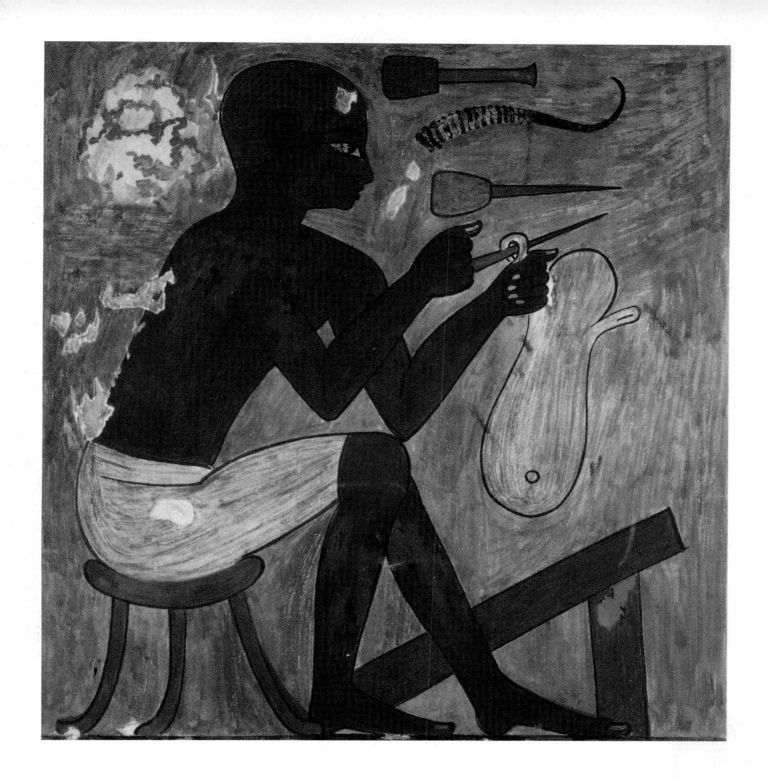

Ancient Egypt

Ancient Egypt was the home of the first sandals. This form of flat shoe with straps arose in response to Egypt's climate and geography.

King Narmer's Palette from around 3100 BC reveals that a servant called a "sandal bearer" walked behind the sovereign carrying the royal sandals on his forearms, indicating the importance henceforth attached to the shoe in ceremonial garb.

Although often depicted barefoot in Egyptian wall paintings, men and women also wore sandals. Egyptian sandals were made of leather, woven straw, strips of palm or papyrus leaves or from the rushes and reeds that grew in the marshes. The Pharaoh and the socially prominent had them made of gold, though sandals were a luxury item for everyone. Tomb excavations have revealed that this object, originally strictly utilitarian, had a social function. The sandal maintained continuity of form throughout Pharaonic civilization and lasted until the Coptic era of Egyptian Christianity. When the pharaoh entered the temple, or when his subjects celebrated the cult of the dead in funeral chapels, they removed their sandals at the sanctuary's entrance, a custom later adopted by Muslims upon entering a mosque. The ritual demonstrates the strong relationship that exists between the shoe and the sacred, a relationship that is also established by specific biblical passages, which will be discussed below. The advent in Egypt of the raised-tip sandal in the second millennium BC is probably a Hittite influence. It is the precursor of the poulaine, or piked shoe, an eccentric medieval fashion introduced to Europe from the East by the Crusades. When sandals are among the items packed for the mummy's afterlife, they are placed in chests or illustrated on horizontal bands decorating the painted interior of the wooden sarcophagi. Evidently, their role was prophylactic.

Texts from the era of the pyramids allude to and reflect the wishes of the dead "to walk in white sandals along the beautiful paths of heaven where the blessed roam."

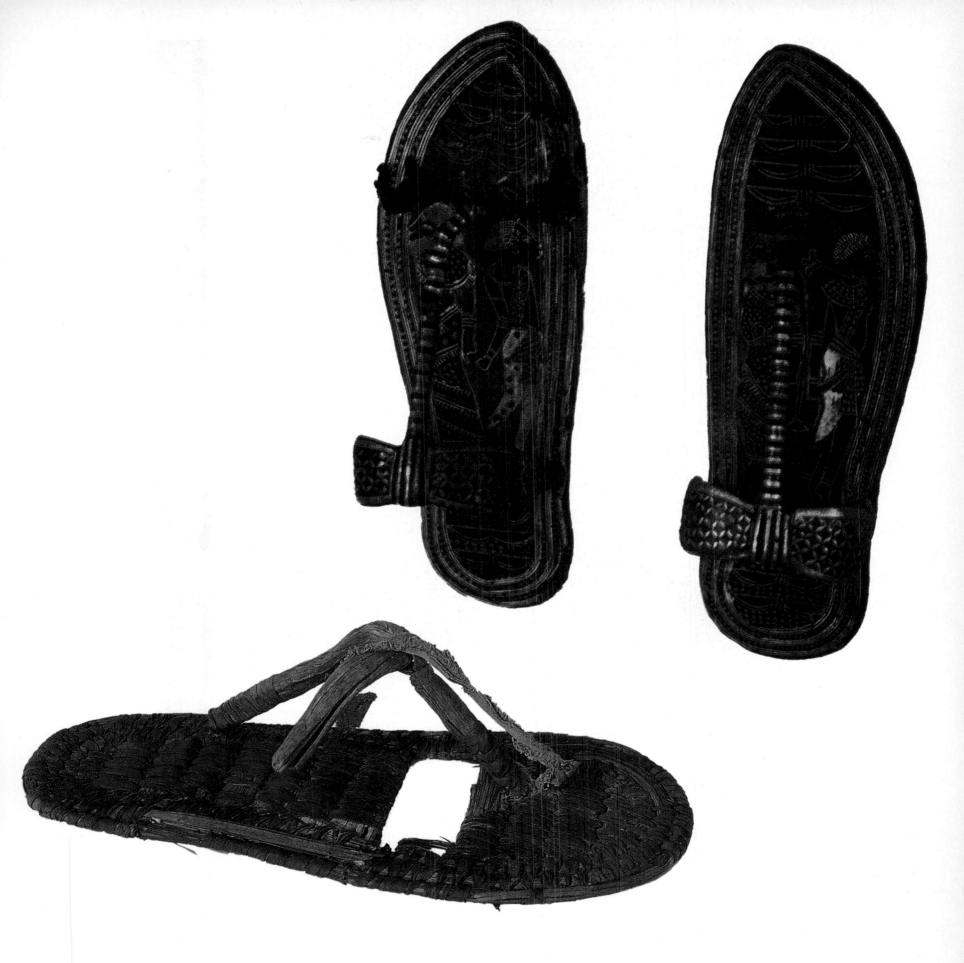

7. Sandals maker, fresco relief. 18th Dynasty, 1567-1320 BC. The Metropolitan Museum of Art, New York.

8. Wooden sandals inlayed with gold, treasure of Tutankhamen. 18th Dynasty, Thebes. Cairo Museum, Cairo.

9. Egyptian sandal of plant fibers. Bally Museum, Schönenwerd, Switzerland.

The Bible: The Shoe in the Old Testament

The earliest written evidence of shoes is considered to be that found in the Bible, although research remains to be done with Chinese, Egyptian, and Mesopotamian texts.

As a rule, Biblical characters wear sandals, whether they are God's chosen ones (the Hebrews), their allies, or enemies, which affirms the Near Eastern origin of this footwear type from earliest antiquity. The Old Testament rarely mentions the design and decoration of the sandal. Apart from its role as an invaluable aid to walking, which is mainly an issue concerning the lives of the Saints, the sandal plays an important symbolic role. Biblical shoe symbolism can be analyzed in its different contexts, which include the removal of shoes in holy places, the shoe in military expeditions, legal actions, and everyday rituals, as well as the shoe as an accessory of seduction when dressing a female foot.

In the most famous example of removing one's shoes in a holy place, the vision of the burning bush, God orders Moses to take off his shoes: "Do not draw near this place. Take your sandals off your feet, for the place where you stand is holy ground" (The Pentateuch, Exodus, III, 5).

The situation repeats itself when the Hebrews come upon the entrance to the Promised Land, as recorded in the Book of Joshua: "And it came to pass, when Joshua was by Jericho, that he lifted his eyes and looked, and behold, a Man stood opposite him with His sword drawn in His hand. And Joshua went to Him and said to Him, 'Are You for us or for our adversaries?' So He said, 'No, but as Commander of the army of the LORD I have now come.' And Joshua fell on his face to the earth and worshiped, and said to Him, 'What does my Lord say to His servant?' Then the Commander of the LORD's army said to Joshua, 'Take your sandal off your foot, for the place where you stand is holy'" (Joshua, 5:13-15).

The order given to Joshua is identical to that given to Moses. Shoes figure in another story from Joshua. The kings, finding themselves beyond the river Jordan, formed a coalition to fight against Joshua and Israel, but the Gibeonites wanted to ally themselves with Israel at any price. So the Gibeonites planned a ruse that would make Israel think they came from a distant land:

"And they took old sacks on their donkeys, old wineskins torn and mended, old and patched sandals on their feet, and old garments on themselves" (Joshua 9:3). Dressed in this fashion they went to find Joshua, who asked them, "Who are you, and where do you come from?" They replied, "From a very far country your servants have come... And these wineskins which we filled were new, and see, they are torn; and these our garments and our sandals have become old because of the very long journey" (Joshua, 9:5, 8, 13).

These old sandals contrast with the ones mentioned in Moses' last sermon when he says to his people: "And I have led you forty years in the wilderness. Your clothes have not worn out on you, and your sandals have not worn out on your feet" (Deuteronomy, 29:5).

The Old Testament mentions footwear in a number of military contexts. The wars against the Philistines are the setting for the Books of Samuel. The rich iconography of the famous battle of David and Goliath, pointing to a much later date than the event itself, which took place between 1010 and 970 BC, usually shows the Philistine giant dressed in sandals and leg armor, but only the leg armor is mentioned in the Bible: "He had a bronze helmet on his head, and he was armed with a coat of mail,

and the weight of the coat was five thousand shekels of bronze. And he had bronze armor on his legs and a bronze javelin between his shoulders" (Samuel, 17:5-6).

The sandal is part of the war imagery evoked in David's exhortations to Solomon, when the king reminds his son that his servant Joab had murdered two of Israel's army commanders: "And he shed the blood of war in peacetime, and put the blood of war on his belt that was around his waist, and on his sandals that were on his feet" (Kings, 2:5). And the messianic prophet Isaiah evokes the sandal when speaking of a military threat from a distant nation: "No one will be weary or stumble among them, No one will slumber or sleep; Nor will the belt on their loins be loosed, Nor the strap of their sandals be broken; Whose arrows are sharp, And all their bows bent" (Isaiah, 5:27-28). Shoes and the lack thereof also figure prominently in Isaiah's prophesy of Egypt's defeat against Assyria, its ancient rival for domination over the Near East: "In the year that Tartan came to Ashdod, when Sargon the king of Assyria sent him, and he fought against Ashdod and took it, at the same time the Lord spoke by Isaiah the son of Amoz, saying, 'Go, and remove the sackcloth from your body, and take your sandals off your feet.' And he did so, walking naked and barefoot. Then the Lord said, 'Just as My servant Isaiah has walked naked and barefoot three years for a sign and a wonder against Egypt and Ethiopia, so shall the king of Assyria lead away the Egyptians as prisoners and the Ethiopians as captives, young and old, naked and barefoot, with their buttocks uncovered, to the shame of Egypt. Then they shall be afraid and ashamed of Ethiopia their expectation and Egypt their glory'" (Isaiah, 20:1-5).

To cast or set down ones shoe in a place symbolized occupancy. In an image reminiscent of the Pharaoh Tutankhamen trampling his enemies underfoot, Psalms 60 and 108 celebrate preparations for a military expedition against Edam: "Moab is My wash pot; Over Edom I will cast My shoe; Philistia, shout in triumph because of Me." "Through God we will do valiantly, For it is He who shall tread down our enemies" (Psalm, 60:8; 12; Psalm, 108:9:13). In the kingdom of Israel, to tag a field with ones foot or to leave ones sandal there symbolized legal ownership. The fundamental text on this tradition is in the Book of Ruth: "Now this was the custom in former times in Israel concerning redeeming and exchanging, to confirm anything: one man took off his sandal and gave it to the other, and this was a confirmation in Israel. Therefore the close relative said to Boaz, 'Buy it for yourself.' So he took off his sandal. And Boaz said to the elders and all the people, 'You are witnesses this day that I have bought all that was Elimelech's, and all that was Chilion's and Mahlon's, from the hand of Naomi. Moreover, Ruth the Moabitess, the widow of Mahlon, I have acquired as my wife, to perpetuate the name of the dead through his inheritance, that the name of the dead may not be cut off from among his brethren and from his position at the gate. You are witnesses this day'" (Ruth, 4:7-10). The sandal's legal symbolism is also evident in the Hebrew law requiring a man to marry his brother's widow if the brother left no male heir. Deuteronomy provides an explicit commentary: "But if the man does not want to take his brother's wife, then let his brother's wife go up to the gate to the elders, and say, 'My husband's brother refuses to raise up a name to his brother in Israel; he will not perform the duty of my husband's brother.' Then the elders of his city shall call him and speak to him. But if he stands firm and says, 'I do not want to take her,' Then his brother's wife shall come to him in the presence of the elders, remove his sandal

10. Domenico Feti. *Moses before the Burning Bush.*

Kunsthistorisches Museum, Vienna.

from his foot, spit in his face, and answer and say, 'So shall it be done to the man who will not build up his brother's house.'

And his name shall be called in Israel, 'The house of him who had his sandal removed'" (Deuteronomy, 25:7-10). To walk barefoot also symbolized mourning. In one ritual, the deceased's relatives went bareheaded and barefoot with their faces partially covered by a type of scarf and ate gifts of bread from their neighbors. Ezekiel mentions the practice in reference to the mourning of the prophet: "Son of man, with one blow I am about to take away from you the delight of your eyes. Yet do not lament or weep or shed any tears. Groan quietly; do not mourn for the dead. Keep your turban fastened and your sandals on your feet; do not cover the lower part of your face or eat the customary food of mourners" (Ezekiel, 24:16-17).

In the 8th century BC Amos evoked the legal rights of the poor and the destitute and railed against the fairness of Israel's courts, corrupted by money. For example, Judges of Israel would issue judgments on insufficient grounds in exchange for a modest gift, a practice the prophet denounced: "I will not turn away its punishment, Because they sell the righteous for silver, And the poor for a pair of sandals" (Amos, 2:6-8).

The sandal symbolizes seduction in the Book of Judith, which recounts the occupation of a small Palestinian village called Bethulia by the armies of the Assyrian king Nebuchadnezzar: "I will cover all the land with the feet of my soldiers, to whom I will deliver them as spoils." (Judith, 2:7)

So Judith, who was a pious widow, got ready to leave town and give herself up to the enemy camp: "She chose sandals for her feet, and put on her anklets, bracelets, rings, earrings, and all her other jewelry. Thus she made herself very beautiful, to captivate the eyes of all the men who should see her." (Judith, 10:4) With her beauty the young woman aroused the passion of Holphernes, the army's leader, eventually taking advantage of his stupor after a banquet to cut off his head. In this way she diverted the attention of his armed forces, which included 120,000 infantrymen and 120,000 horsemen. In the hymn of thanksgiving sung by this biblical Joan of Arc, the victorious sandal counts among the accessories of feminine seduction: "Her sandals caught his eyes, and her beauty captivated his mind. The sword cut through his neck" (Judith, 16:9 New American Bible).

The Bible is mostly reticent concerning the aesthetics of the shoe. Ezekiel alludes to it discretely in the guilty loves of Jerusalem: "I clothed you with an embroidered dress and put leather sandals on you. I dressed you in fine linen and covered you with costly garments" (Ezekiel, 16:10). And if the word boot only appears once in Isaiah ("Every warrior's boot used in battle" (The Birth of the Prince of Peace, Isaiah, 9:5, New International Version), the sandal is primarily recognized as a symbol. This symbolism endures in the Muslim ritual of removing shoes before entering a mosque, a ritual that continues in the Muslim world day.

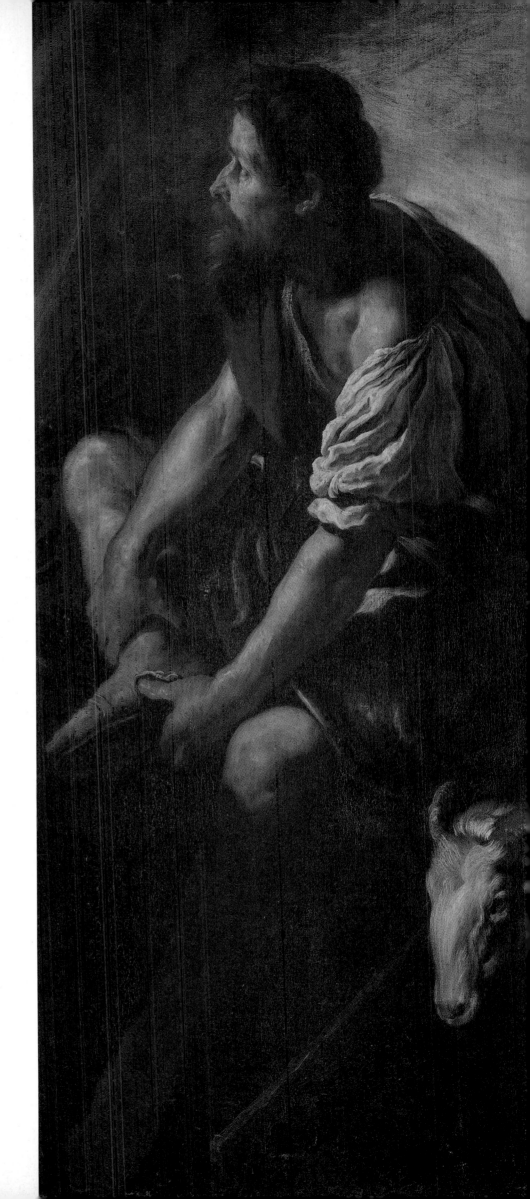

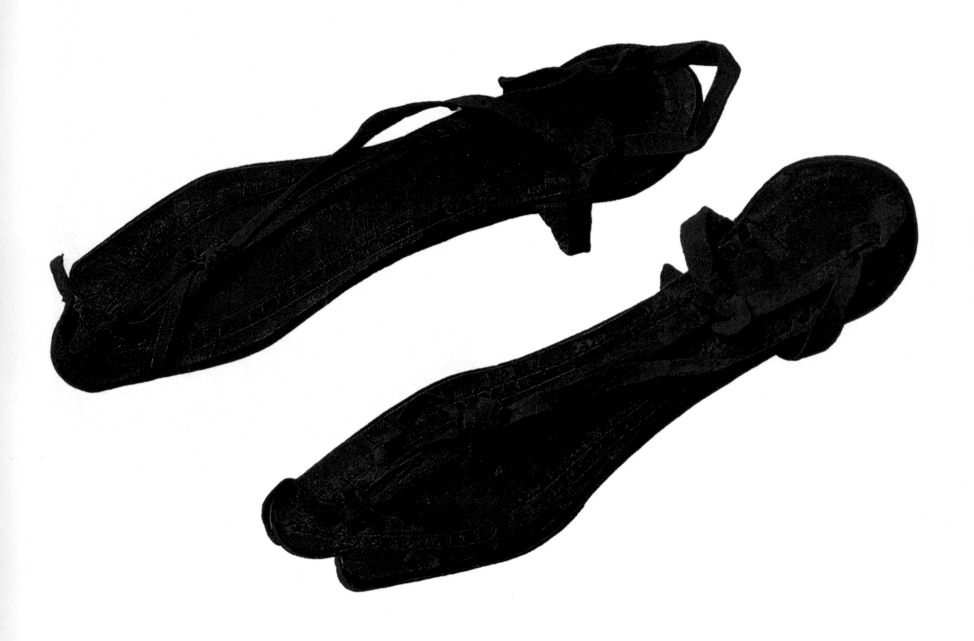

11. Sandals found in the fortress of Massada.

12. François Boucher, *Saint Peter Trying to Walk on Water*, 1766.

Saint-Louis Cathedral, Versailles.

The Shoe in the New Testament:

The Sandals of Jesus

The writings of the apostles Matthew, Mark, Luke, and John confirm the prediction John the Baptist made while baptizing people with water in Bethania, beyond the River Jordan: each evoke Jesus' shoes through the voice of the prophet: "...but He who is coming after me is mightier than I, whose sandals I am not worthy to carry" (Matthew, 3:11). "And he preached, saying, 'There comes One after me who is mightier than I, whose sandal strap I am not worthy to stoop down and loose" (Mark, 1:7).

"I indeed baptize you with water; but One mightier than I is coming, whose sandal strap I am not worthy to loose" (Luke, 3:16).

"...but there stands One among you whom you do not know. It is He who, coming after me, is preferred before me, whose sandal strap I am not worthy to loose" (John, 26-27).

This statement (repeated four times) refers to sandals that were attached to the foot with a strap. These were typical during the Roman occupation of Palestine and were worn by Jesus' contemporaries. The New Testament mentions them on numerous occasions. If we look at the story of Mathew and Luke in the calling of the seventy-two disciples, Jesus advises them to walk barefoot: "Provide neither gold nor silver nor copper in your money belts, nor bag for your journey, nor two tunics, nor sandals, nor staffs... (Matthew, 10:9-10) And whoever will not receive you nor hear your words, when you depart from that house or city, shake off the dust from your feet" (Matthew, 10:14) "...behold, I send you out as lambs among wolves. Carry neither moneybag, knapsack, nor sandals..." (Luke, 10:3-4).

But Mark gives a different version: "He commanded them to take nothing for the journey except a staff – no bag, no bread, no copper in their money belts – but to wear sandals, and not to put on two tunics..." (Mark, 6:8-9).

Although it emphasizes asceticism, Mark's version retains the shoe as a symbol of travel, as Jean-Paul Roux explains in an article in the journal of the Institute of Calceology entitled, "The symbolism of the shoe in the religions descended from Abraham: Judaism, Christianity, and Islam." In Luke's parable of the prodigal son, the father says of his newly found son, "Bring out the best robe and put it on him, and put a ring on his hand and sandals on his feet" (Luke, 15:22). Only free men could enjoy sandals, as slaves did not have the right to wear shoes. Elsewhere in the New Testament, the account of Saint Peter's deliverance in the Acts of the Apostles contains a story about sandals: "That night Peter was sleeping, bound with two chains between two soldiers; and the guards before the door were keeping the prison. Now behold, an angel of the Lord stood by him, and a light shone in the prison; and he struck Peter on the side and raised him up, saying, 'Arise quickly!'

And his chains fell off his hands. Then the angel said to him, 'Gird yourself and tie on your sandals'; and so he did. And he said to him, 'Put on your garment and follow me'" (Acts, 12:6-8).

In the later iconography of Philippe de Champaigne's seventeenth-century painting, Christ Nailed to the Cross (Augustins Museum, Toulouse), sandals like the strapped versions evoked in the prophesy of John the Baptist are depicted carelessly strewn on the ground. Finally, if we turn to the Gospel of Saint Matthew, we read: "Now in the fourth watch of the night Jesus went to them, walking on the sea. And when the disciples saw Him walking on the sea, they were troubled, saying, 'It is a ghost!' And they cried out for fear. But immediately Jesus spoke to them, saying, 'Be of good cheer! It is I; do not be afraid.' And Peter answered Him

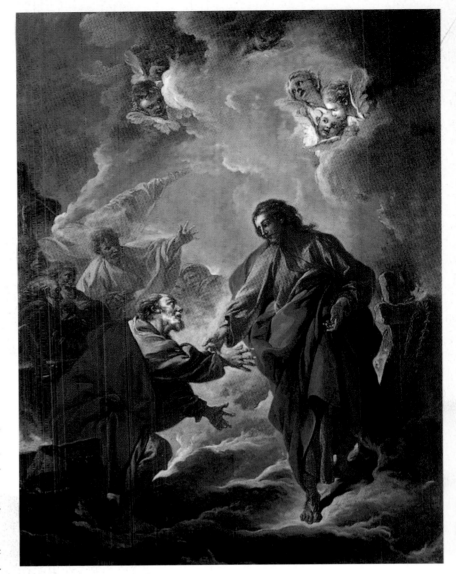

and said, 'Lord, if it is You, command me to come to You on the water.' So He said, 'Come.' And when Peter had come down out of the boat, he walked on the water to go to Jesus. But when he saw that the wind was boisterous, he was afraid; and beginning to sink he cried out, saying, 'Lord, save me!'" (Matthew, 14:25-30). This evangelical testimony was the subject of Boucher's eighteenth-century painting, Saint Peter Walking on Water, remarkable in that the apostle is shoeless, whereas Jesus is depicted in magnificent sandals based on the type worn by Roman patricians.

In conclusion, the simpler shoes (conceived for walking rather than for ceremonial use) discovered in the fortress of Massada built by Herod in the desert of the Dead Sea provide a good indication of the shoes worn by Christ and his contemporaries mentioned by the Apostles. These shoes are also more in keeping with Christ's spirit of poverty. Because of their surprisingly modern concept, their use will span the centuries, particularly in Africa, and they can be found in many third-world countries today, often reduced to a simple sole cut out from a salvaged tire with a y-shaped thong. The sandal of Jesus moreover heralds the work of certain 21st-century designers who would take inspiration from the sandal and update its appearance.

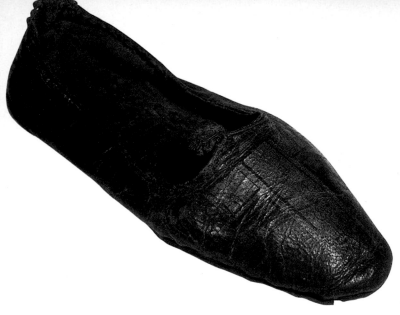

Antiquity – The Copts

Coptic civilization was a bridge between Antiquity and the Middle Ages. Direct descendants of the Pharaohs, the Copts were Egyptians that practiced Christianity. Our knowledge of their shoes comes from archaeological digs undertaken in the 19th century, in particular at Achmin.

Additional information is available from mummy textiles and sarcophagi tops from the 1st to 4th centuries AD, which usually depicted people wearing sandals, although sometimes people appear barefoot. Funeral customs changed in the 4th century when the dead were buried dressed in their most precious clothing. From that time forward, painted textiles having disappeared, steles only offer rare images that show a type of shoe with a pointed toe.

As was the case throughout Egyptian antiquity, the heel was unknown to the Copts: shoes, boots and sandals were always flat-soled. The use of full boots and ankle boots remains exceptional and reserved for men. These forms of footwear show little variety, but Coptic shoemakers demonstrated imagination in the decorative techniques they employed, using red and brown leather, leather piping curled into spirals, geometric motifs cut out of gold leather, and even sculpted leather soles.

Greece

As in Egypt, the most popular shoe in Greece was the sandal. The Homeric heroes of the Iliad and The Odyssey wear sandals with bronze soles, while the gods wear sandals made of gold. Agamemnon, legendary king of Mycenae, protected his legs with the help of leg armor fastened with silver hooks.

Sandals figure in a story about the Greek philosopher Empedocles, born around 450 BC in Agrigentum. As the story goes, Empedocles wanted people to believe he had ascended into heaven, so he dove into the opening of Mt. Etna. The volcano swallowed him, but ejected his sandals intact, in this way revealing the suicide's hoax.

Archaeological discoveries in the tombs at Vergina confirm that wealthy Macedonians during the reign of Phillip II (382 BC-336 BC) wore sandals with soles of gold or gilded silver. The Greek sandal, worn by men and women alike, had a leather or cork sole of variable thickness, differentiated right and left feet, and attached to the foot with straps. Originally simple shoes, sandals later displayed elegant complexity. Examples are found on sculptures from the period, such as the sandals worn by Diana of the Hunt (Louvre Museum, Paris). Attic vases show certain figures wearing laced boots called endromides, also known as embas when trimmed with a flap.

As for other models of Greek footwear, the pointed shoe of the Hittite variety, with which the Ionians were long familiar, never reached mainland Greece, although it was depicted by Greek vase painters who wanted to give an oriental character to their figures. Aeschylus (525 BC-456 BC) is credited with inventing the cothurne. Worn by the actors in Greek tragedies who played the roles of heroes and gods, the cothurne had an elevated cork sole that increased height at the expense of stability. This theatrical shoe adjusted equally to fit both feet, whence the expression "more versatile than a cothurne." It is interesting to note that the cothurne, because of its height, represents the beginnings of a heel, which would remain unknown to Antiquity, but would appear later in Italy at the end of the 16th century.

One Greek custom was reserved for courtesans: the wearing of sandals embellished with precious stones. It was said that their studded soles left an unambiguous message in the sand that said, "follow me." The rich variety of Greek footwear goes against the advice of Plato (428 BC-348 BC), who advocated walking barefoot.

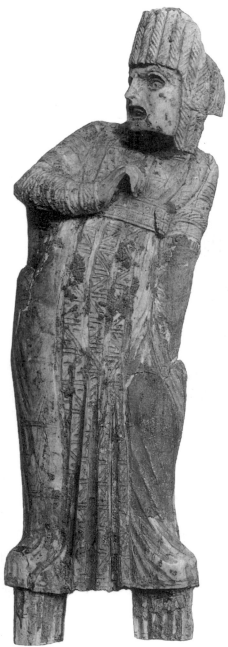

13. Man's slipper, vamp decorated with motifs gilded with gold leaf.

Egypt, Coptic era. International Shoe Museum, Romans.

14. Ivory statuette of a Greek actor wearing cothurnes. Petit-Palais Museum, Paris.

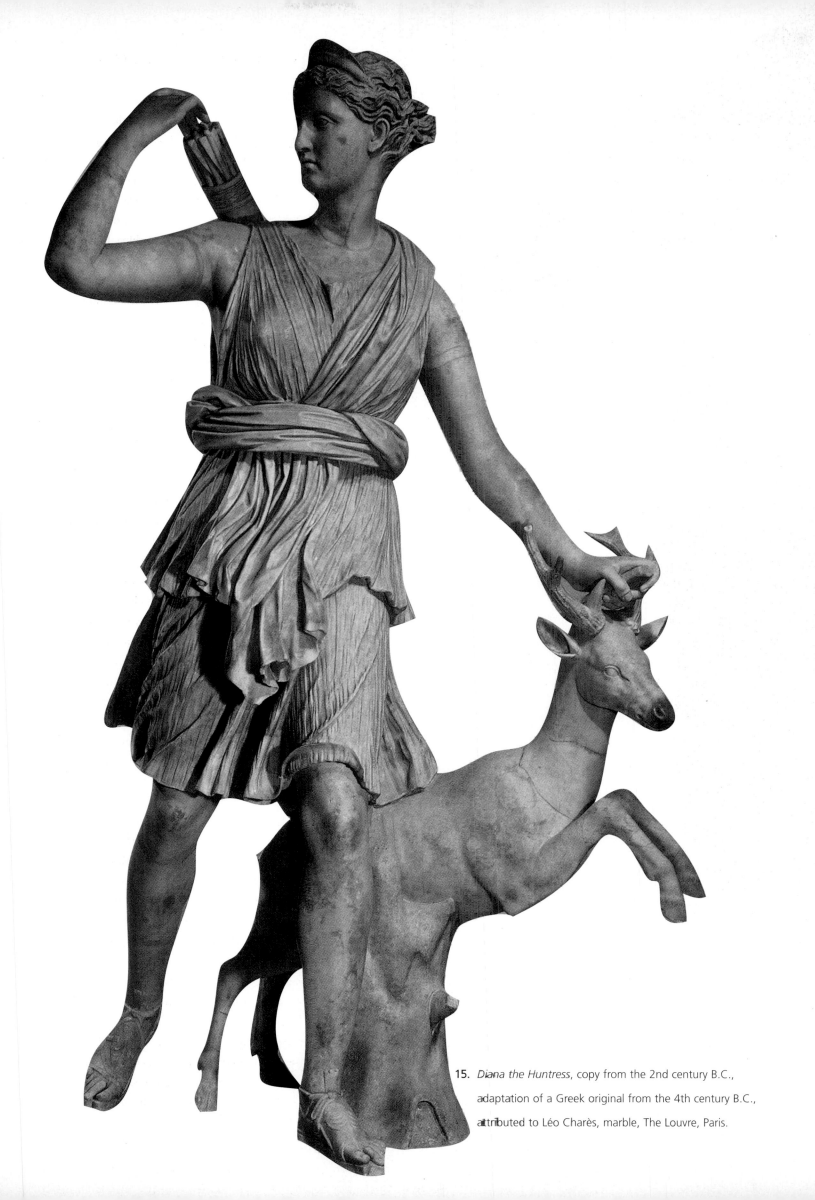

15. *Diana the Huntress*, copy from the 2nd century B.C.,
adaptation of a Greek original from the 4th century B.C.,
attributed to Léo Charès, marble, The Louvre, Paris.

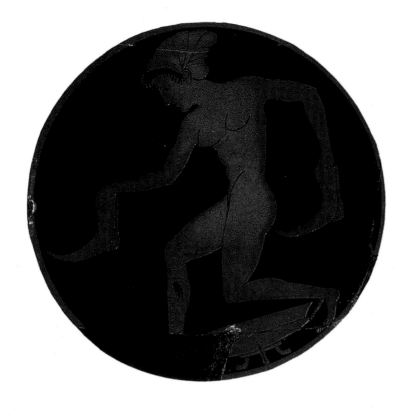

The Etruscans

The Etruscans probably originated in Asia Minor, appearing in Italy in what is now Tuscany at the end of the 8th century BC. Realistic paintings decorating their tombs and cemeteries (Triclinium, Tarquinia, Caere) portray gods and mortals dressed in raised-toe shoes of the Hittite variety. Strapped sandals, cut shoes, and laced boots emerged in Etruria in the 4th century BC and represent established contacts with other peoples around the Mediterranean basin.

Rome

Rome was the direct heir to Greek civilization and felt its influence in the area of footwear: Roman shoes are mainly imitations of Greek models.

In ancient Rome, shoes were indicators of social status and wealth. Some patricians wore shoes with soles of silver or solid gold, while plebeians were content to wear clogs or rustic footwear with wooden soles. Slaves lacked the right to wear shoes and walked barefoot, their feet covered in chalk or plaster. When high-ranking Roman citizens were invited to a feast, they had someone carry their sandals at the home of their host. The less fortunate had to carry their own shoes, because it was considered rude to keep ones walking shoes on. As a bed was used for dining in Rome, shoes were removed before the meal and put back on when leaving the table.

Roman shoes fall into two categories: the solea, a form of sandal, and the calceus, a closed toe shoe worn with a toga. Other types evolved with variation in colour, form, and construction. Magistrates wore strange-looking shoes with curved toes made out of black or white leather and decorated on the side with a gold or silver crescent. As in Egypt and Greece, the difference between the left and right foot was well differentiated. Shoemakers were citizens who worked in shops, rather than slaves. This is a crucial distinction in understanding the status of the shoe as an object.

In ancient Rome, the shoe began to acquire much importance in the military arena. The caliga, the Roman soldier's shoe, was a type of sandal. Strapped to the foot, it had a thick leather sole with pointed studs. It was up to the soldiers to acquire the studs; under certain circumstances, however, they were distributed free of charge as part of a ceremony called the clavarium.

It is said that as a child the Emperor Caligula was so fond of wearing the caliga he was named after the shoe, a delightful and telling anecdote. The mulleus, a closed shoe that was red in colour, differed little from the calceus. Worn by emperors, magistrates, and the children of senators, it got its name from the seashell from which bright crimson was extracted. The campagus took the form of a boot that exposed the foot. Trimmed in fur, and often decorated with pearls and precious stones, it was intended for generals to wear. A crimson version was exclusively reserved for emperors.

As in ancient Greece, the sandal and the slipper were mainly intended for women to wear indoors. The soccus, a type of slipper with a raised tip and identical for both feet, was apparently of Persian origin; it would become a traditional shoe in Turkey. These delicate little shoes aroused the concupiscence of the era's fetishists.

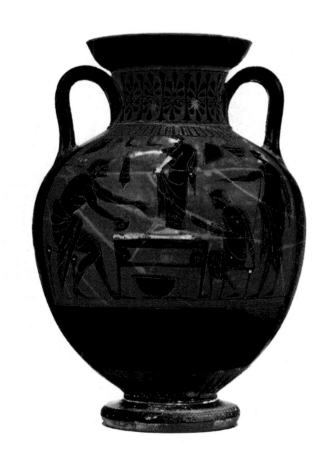

16. Attican cup with red figures, attributed to Epiktétos.
    Around 500 BC. Agora Museum, Athens.

17. Attica urn with black figures, representing a shoe repairer's workshop.
    Around 520-510 BC. Boston Museum of Fine Arts, Boston.

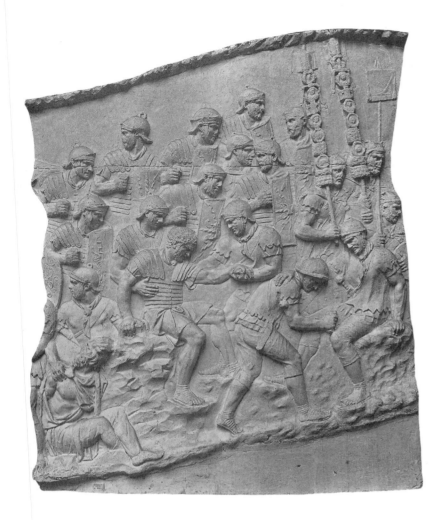

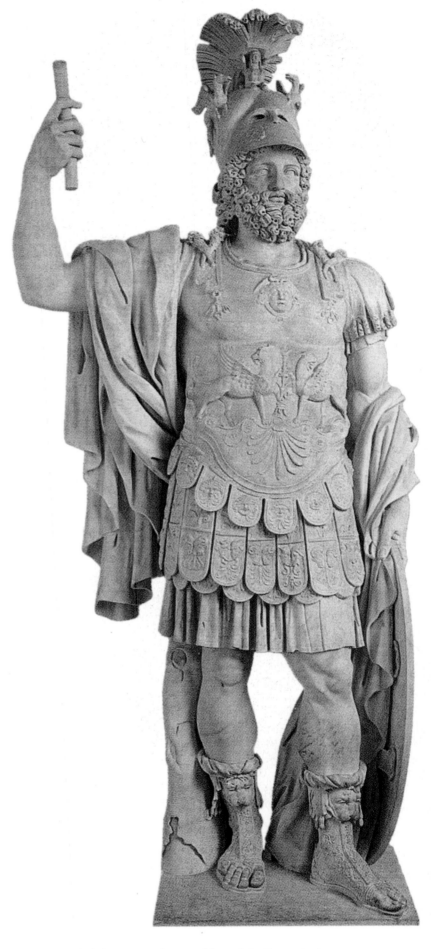

Suetonus (70-128) tells how the Roman senator Lucius Vitellus, who carried under his tunic the slipper that his mistress wore on her right foot, without the slightest embarrassment, would remove the shoe in public and cover it with kisses. Red shoes had long been the privileged attribute of Roman courtesans before all women dared to wear them.

After the emperor Aurelius (212-275) wore them, red shoes became an Imperial symbol, giving birth to a tradition that was later taken up by the Papacy, and subsequently by all the courts of Europe, which wore red-heeled shoes.

We know from the writings of Juvenal (55-140) that to give a spanking with a shoe was a serious punishment commonly administered to children and slaves.

Romantic Romans put their shoes to more gallant use by inserting amorous messages between the sandal and the foot of their confidant. In this way, sandals became a drop box for love notes as advocated by Ovid (43 BC-17 AD) in *The Art of Love*.

18. Low-relief of the Trajan column, soldiers of the Roman legions (military shoes). Rome, 113 AD. Marble.

19. Colossal statue of the god Mars (shod in *campagus*). 1st century AD. Capitole Museum, Rome.

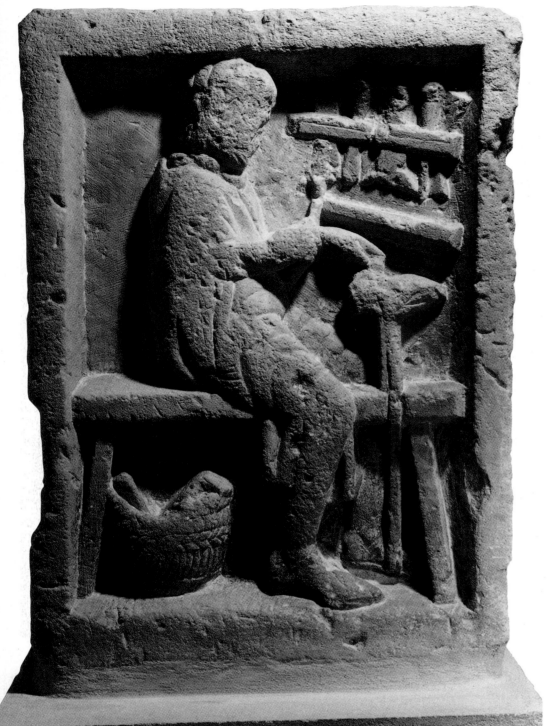

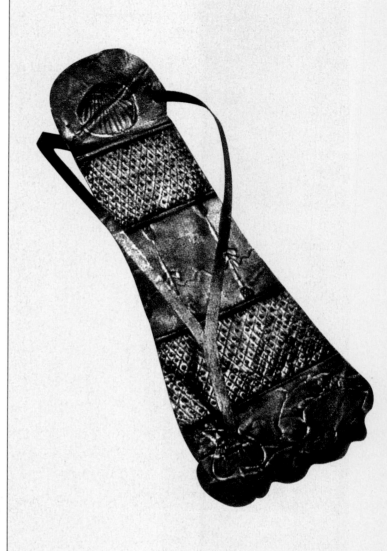

The Gallo-Romans

The Gallo-Romans wore various versions of flat shoes with rounded toes. The most popular were ordinary sandals for men and women based on Roman models.

The gallica was a closed shoe with a wooden sole and was the ancestor of the galoshes (a later overshoe with a wooden sole).

An 11th-century monument to a shoemaker confirms the existence of the shoemaker's industry and the respect these artisans enjoyed.

20. Funerary stele of a cobbler. Reims, Marne, faubourg Cérès, Gallo-Roman, 2nd century AD. Collection of the Saint-Rémi Museum of Reims. Photo by Robert Meulle.

21. Sliver sandal. Byzantine period. Bally Museum, Schönenwerd, Switzerland.

22. Mosaics from the churches of Saint Vital and Saint Apollinaire in Classe de Ravenne. Around 547 AD. The Emperor Justinien and his servents.

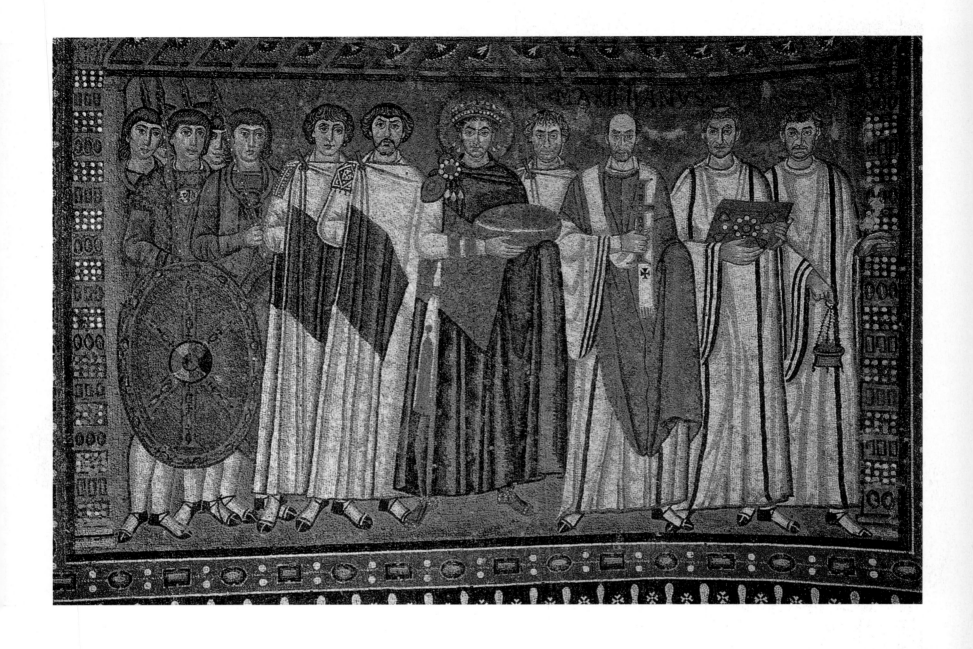

The Byzantine empire

Byzantine civilization extended from the 5th to the 15th century, producing throughout this period a wealth of crimson leather shoes trimmed in gold reminiscent of embroidered Persian-style boots, as well as the Roman soccus and mulleus.

Byzantine mules and slippers were objects of luxury and refinement initially reserved for the Emperor and his court. Crimson or gold slippers were worn in the eastern Mediterranean basin, in particular in the area around Alexandria and in the Nile valley. Excavations at Achmin have yielded many examples that belonged to women. The arrival of Christian shoemakers in this region revived the craft of shoemaking, as Christian symbols were added to the geometric decorative tradition. A silver sandal discovered in an Egyptian tomb and now in the collection of the Bally Museum is a good example. Dating to the 6th century AD, it is embellished with the image of a dove symbolizing Christ.

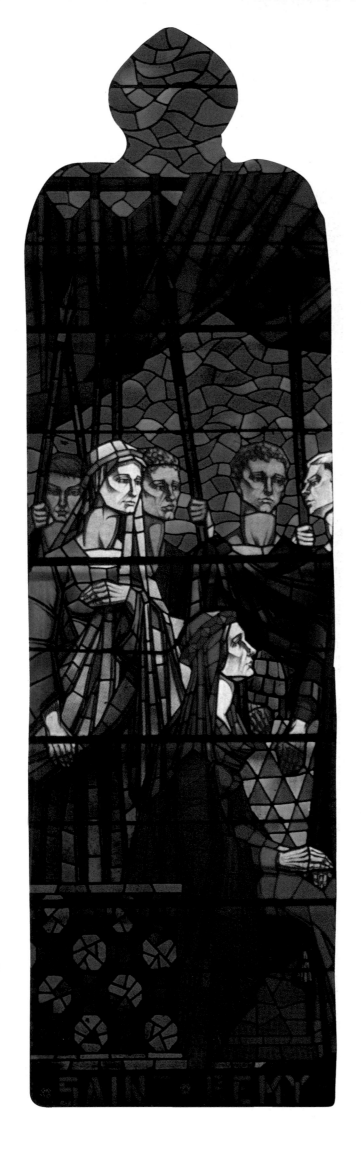
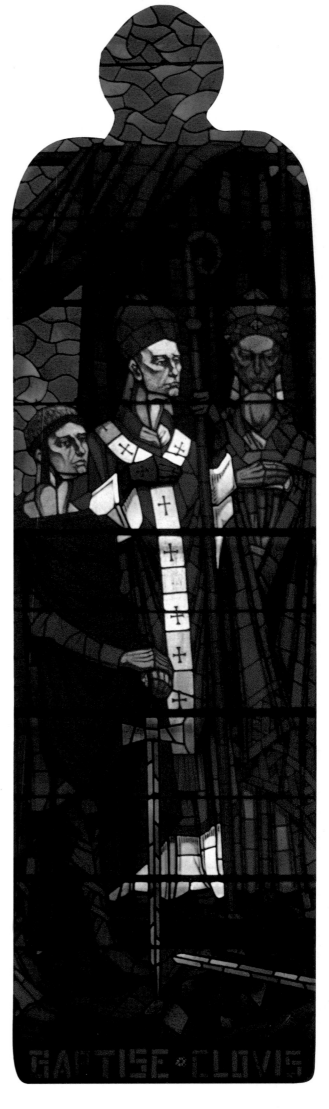

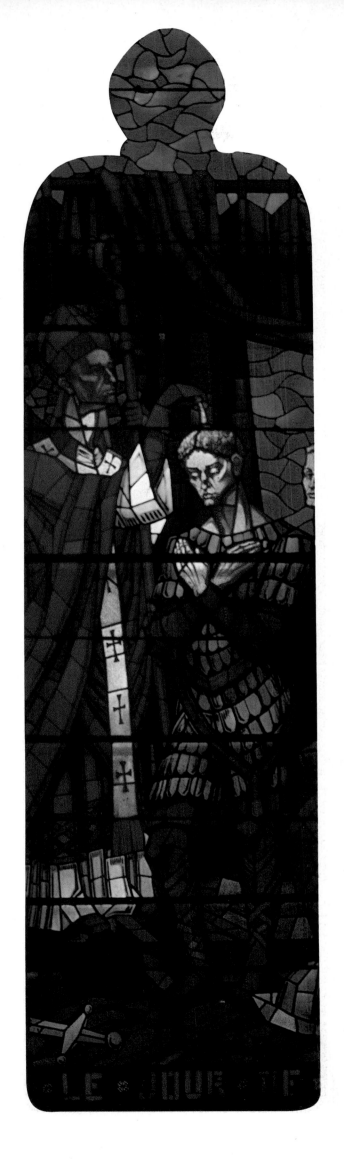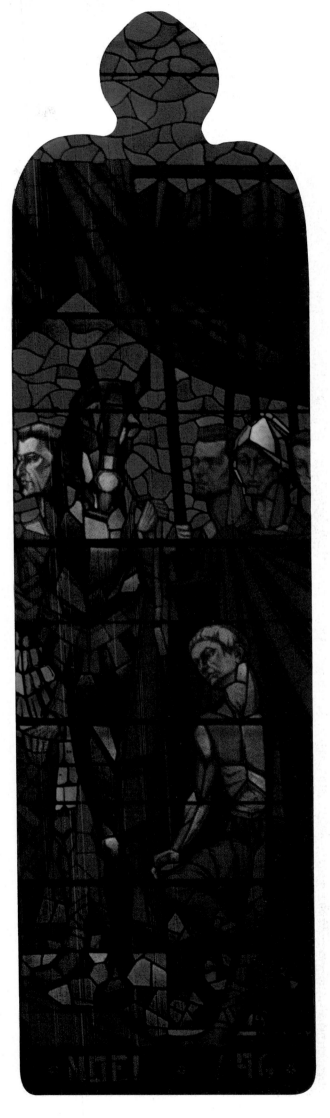

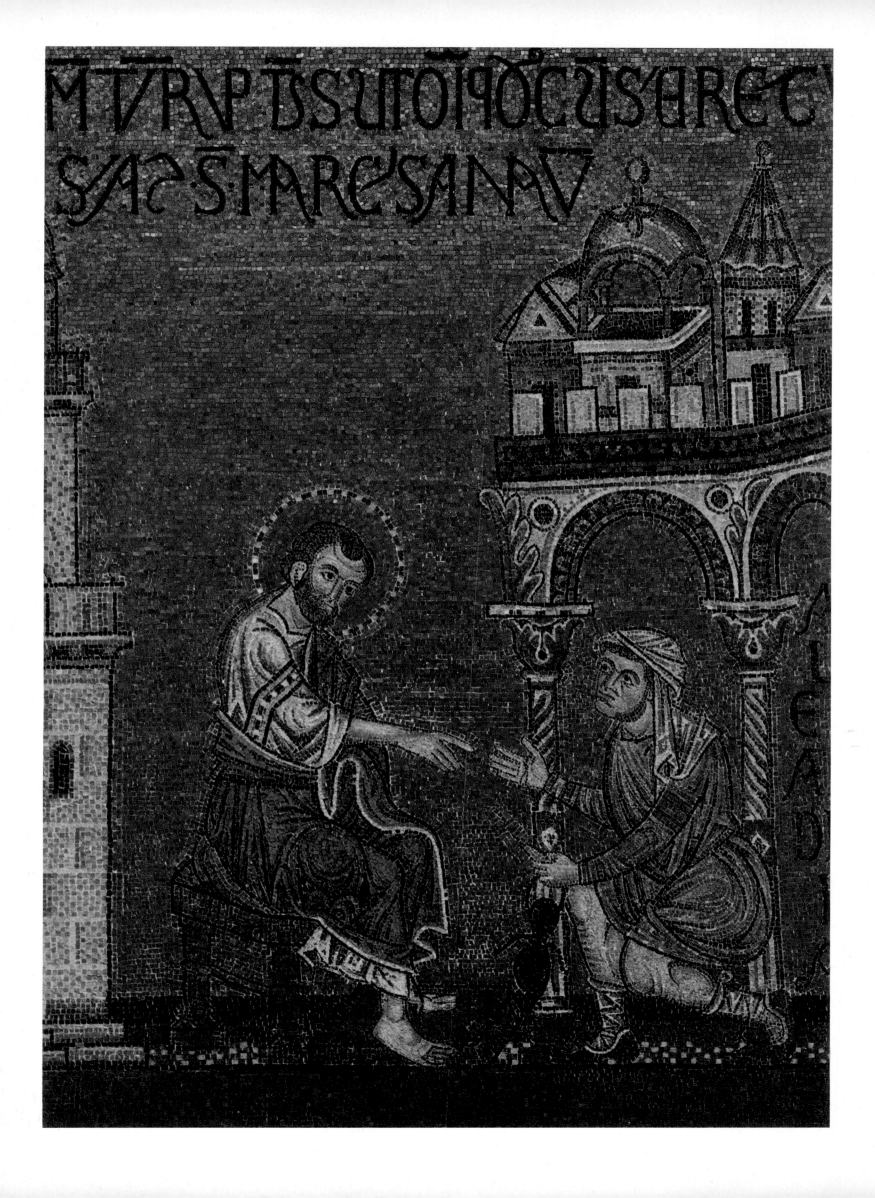

The Middle Ages

As the Middle Ages dawned in the West, footwear remained under the influence of ancient Roman models. The Francs wore shoes equipped with straps that rose to mid-thigh. Only their leaders wore shoes with pointed tips.

Thanks to the extraordinary degree of preservation of certain burials, we have an idea of what Merovingian shoes looked like. The tomb discovered at Saint-Denis of Queen Arégonde, wife of King Clotaire I (497-561), has enabled us to reconstruct an image of her shoes as supple leather sandals with straps intertwining the leg. Elsewhere, gilded bronze shoe buckles decorated with stylized animals discovered in a leader's tomb at Hordaim, are proof of the attention given to shoe ornamentation during this period. Shoes were very costly during the Middle Ages, which is why they appear in wills and are among the donations made to monasteries. Costliness also explains why a fiancé would offer his future wife a pair of embroidered shoes before marriage, a lovely tradition dating to Gregory of Tours (538-594). We can get a sense of the opulence of this gift from the shoes of this era preserved in the museum of Chelles near Paris.

The strapped or banded shoe continued into the Carolingian period, although the woman's model became more embellished. As for the wooden-soled gallique or galoche, it too remained in use.

From this time forward, soldiers protected their legs with leather or metal leggings called bamberges. In the 9th-century, a shoe called the heuse made out of supple leather extending high on the leg announced the arrival of the boot.

We known from the monk of the Saint Gall monastery that emperor Charlemagne wore simple boots with straps intertwining the legs, although for ceremonies he wore laced boots decorated with precious stones. But frequent contact between France and Italy helped develop a taste for regalia and increasingly the shoe became an object of great luxury.

At the same time, religious councils were ordering clerics to wear liturgical shoes while performing mass. Called sandals, these holy shoes were of cloth and completely covered the cleric's foot. Pope Adrian I (772-795) instituted the ritual of kissing feet. When some clergy members deemed this rite undignified, a compromise was established. Henceforth, the papal mule would be embroidered with a cross. Kissing this cross was no longer a sign of servitude, but one of homage to Christ's representative on earth. Regarding shoemaking, the French word cordouanier (which became cordonnier or shoemaker) was adopted in the 11th century and signified someone who worked with Cordoba leather and by extension, all kinds of leather. As in Antiquity, shoes were patterned separately for the right and left foot. Shoes made out of Cordoba leather were reserved for the aristocracy, whereas those made by çavetiers, or cobblers (shoe repairmen) were more crudely fashioned. The wearing of shoes began to expand in the 11th-century. The most common medieval type was an open shoe secured by a strap fitted with a buckle or button.

Other types included estivaux, a summer ankle boot of supple, lightweight leather that appeared in the second half of the 11th century; chausses with soles, a type of cloth boot reinforced with leather soles worn with pattens (supplemental wooden under soles) for outdoor use; and heuses, supple boots in a variety of forms originally reserved for gentlemen, but which became common under the reign of Philippe Auguste (1165-1223). In the early 12th century, shoes became longer. Called pigaches, these shoes were forerunners of the poulaine style a knight named Robert le Cornu is credited with introducing.

The Crusaders brought the exaggerated style with its inordinately long tip back from the East. It is based on the raised-toe model of Syrian, Akkadian, and Hittite culture, and reflects the vertical aesthetic of gothic Europe. When people of modest means imitated this eccentric fashion initially reserved for the aristocracy, the authorities responded by regulating the length of the shoe's points according to social rank: $1/2$ foot for commoners, 1 foot for the bourgeois, 1 and $1/2$ feet for knights, 2 feet for nobles, and 2 and $1/2$ feet for princes, who had to hold the tips of their shoes up with gold or silver chains attached to their knees in order to walk. The shoe length hierarchy led to the French expression "vivre sur un grand pied," (to live on a large foot), denoting the worldly status represented by shoe length.

The poulaine was made of leather, velvet, or brocade. The uppers could sport cutouts in the form of gothic church windows, although obscene images were sometimes used. A small round bell or an ornament in the shape of a bird beak often dangled from the tip of the shoe. There was even a military poulaine to go with a soldier's amour. Interestingly, during the battle of Sempach between the Swiss confederates and the Austrians in 1386, knights had to cut off the points of their poulaines because they interfered with combat.

Worn throughout Europe by men and women alike, as well as by certain clerics, the poulaine was condemned by bishops, excommunicated by religious councils, and forbidden by kings. But its immoral status only made the poulaine more seductive, and it was all the rage in the Burgundian court. Indeed, the poulaine would only disappear in the early 16th century, after a four century run.

Flat-soled shoes lasted the entire medieval period, but a heel was beginning to emerge as evidenced in Jan van Eyck's *Arnolfini Couple*. The protective wooden pattens, depicted carelessly strewn on the floor in the left of the painting, exhibit an incline: the rear heel is higher than the front support.

Shoes were scarce and costly items in the middle ages, so protective wooden soles were used for going out in muddy backstreets. But the under soles made the shoes too noisy: it was strictly forbidden to wear them in church.

Previous pages:

23. Stained-glass window of the baptism of Clovis by Saint-Rémy (496).

Sanctuary of Saint Bonaventure, Lyon 2nd, by L. Charat and

Mrs. Lamy-Paillet in 1964.

Photo by J. Bonnet, Imp. Beaulieu Lyon.

24. *Saint Mark Healing Aniane the Cobbler*, detail from a mosaic.

13th century. Saint Mark Basilica, Venice.

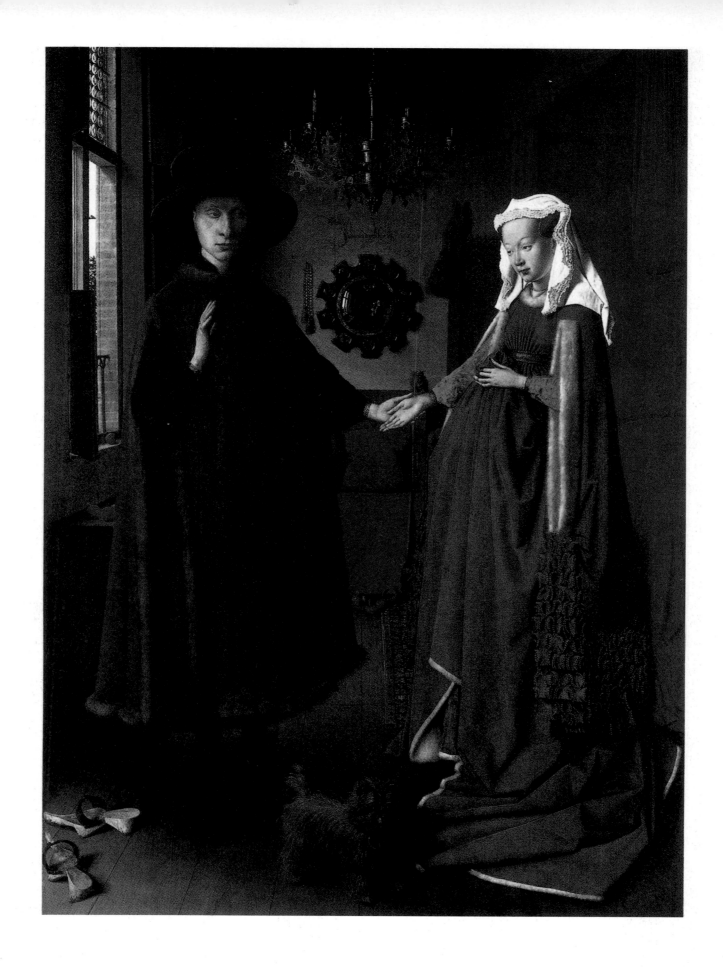

29. Jan van Eyck. *The Arnolfini Portrait*, 1434.

Oil on panel. 83.8 x 57.2 cm. National Gallery, London.

30. *Philippe VI de Valois Receives Tribute from His Vassal Edward III of England*,

detail of an illumination from the Chronicles of Jehan Froissart. 15th century.

National Library of Paris, Paris.

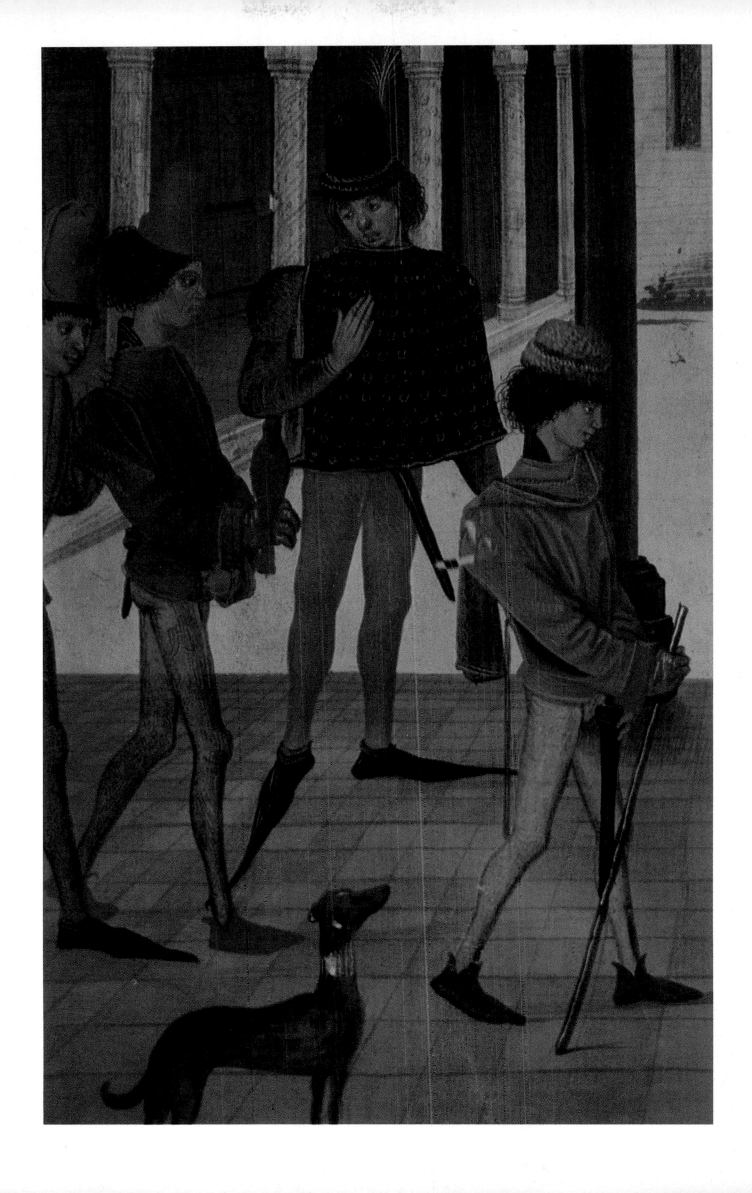

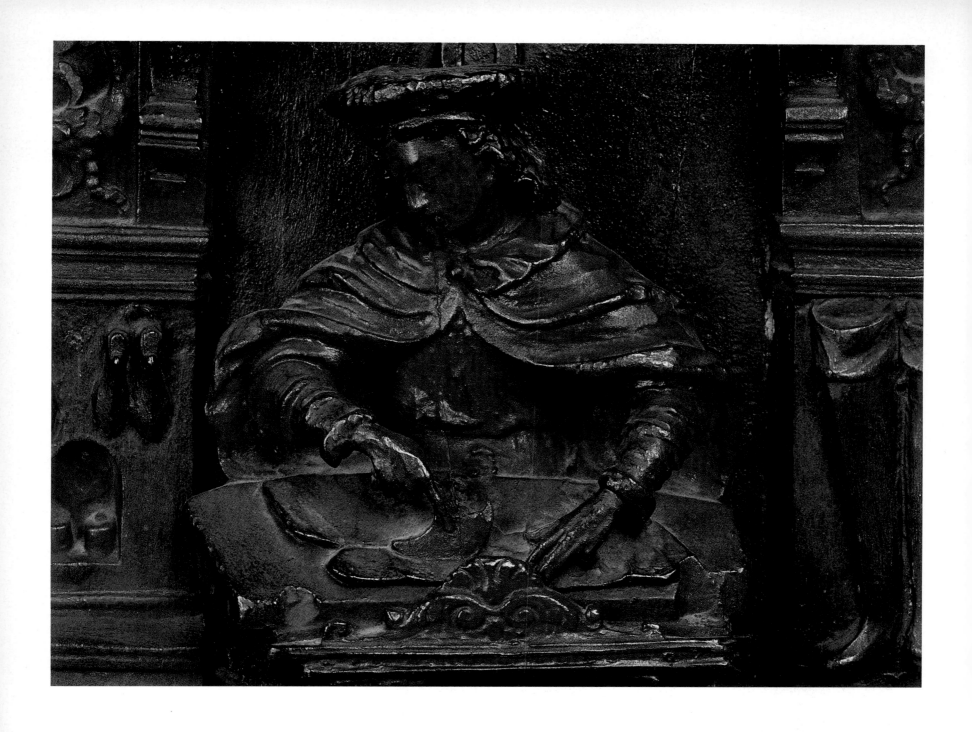

The Legend of Saint Crispin and Saint Crispinian

Crispin and Crispinian were two brothers from a patrician Roman family who converted to Christianity under the reign of Diocletian (245-313). Pope Caius (283-296) gave them the task of converting Gaul and in 285 AD they settled in Soissons to work as shoemakers and to preach the word of God. When the Roman general Maximianus Herculeus asked them to renounce their faith and to worship pagan idols, the brothers refused, which led to their frequent and cruel persecution. They were flagellated, pierced with awls, burned with boiling oil and molten lead, and finally thrown into the river Aisne with a millstone around their neck. Then a miracle occurred: the stone came loose and the shoemakers reached shore safe and sound, praising God. When Maximianus got the news, he had their heads cut off in 287.

Although their remains were left for vultures, the shoemakers' bodies remained in tact; two old beggars gave the martyrs a proper burial. In 649, the Bishop of Soissons, named Ansérik, moved the two brothers' remains into the crypt of his basicala, which later came to be called the Abbaye Saint-Crépin-le-Grand. When the shoemaker's guild was established in the cathedral of Paris in 1379 by king Charles-le-Sage (1338-1380), the shoemakers chose Saint Crispin and Saint Crispinian as their patrons, whom they formally celebrate on October 25th. Many images of Saint Crispin and Saint Crispinian are still preserved in the chapels of parish churches where late medieval guilds paid tribute to their patron saints and dedicated altars.

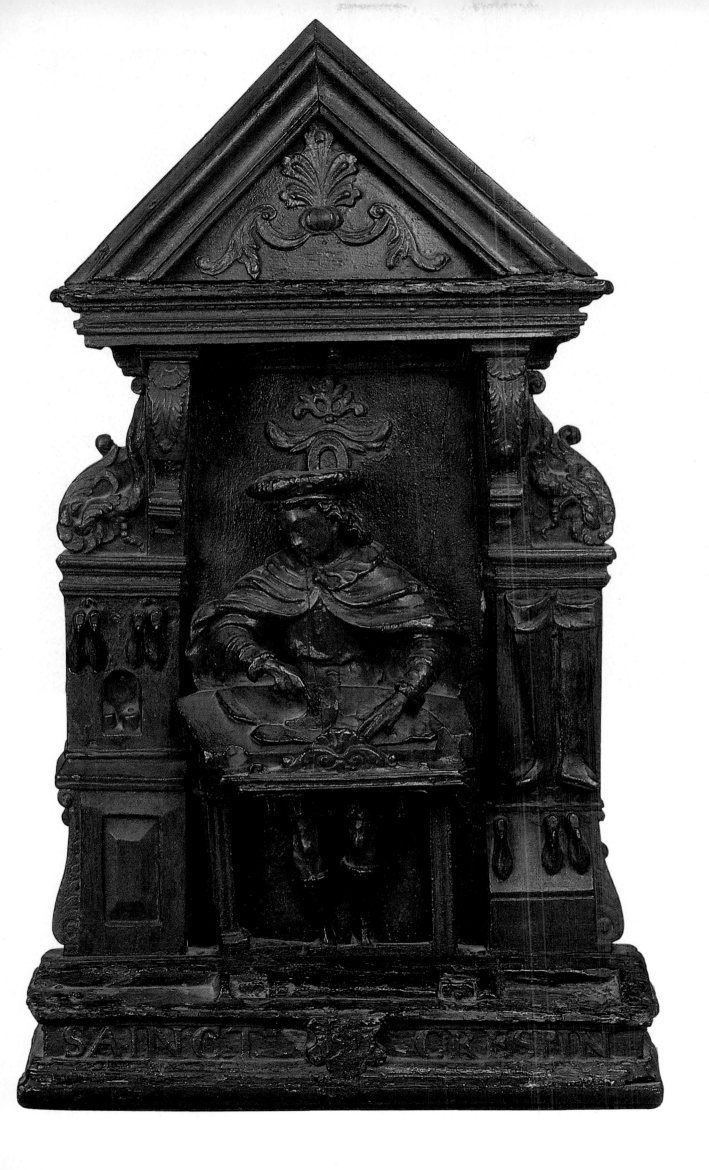

31. Sign of shoemaker-bootmaker,
"To Saint Crispin". 1593.
Carnavalet Museum, Paris.

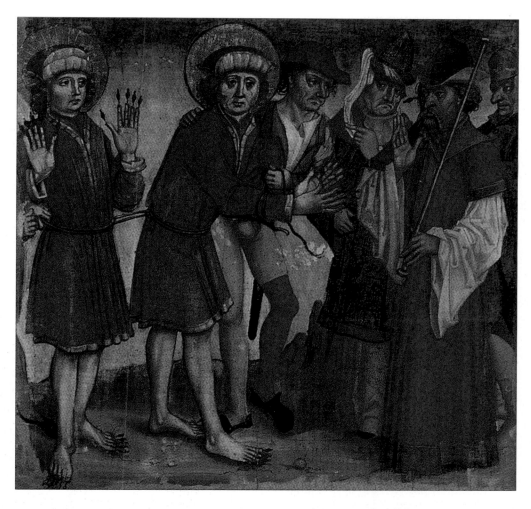

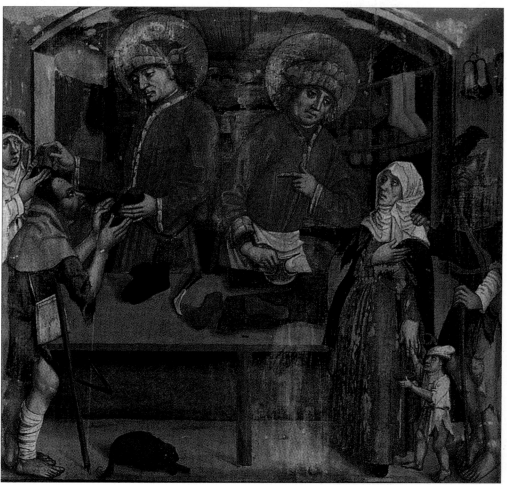

32. Retable of the "Master at the Eyelets" (1500-1510):
two scenes in the life of Saint Crispin and Saint Crispinian.
Scweizerisches Landesmuseum, Zurich.

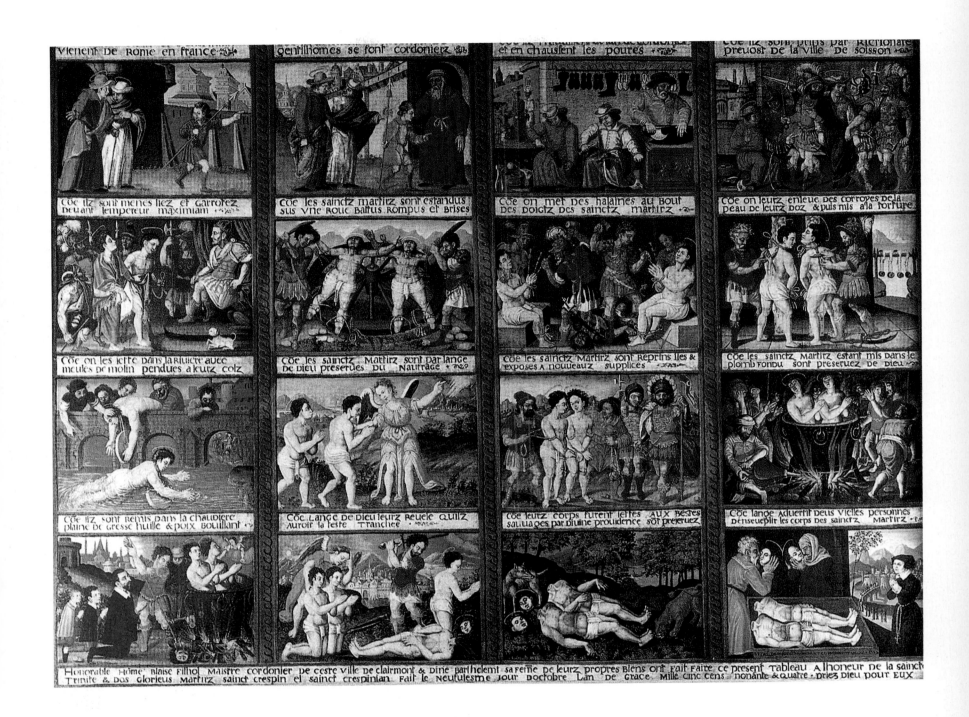

33. *The Martyr of Saints Crispin and Crispinian,*

votive offering of 1594 by painter Vital Despigoux.

Panel on wood. Clermont-Ferrand Cathedral, Puy-de-Dôme.

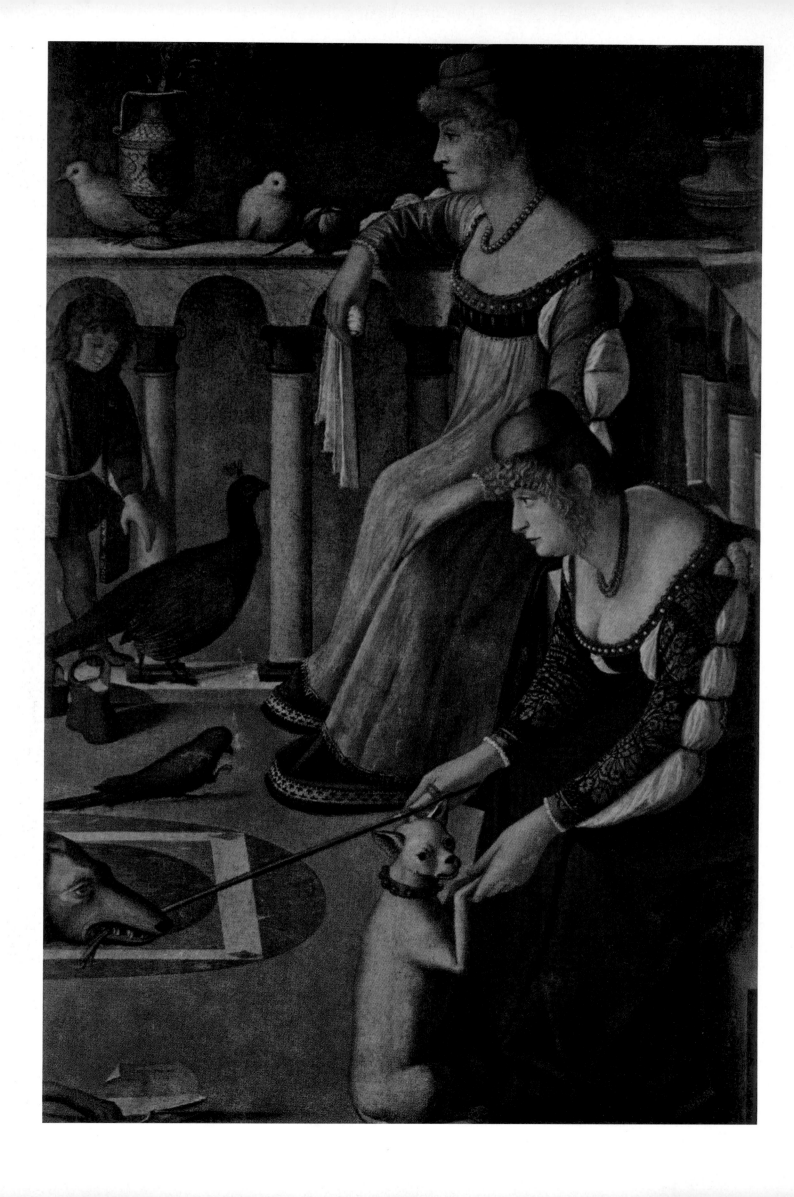

The Renaissance

At the end of the 15th century, poulaines fell victim to their own success and ended up popularized for common use. They were succeeded, without the slightest transition, by extremely wide, square-toe shoes designed for the fashion-conscious. As incongruous with fashion history as it may seem, this shoe was actually inspired by a congenital malformation: King Charles VIII had six toes on each foot, hence the very large toes of his custom-made shoes. The reaction against the previous fashion quickly went too far in the opposite direction. The Valois shoe worn during the reign of Louis XII (1462-1515) occasionally reached widths of thirty-three centimeters. The tip of the shoe, which was stuffed and decorated with animal horns, resembled a cow's head, leading to nicknames such as mufle de vache (cow muzzle), pied d'ours (bear foot), and bec de cane (duck bill). The shoe's eccentric form meant people had to straddle wide in order to walk, which naturally provoked sarcastic remarks.

During this same period, Venetians were wearing shoes called chopines, also known as mules échasses (mules on stilts) or pied de vach (cow feet). Attached to the foot with ribbons, these bizarre shoes displayed exaggerated platforms that could reach fifty-two centimeters high. The platforms themselves were of wood or cork and covered in velvet or richly decorated leather. Hidden under skirts, the shoes remained safe from scrutiny, but they resulted in a very comical walk. Hoisted upon such shoes, noblewomen had to support themselves between the shoulders of two servants in order to get around safely. This eccentric fashion certainly originated in Turkey, a country with which the Doges of the Republic traded. Turkish women were known to go to the bath on raised soles. Through the modified form of the chopine a Turkish harem shoe thus entered the palaces of Venetian aristocrats.

The wearing of chopines was banned in Spain by the archbishop of Talavera, who labeled women who wore them "depraved and dissolute." The more tolerant Italian church, on the other hand, failed to blacklist the shoe. Quite contrarily, the church, in collusion with jealous husbands, saw a way to immobilize fickle wives at home, and thereby stymie illicit affairs. Although all the courts of Europe were taken with the chopine, the shoe was never more than a limited fashion. It nevertheless managed to reach England, where Shakespeare's Hamlet says: "Your ladyship is nearer to heaven than when I saw you last by the altitude of a chopine" (Hamlet, Act II, Scene II).

The pantoufle, or mule, was a more moderate style imported from Italy that was first adopted in France in the early 16th century. Made of a thick cork sole without rear quarter, its lightness made it especially suitable for women to wear indoors.

From the reign of Francis I (1494-1547) to Henry III (1551-1589), men and women wore shoes called escarfignons. Also known as eschappins, these were flat slippers of satin or velvet with low-cut uppers and slashes. The horizontal and vertical slashes revealed the precious fabric of the stockings underneath. Rabelais (1494-1553) describes the shoes exactly in Gargantua, when he recounts the costumes of the Abbey of Thélème: "The shoes, slippers and mules of crimson, red, or purple velvet, resembled a jagged crayfish's beard." Like other articles of clothing during this period, shoes took after Germanic styles and were decorated with slashes called crevés. Nevertheless, the invention of the slashed shoe is credited to the soldiers of Francis I during the wars with Italy who, sustaining injuries from marching or from combat, had to adapt their shoes to fit their bandaged feet. As for protecting delicate shoes from filthy streets, wooden pattens remained popular for outdoor use.

Leonardo da Vinci is said to have invented the heel, but it did not appear until the end of the 16th century, when it began to rise, most likely in response to the flattering effect of greater height produced by the chopine. The first heels were attached to the sole by a piece of leather, as can be seen in the painting from the French School, entitled A Ball at the Valois Court (c.1582) in the Museum of Fine Arts, Rennes.

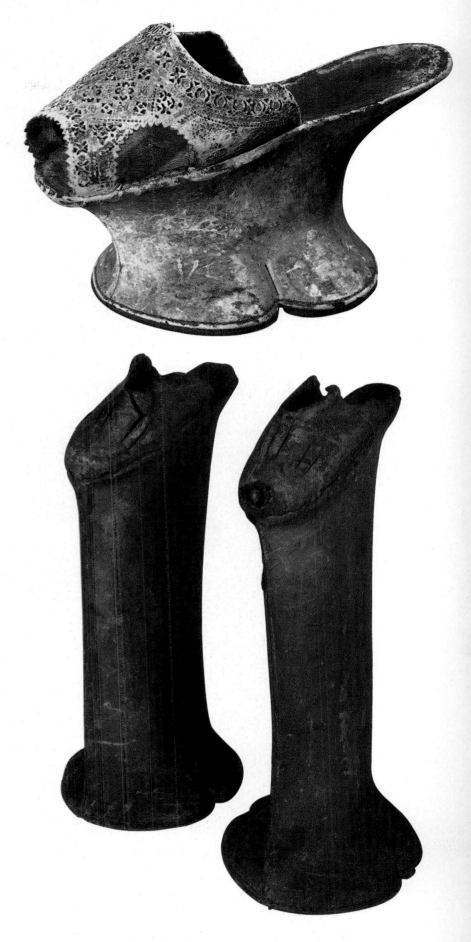

34. Carpaccio. *Two Venetian Courtesans*, 1500. Correr Museum, Venice.

35. Chopine. Venice, 16th century. International Shoe Museum, Romans.

36. Wooden chopine covered in hide worn by the Venetians. Italy, 16th century. Height: 49 cm. Jacquemart Collection, depot of the National Museum of the Middle Ages, Thermal Baths of Cluny in Paris, International Shoe Museum, Romans.

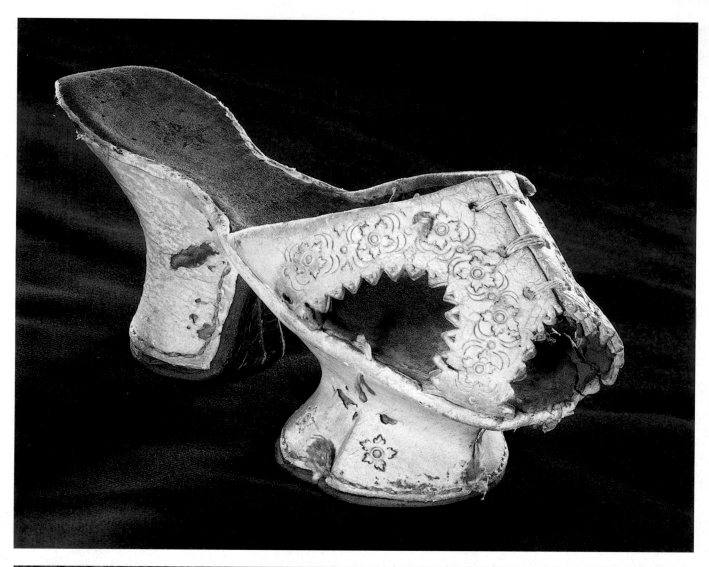

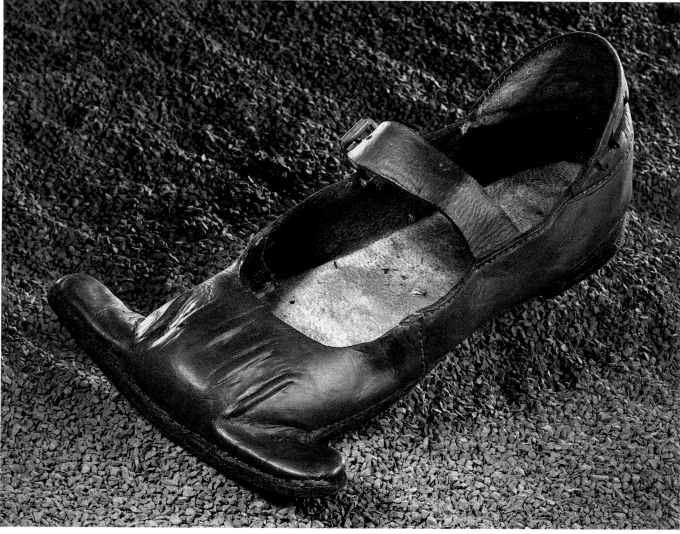

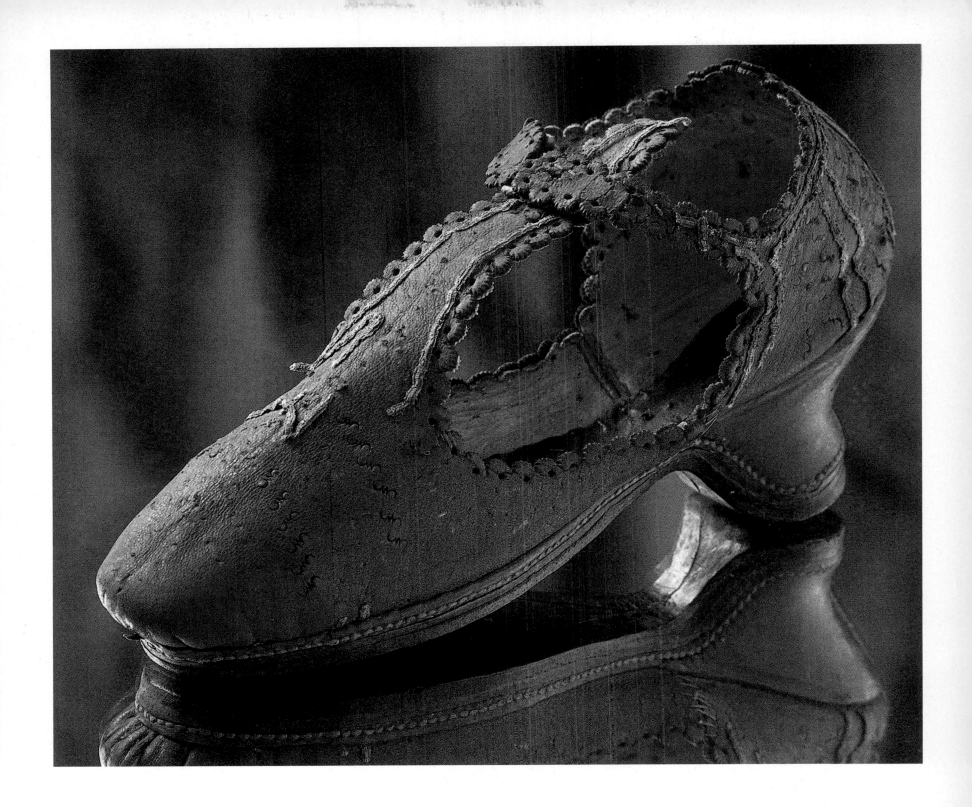

37. Chopine having been worn. Venice, Italy, around 1600.

Weissenfels Museum, with the authorization of Irmgard Sedler.

38. Man's leather shoe. Around 1530-1540.

Weissenfels Museum, with the authorization of Irmgard Sedler.

39. Woman's shoe. Henri III period, France, 16th century.

International Shoe Museum, Romans.

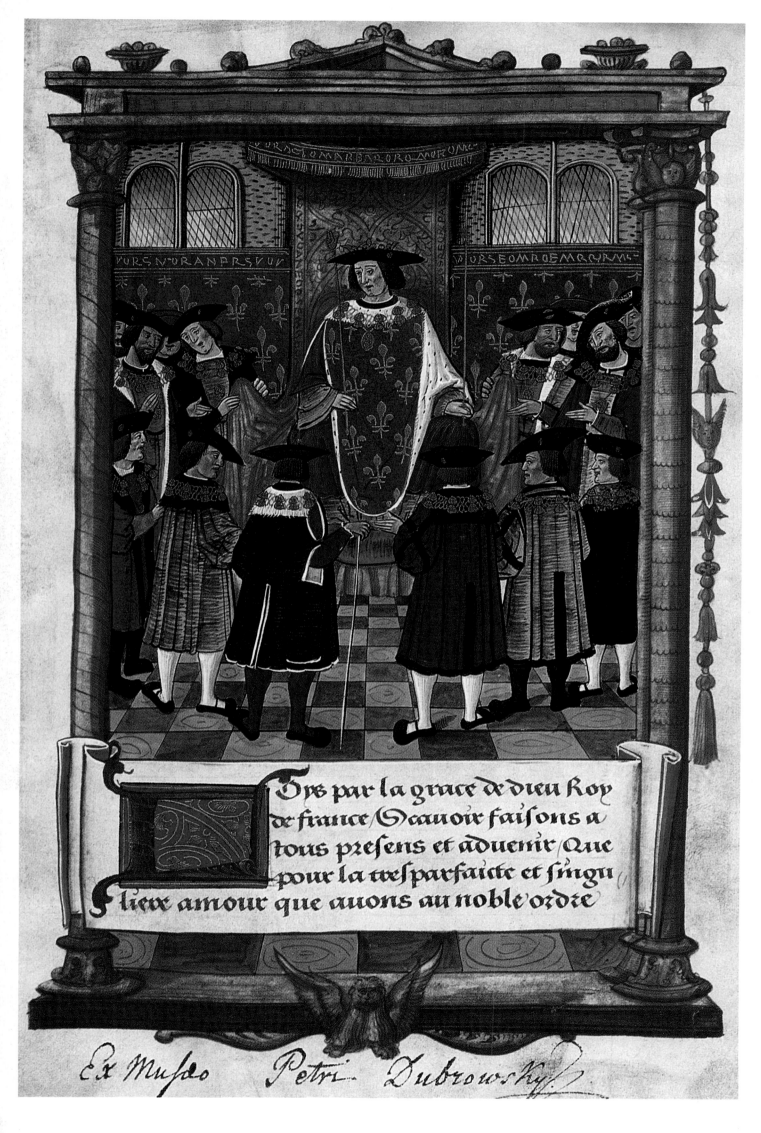

Frs par la grace de dieu Roy
de france Scauoir faisons a
tous presens et aduenir Que
pour la tresparfaicte et singu
lier amour que auons au noble ordre

Ex Musœo Petri Dubrowsky

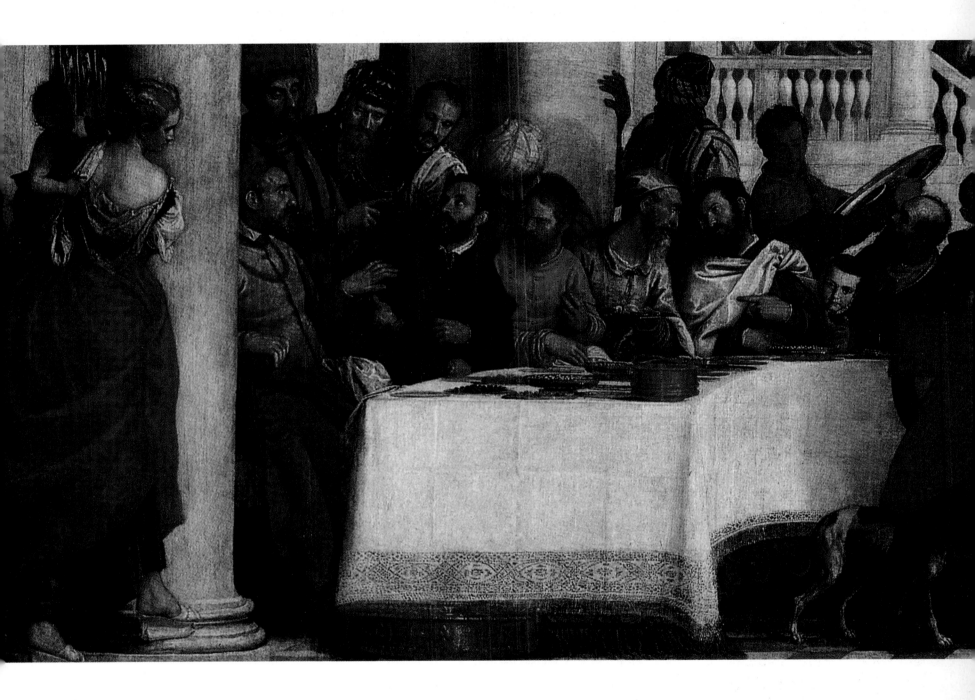

40. *King Louis XI Seated on a Throne, Surrounded by the Knights of the Order of Saint Michael.* 16th century, F° 9. The Hermitage Museum, Saint-Petersburg.

41. Paolo Caliari, known as Véronèse. *The Meal at Simon's House*, detail, around 1570. Château de Versailles.

Following pages:

42. Anthony van Dyck. *Portrait of Charles I*, around 1635. Oil on canvas. 266 x 207 cm. Louvre Museum, Paris.

43. Frans Pourbus. *Henri IV*, 1610. Louvre Museum, Paris.

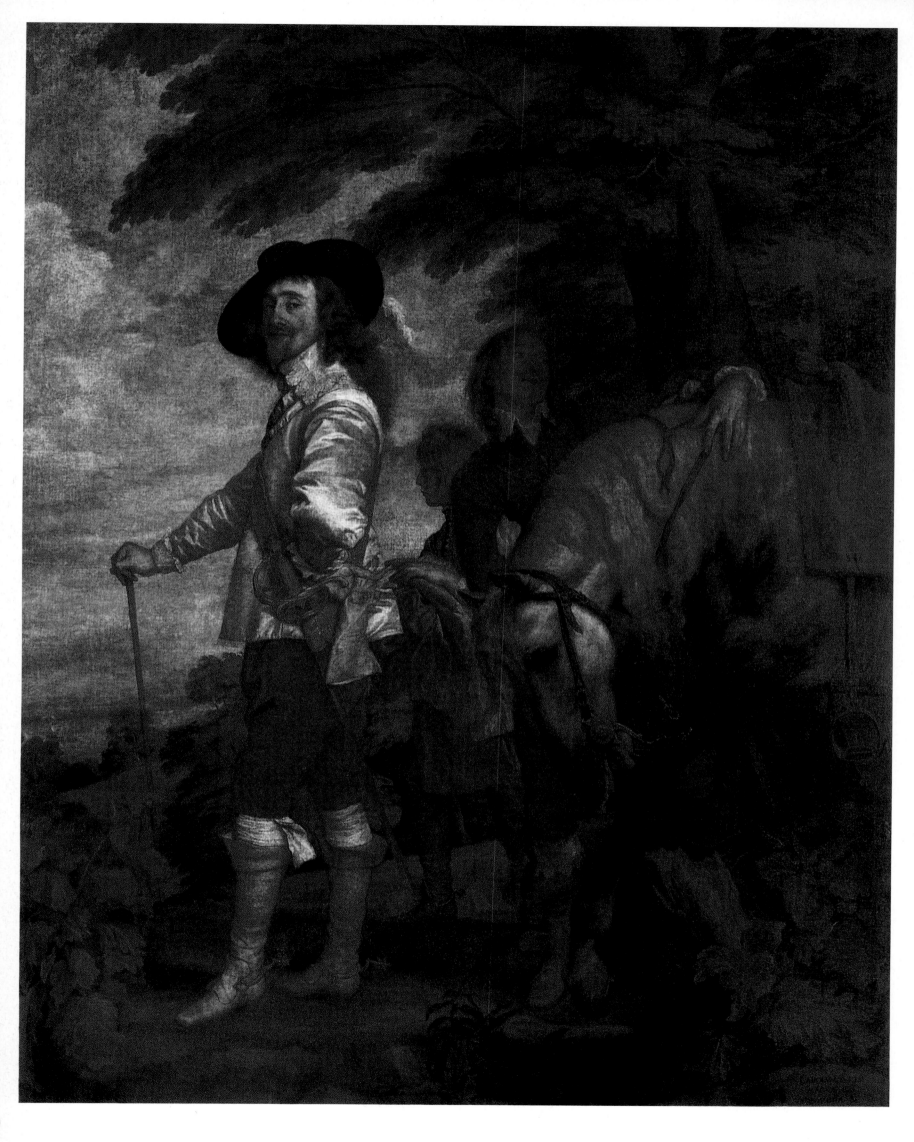

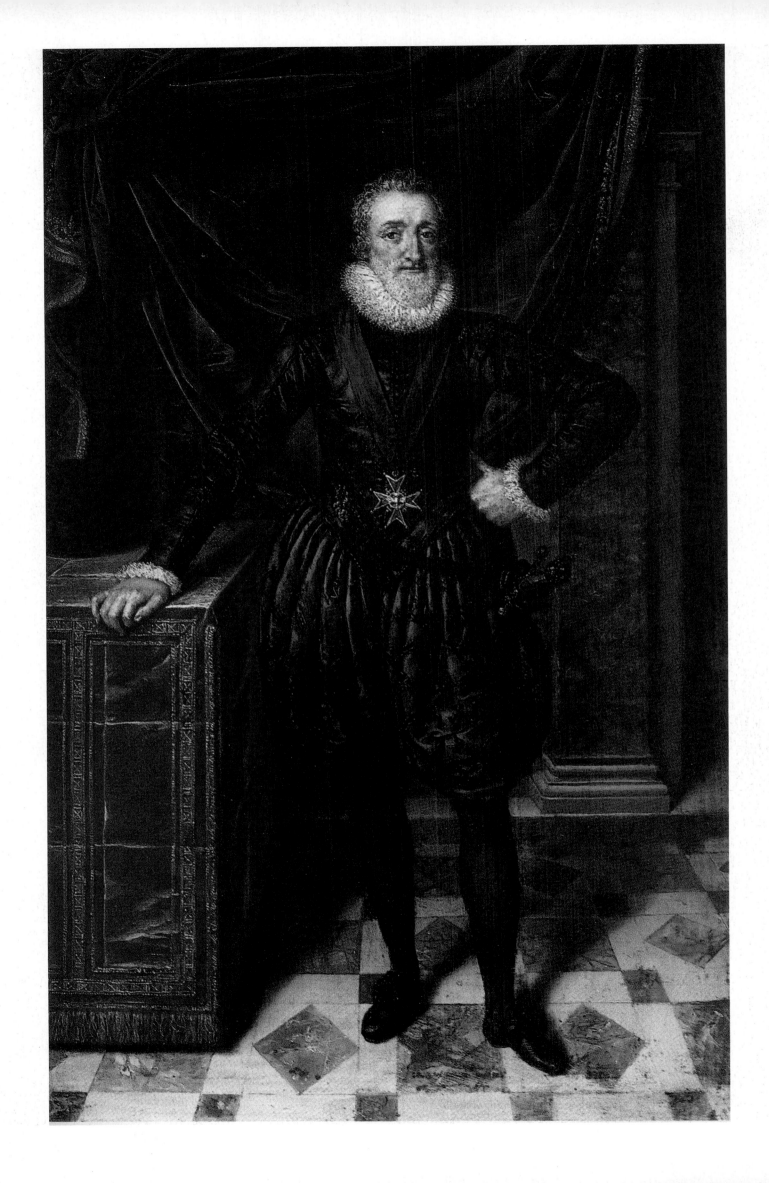

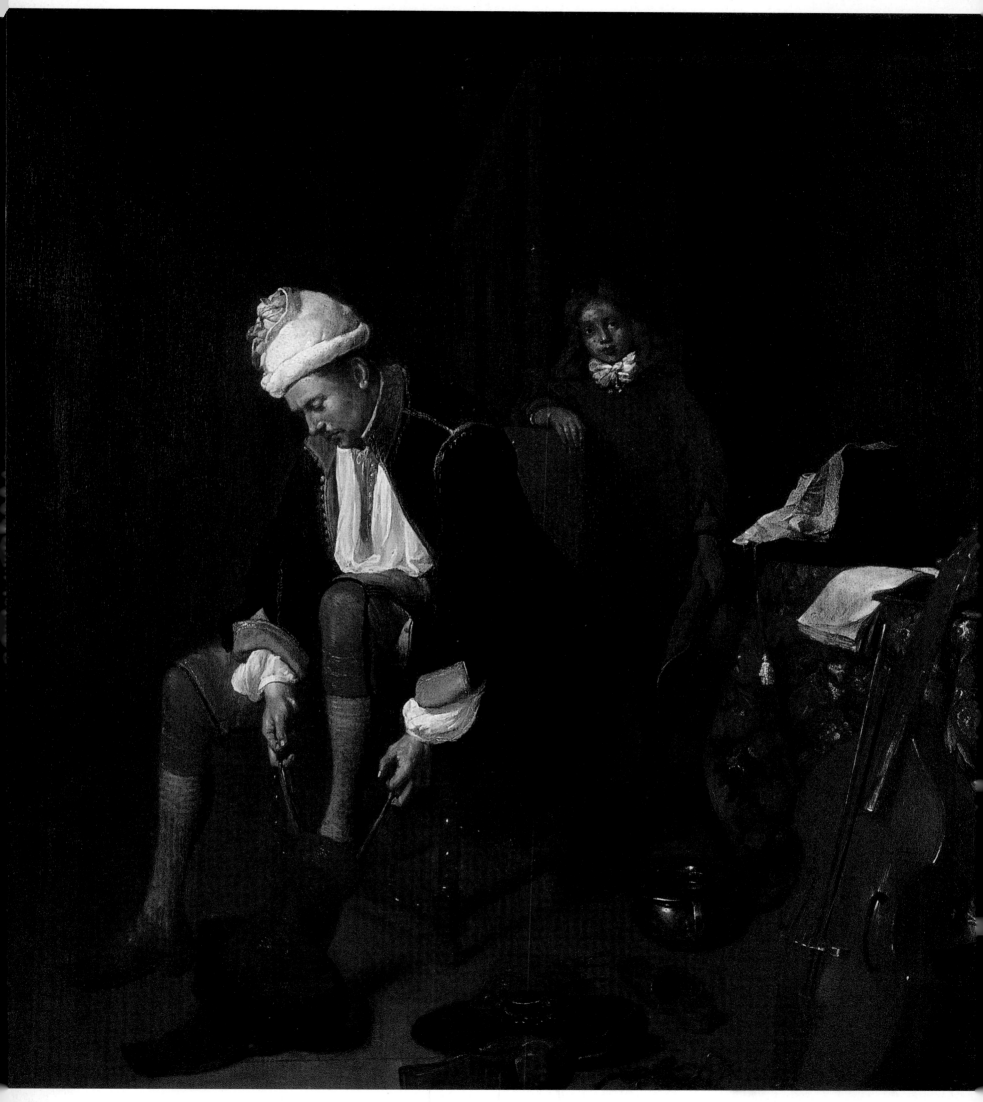

17th century

The 17th century witnessed the export of French style throughout Europe. The fragile eschappins of the Renaissance began to disappear during the reign of Henry IV (1553-1610), replaced by sturdy shoes whose uppers slightly exceeded the sole. The toe of 17th-century shoes, at first rounded, became square under Louis XIII (1601-1643). All shoes of the period revealed side openings. The method of fastening the shoe on top was hidden by a buckle or large bow. But the greatest novelty of the period was the heel, which imparted men and women with a form of bearing that would become the customary posture of European courts in the 17th century.

The new 17th-century shoe had an opening between the heel and the sole, from which it acquired the name soulier à pont-levis (raised bridge shoe). It was also called the soulier à cric (referring to a jack), a French onomatopoeia associated with the sound one made when walking in the shoe, according to Agrippa d'Aubigné's pamphlet (1552-1630), *Le Baron de Fenestre*. Around 1640, shoe length exceeded the foot, but the square toe was retained. Early in the 17th century, Henri IV sent a tanner named Roze to Hungary to study their method of leather preparation. His return heralded the rebirth of the Hungarian leather craftsmen and they began producing a soft leather used for boot making that clinged to the calf and the thigh. In boot making, the boot's over foot, was held by a soulette, which was attached under the foot and held the spur. After 1608, when boots were permitted at court, salons, and balls, the spur was covered with a piece of cloth to prevent damage to ladies' dresses.

Beginning in 1620, boots called bottes à entonnoir or bottes à chaudron (caldron boots) could be pulled up over the knee for horseback riding, or allowed to fall around the calf for other occasions. The purely utilitarian heel was positioned under the boot to better support the foot in stirrups. Special fabric boot stockings decorated with lace were worn to preserve the silk ones. Boot stockings were worn with entonnoir boots, which had the disadvantage of becoming a receptacle for water when worn in inclement weather. Lazzarines and ladrines were shorter, lighter boots with an ample cuff that were very popular during the reign of Louis XIII. But boots began to disappear from the salons and from court during the reign of Louis XIV (1638-1715), although they were still worn for hunting and in war. Even the heavy boot worn by soldiers until the beginning of the 19th century was gradually replaced in elegant surroundings by a softer version. In 1663, a shoemaker named Nicolas Lestage, established in Bordeaux under the trade name Loup Botté, presented the king with a pair of seamless boots. The shoemaker's masterpiece earned him great fame and prestige, including a coat of arms that contained a gold boot, a gold crown, and the lily of the house of France, but his trade secret would only be revealed much later: he worked from the skin of a calf's foot that remained intact. At Versailles, the royal residence since 1678, Louis XIV wore mules tended by the first valet during the ceremonial rising required by rituals of etiquette. The king's mules became the property of the outgoing chamberlain or the valet at the end of the year. A number of developments in footwear took place during the reign of Louis XIV: lateral openings were eliminated from shoes and wooden heels became the province of a specialized craftsman called le talonnier (heelpiece maker). The Sun King had his own heels trimmed in red leather and his courtiers hastened to imitate him. Red heels remained the mark of aristocratic privileges until the French Revolution, and were only worn by nobles admitted to the court. The height of these heels was noted as a symbol of society's vanity in a letter written to Cardinal Montalto by the disparaging courtier Marigny: "I wear pointed shoes with a pad under the heel making me high enough to aspire to the title Royal Highness."

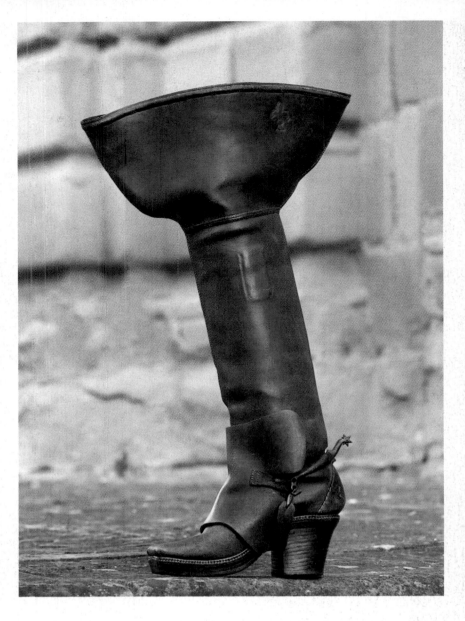

44. Gerritsz van Brekelenkan. *A Gentleman Slipping on a Boot*, Dutch School, 1655. International Shoe Museum, Romans.

45. Musketeer boot. France, 17th century.

Following pages:

46. Hiacynthe Rigaud. *Louis XIV*, 1701. Canvas, 277 x 194 cm. Louvre Museum, Paris.

47. Anonymous. *The Count of Toulouse Dressed as a Novice of the Holy Spirit*, around 1694. Condé Museum, Chantilly.

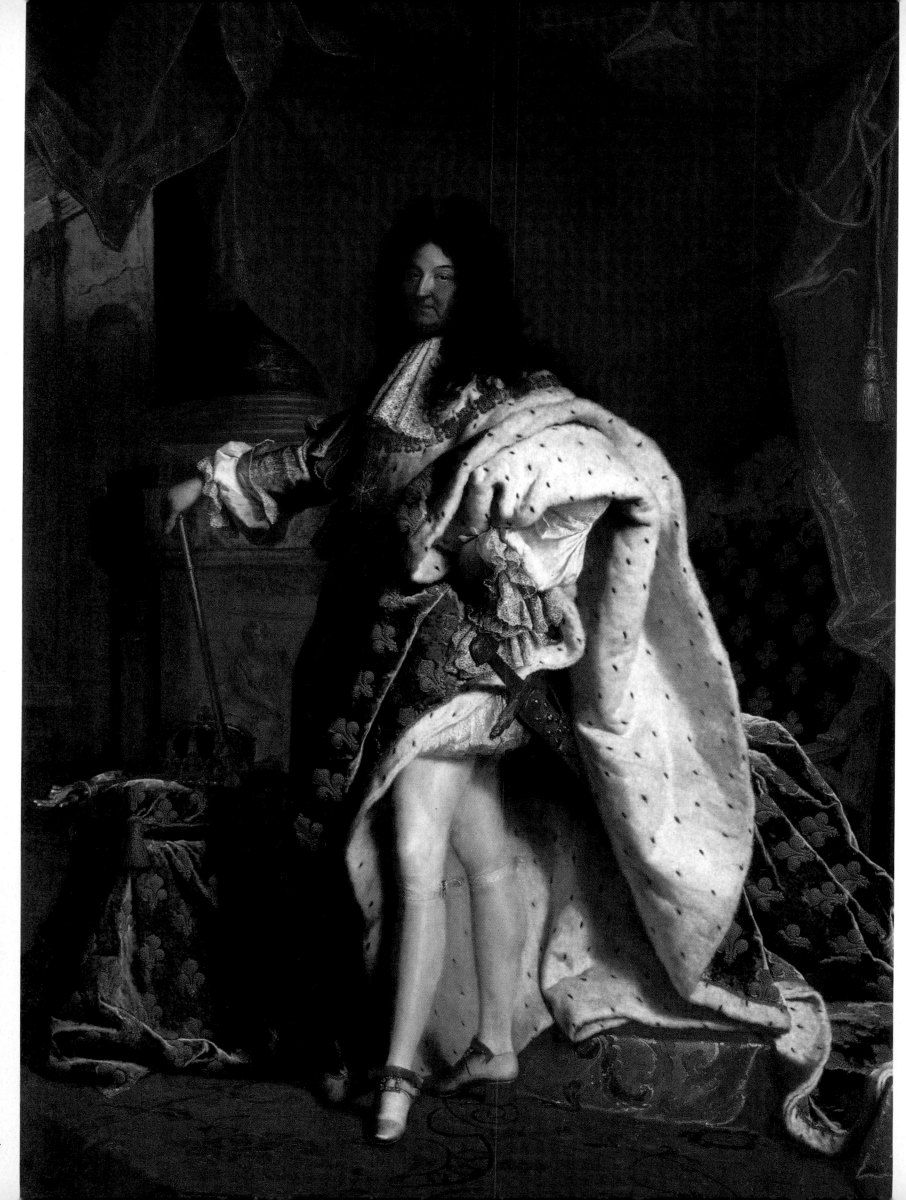

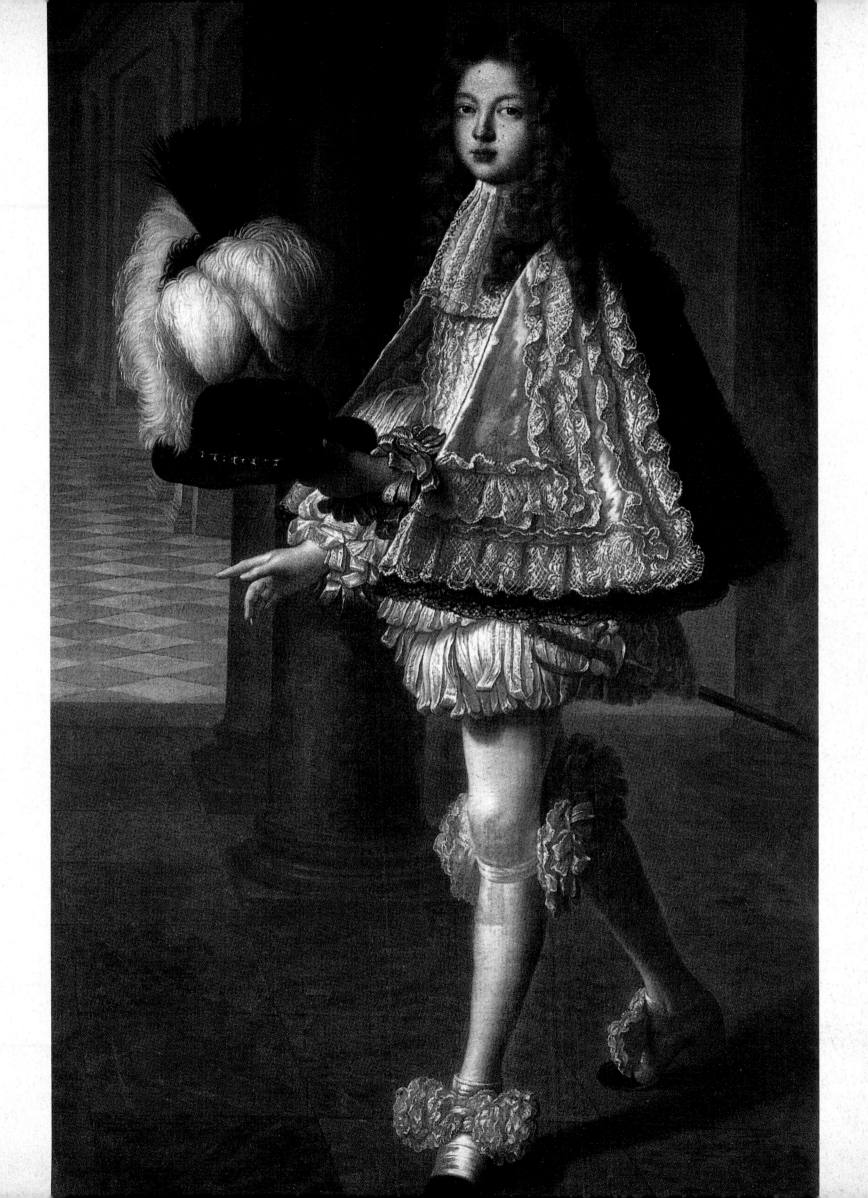

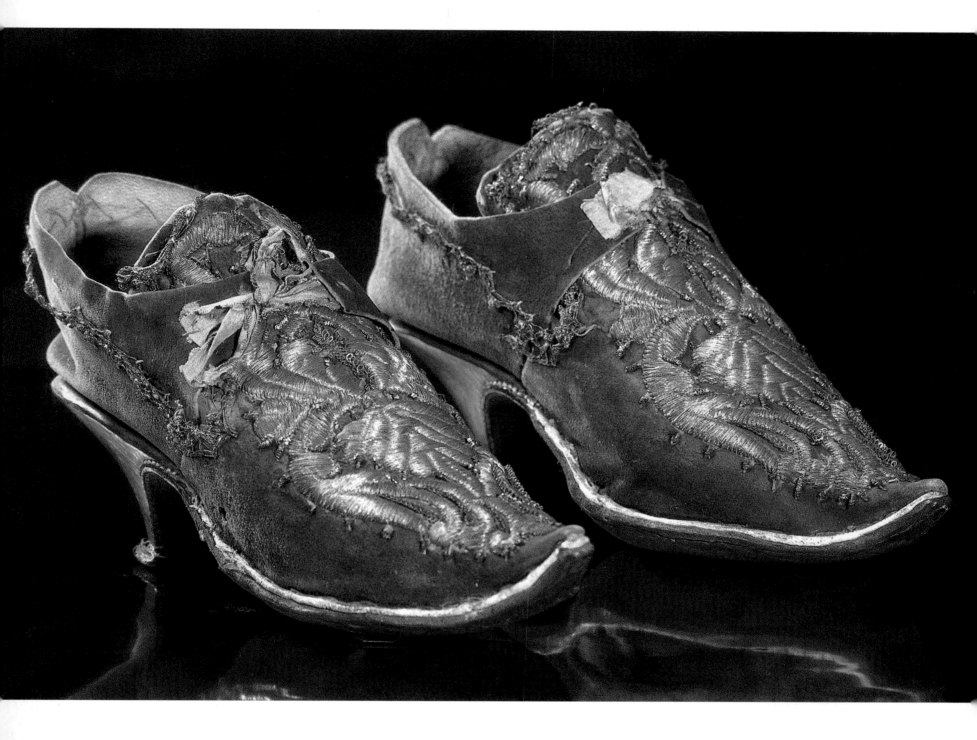

Jean de la Fontaine (1621-1695) was well aware of the dilemma women faced walking on awkward high heels. In his fable called *The Milkmaid and the Jug of Milk*, he has Perrette the milkmaid wear flats so that she can take big steps, move with greater agility, and get to town without incident. Around 1652, the fashion was pointed shoes; later they became square. Women's shoes were based on masculine forms, but always utilized more refined materials, primarily silk brocade, velvet, and brocart, a rich silk brocade sewn with silver and gold thread. Leather on women's shoes was sometimes trimmed with fine silk embroidery. Overshoes called galoches were worn to protect these smart-looking and delicate shoes from muddy streets. Some shoes exhibited a unique feature whereby the quarter terminated with two tabs attached to the throat of the shoe with a buckle. The throat lay as a flap over the top of the shoe; in French it was called the oreillle.

These shoes were originally decorated with a large ornament made out of two ribbon loops called ailes de moulin à vent, or windmill sails. This was the look Molière (1622-1673) derided in *The School for Husbands* when Sganarelle Scoffs, "Those little ribboned shoes make you look like you have big feathery pigeon feet."

Between 1670 and 1680, buckles embedded with a combination of real and fake pearls and diamonds replaced bows on tops of shoes. Unembellished bronze buckles were worn during mourning. Buckles were stored in jewelry boxes and adapted for use on different shoes. Children's shoes were smaller versions of adult models. Children of the wealthy wore shoes made of tripe blanc, a type of wool velour.

Shoes worn by the lower classes exhibited little development. The masses wore wooded clogs or big leather shoes until they were completely deteriorated. Examples are depicted in paintings of the period by the Le Nain Brothers.

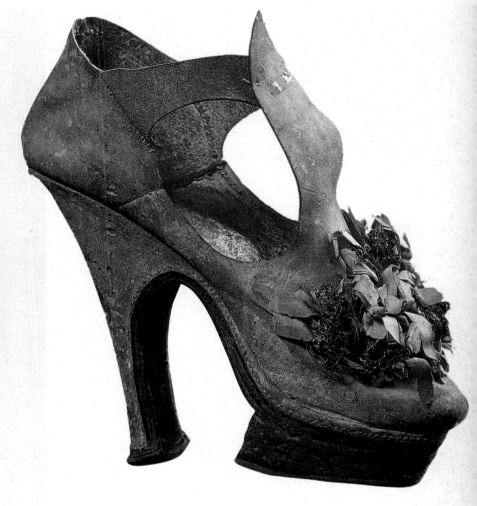

amey hth

F Séré direxit

ARMOIRIES

Concedées par LOUIS XIV, à son Cordonnier ordinaire,

Maître Nicolas LESTAGE de Bordeaux

Inventeur de la Botte incomparable sans couture.

48. Woman's shoe in blue leather with decoration embroidered in silver.
Italy, 17th century. International Shoe Museum, Romans.

49. Coat of arms granted by Louis XIV to his standard shoemaker,
Master Nicolas Lestage, inventor of the incomparable boot without seams.

50. Woman's shoe. Italy, 17th century. International Shoe Museum, Romans.

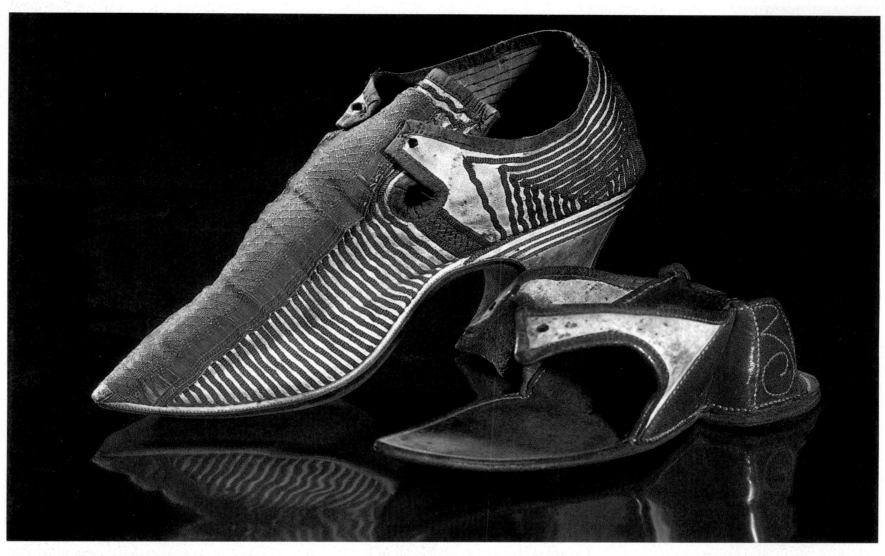

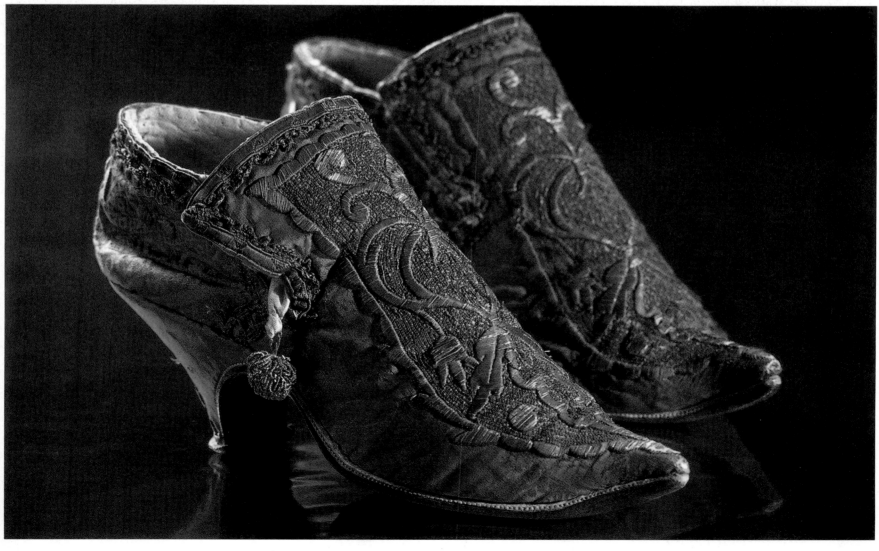

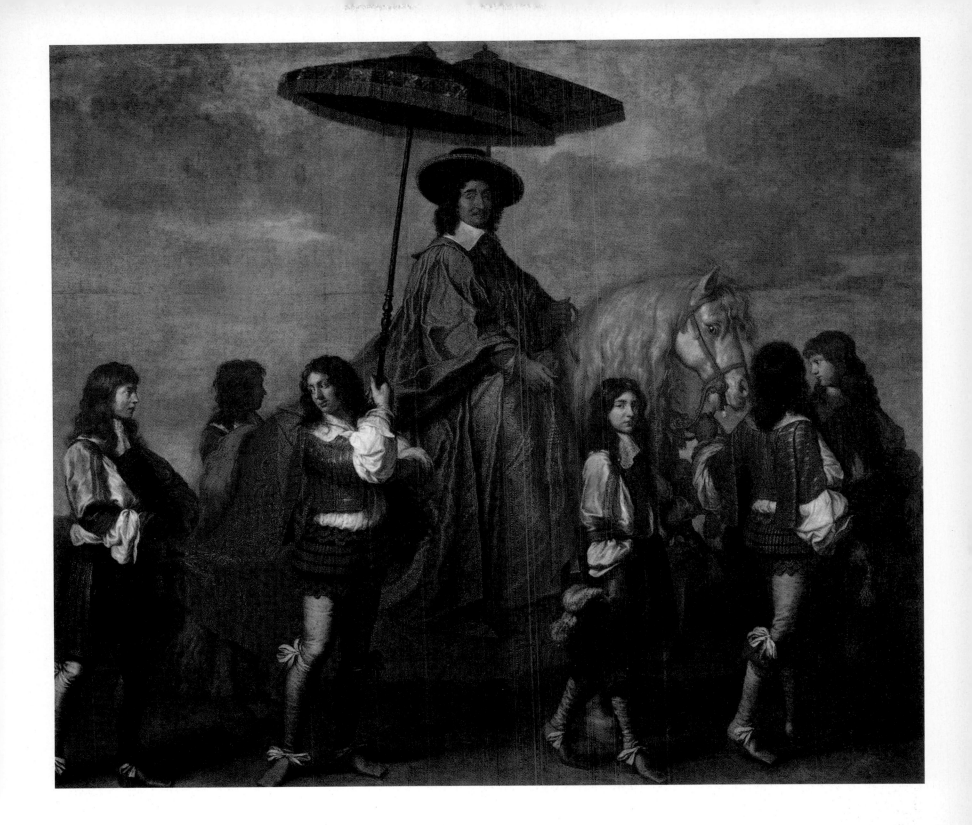

51. Woman's shoe with its protective clog. Louis XIV period, 17th century. The fragility of these shoes necessitates the wearing of protective clogs to walk outside or face muddy grounds. The protective clog has a notch to place the heel. International Shoe Museum, Romans.

52. Woman's shoe in damask embroidered with threads of gold and silver. Louis XIV period, 17th century. International Shoe Museum, Romans.

53. Le Brun, *The Chancellor Séguier*, 295 x 351cm, The Louvre, Paris.

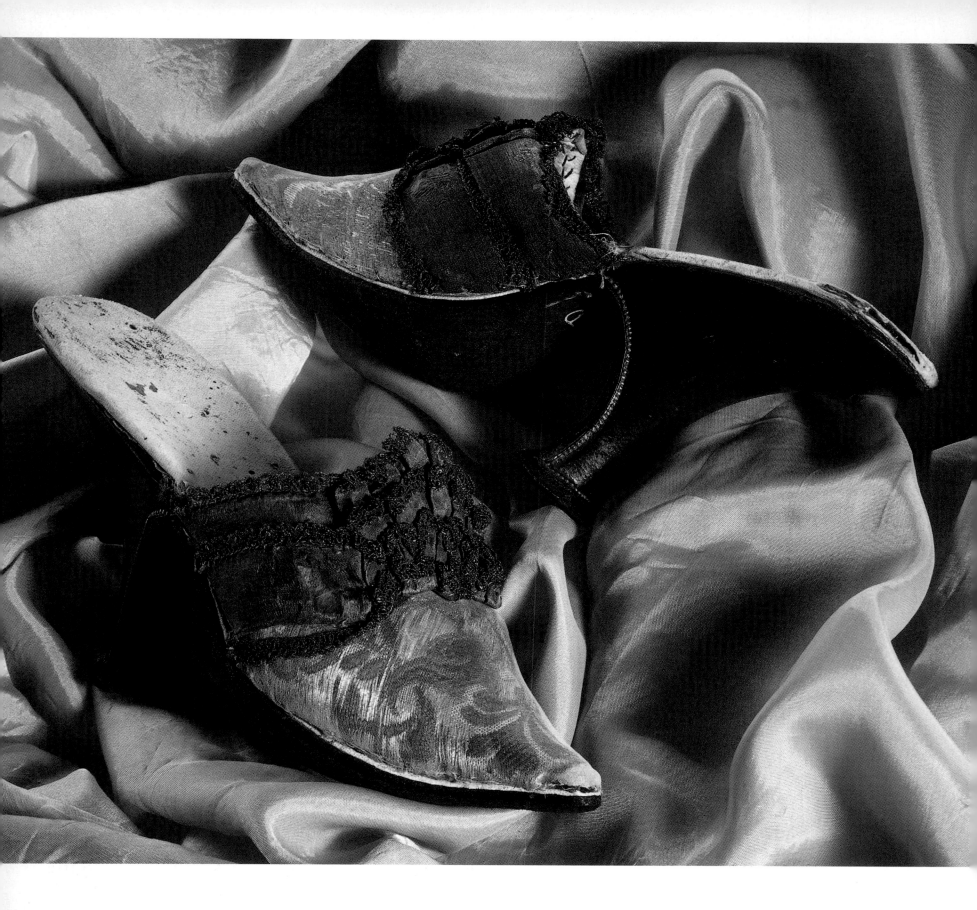

54. Woman's mules. Around 1720-1730. Weissenfels Museum,
   with the authorization of Irmgard Sedler.

55. François Boucher. *La Toilette*, 1742. Oil on canvas. 52.5 x 65.5 cm.
   Thyssen-Bornemisza Collection, Madrid.

56. William Hogarth. *Mariage à la Mode. After the Marriage*, 1734-1735.
   Oil on canvas. 70 x 91 cm. National Gallery, London.

18th century

At the beginning of the 18th-century, France still held sway over the world of elegance.

From the Regency to the French Revolution (1715-1789), there was little variation in shoe shapes. The toe could be round or pointed and was sometimes raised, but never square. A heel was named after Louis XV le Bien-Aimé (1710-1774). Elegant ladies favored two different styles: the mule for indoors and high-heeled shoes for more formal outfits. Mules with heels of variable height had uppers of white leather, velvet, or silk, which was usually embroidered. Many models of mules and shoes are depicted in the work of the period's artists, including the prints of Beaudoin and Moreau le Jeune and the paintings of Quentin de Latour, Boucher, Gainsborough, and Hogarth, among others. Fragonard's *The Swing* shows a mischievous young woman in a wind-swept skirt carried high by her swinging, which sends her pink mule towards the nose of her suitor stretched out among the branches beneath the lovely creature.

The curved lines of the Louis XV style are also recognizable in the period's heeled shoes, which now attain their maximum height. The curved heel, positioned under the arch of the foot, served as a shank and stabilized the shoe's balance, although walking in them remained precarious – like walking in Venetian chopines during the Renaissance. To overcome this drawback, fashionable women began using canes in 1786, as the Count de Vaublanc noted in his memoirs: "If she wasn't holding her weight back with a cane, the doll would fall on her nose."

The pinnacle of 18th-century refinement would come to be nestled in diamond-encrusted heels, which in this instance were referred to as *venez-y voir* (take a look), although the coquetry was secret, due to the fact that dresses almost touched the floor. Restif de la Bretonne (1734-1806), whose glorification of the feminine foot and shoe is well known, is clearly referring to the shoe in the following description:

"It was a shoe of mother-of-pearl with a flower made of diamonds: the edges were trimmed in diamonds, as was the heel, which was quite slender in spite of this ornament. This pair of shoes cost two thousand écus, not counting the diamonds in the flower, which were worth three or four times this amount: it was a gift from Saintepallaire" (*The Pretty Foot*, p. 240). These enchanting shoes were of white embroidered leather or precious silks to match dresses and were finished with a buckle that could be changed for each outfit. As in the previous century, polished silver buckles, decorated with glass gems or precious stones, were stored in jewelry boxes and passed down through inheritance. Women continued to protect their shoes when going out by wearing the wooden pattens, which were now secured with two leather straps fastened to the top of the foot; the sole was fitted with a notch for the heel. 18th-century France experienced a passion for the East, as evidenced in historical, economic, and cultural contexts. In the context of footwear, the taste for the exotic led to a craze for pointed shoes with raised toes, variously referred to as shoes à la turque (Turkish) en sabot chinois (Chinese), or à l'orientale (Eastern).

Men wore simple, flat-heeled shoes embellished with a buckle. Made of dark-coloured or black leather, these shoes emphasized the light-coloured stockings men wore with silk pants. Certain shoes of this type made of silk or velvet to match men's doublets enjoyed great popularity. A taste for imported English boots (and many other English fashion details) was revived around 1779. A new type of soft leather boot with cuffs to be worn with hunting outfits and court uniforms began to gain popularity during the last twenty years of the 18th-century and would remain common until the 19th century.

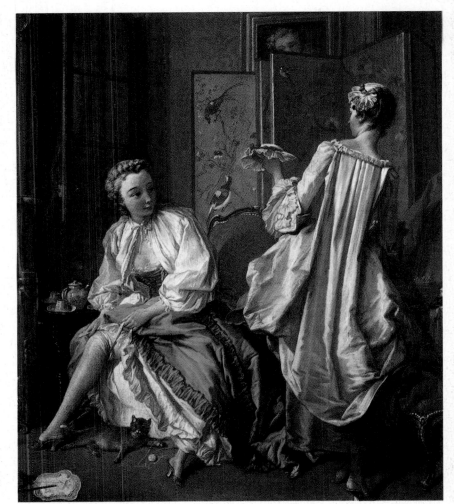

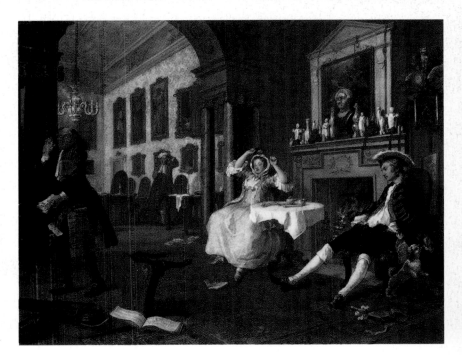

Following pages:

57. Fragonard. *The Swing*. Oil on canvas. 81 x 64.2 cm. Wallace Collection, London.

58. Woman's shoe. Louis XV period, France, 18th century. Silver buckle accentuated with stones from the Rhine. International Shoe Museum, Romans.

59. Woman's shoe, toe upturned in the eastern style. Louis XV period, France, 18th century. International Shoe Museum, Romans.

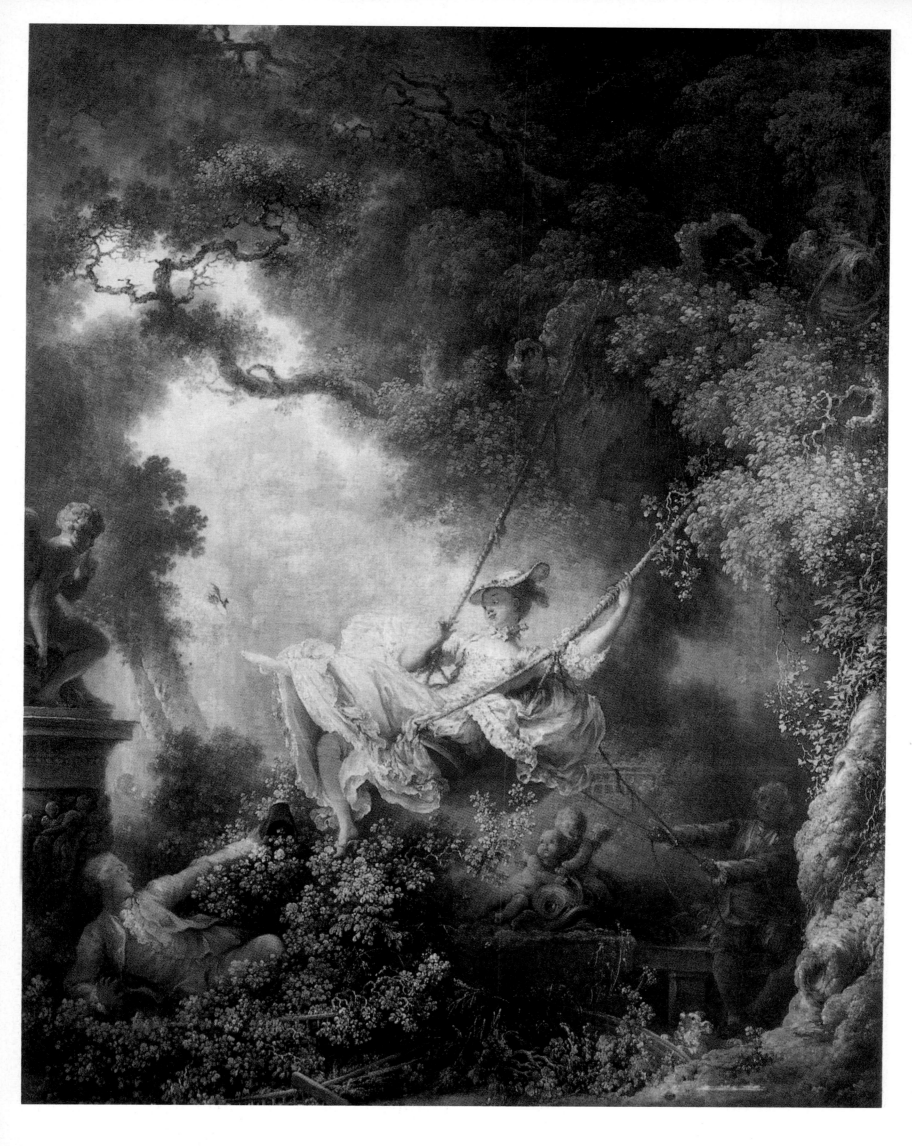

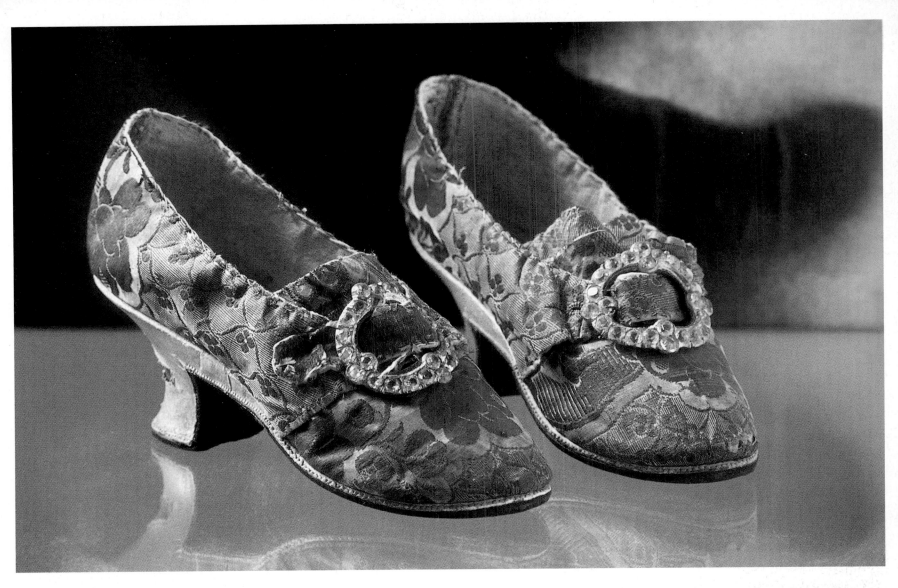

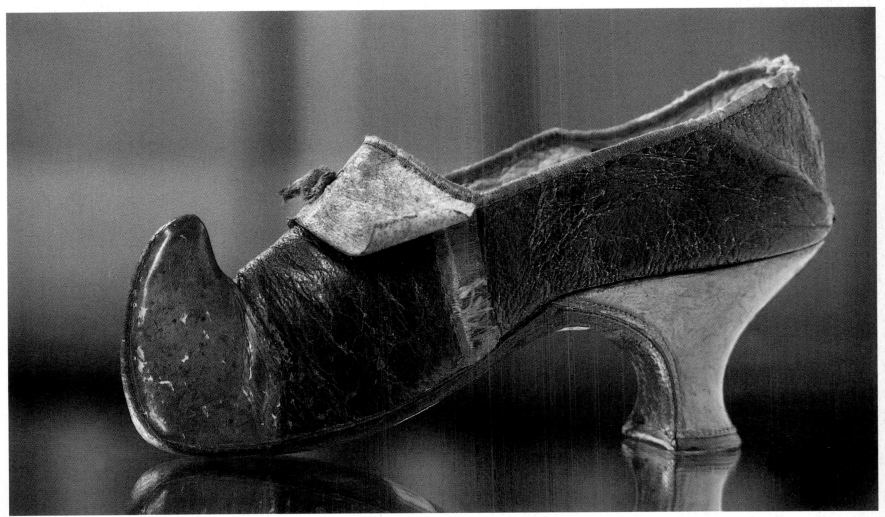

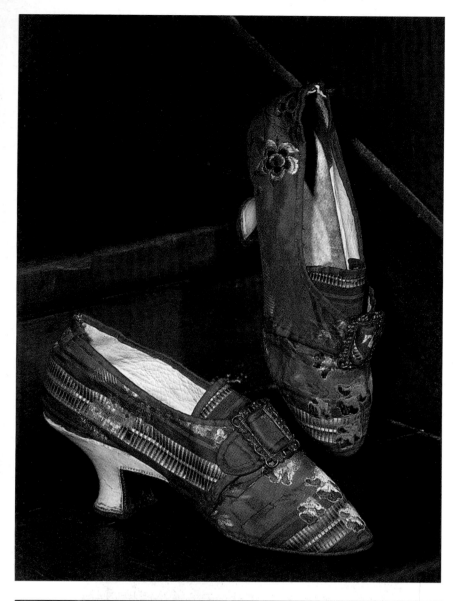

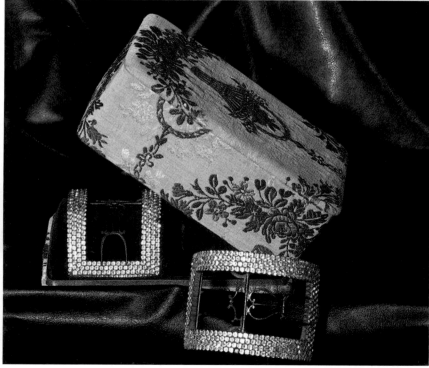

The return to greater simplicity and to straight lines preferred during Louis XVI's reign had its counterpart in footwear. For example, the buckle on men's shoes assumed greater prominence and women's heels became shorter. Additionally, women's heels were sheathed in white leather, while their shoe buckles were usually superceded by an ornament made of gathered fabric called a bouillonné, which was placed on the shoe's upper and matched the dress.

Shoemakers had stopped making shoes differentiated for the left and right foot during the Renaissance, but the practice made a limited comeback at the end of 18th century. By the second half of the 19th century it would become a standard manufacturing technique as shoemaking was industrialized.

In the years before the French Revolution, shoemakers managed thriving shops. The writer Sébastien Mercier records that, "in their black outfit and powdered wig, they look like Clerks of the Court." But when the Revolution came, shoemakers sympathized with the spirit of the new era: seventy-seven shoemakers participated in the storming of the Bastille.

In Arras, Robespierre drafted the shoe repairmen's official grievances, while in Vierzon, an appointee to the Public Safety Committee wrote to representative Laplance in September 1793 that he had replaced the court "made up of old wigged heads" and appointed a shoemaker to it. When the revolutionary Saint Just saw that ten thousand soldiers in the Rhine army were going barefoot, he ordered the city of Strasbourg to remove the shoes of ten thousand aristocrats with instructions to deliver the shoes to the soldiers before ten o'clock the next morning. To avoid the guillotine, everything reminiscent of aristocratic luxury had to be eliminated, making way for a simpler, but still elegant style. Even shoes sported a revolutionary cockade, the symbol of the new patriotic religion. Men dared not wear fine shoes with buckles out of fear of being labeled an aristocrat, although Robespierre himself risked wearing them. The masses generally wore clogs.

It was at this time that Antoine Simon was working as an obscure shoemaker on the rue des Cordeliers in Paris. A Jacobin and later a member of the Paris Commune, he was chosen by the Convention to look after the young dauphin in the Temple after the child was separated from his mother, Queen Marie-Antoinette, on July 3, 1793. Himself an illiterate, the new tutor to the Capet son had orders to make the child forget his social status. And with the help of his wife, the shoemaker succeeded in transforming the child into a perfect little sans-culotte, teaching his nine-year-old pupil a repertoire of invectives against God, his family, and the aristocracy, as well as revolutionary songs, such as "ça ira, ça ira" and "la Carmagnole."

Unlike the tormenter he is often depicted as, the coarse, uneducated shoemaker grew fond of little Louis XVII, as did Madame Simon. To amuse the child, Simon bought him a dog named Caster, followed by birds that he set up in a large aviary with seventeen bars where the child raised pigeons, a fact affirmed by the Temple's own accounts, which record the purchase of feed for the young Capet's pigeon. But in January 1794, by order of the Committee for Public Safety, Simon was relieved of his duties. It was against his will and against the will of the child, who begged the shoemaker to take him away and teach him how to make shoes. Alas, Simon the shoemaker was guillotined after 9 thermidor (the fall of Robespierre on July 27, 1794).

From 1795 to 1799, footwear under the Directory began to evolve into the early neo-classical style favored by Napoleon I. The light, flat, and pointed new style, for both men and women, confirmed the end of the former regime's heel. The most elegant and striking women of this period, known as les merveilleuses, wore sandals equipped with ribbons which they wore intertwined around their legs.

60. Woman's shoes. Louis XV period. Jacquemart Collection, International Shoe Museum, Romans.

61. Man's shoe buckle and its original case. 18th century.

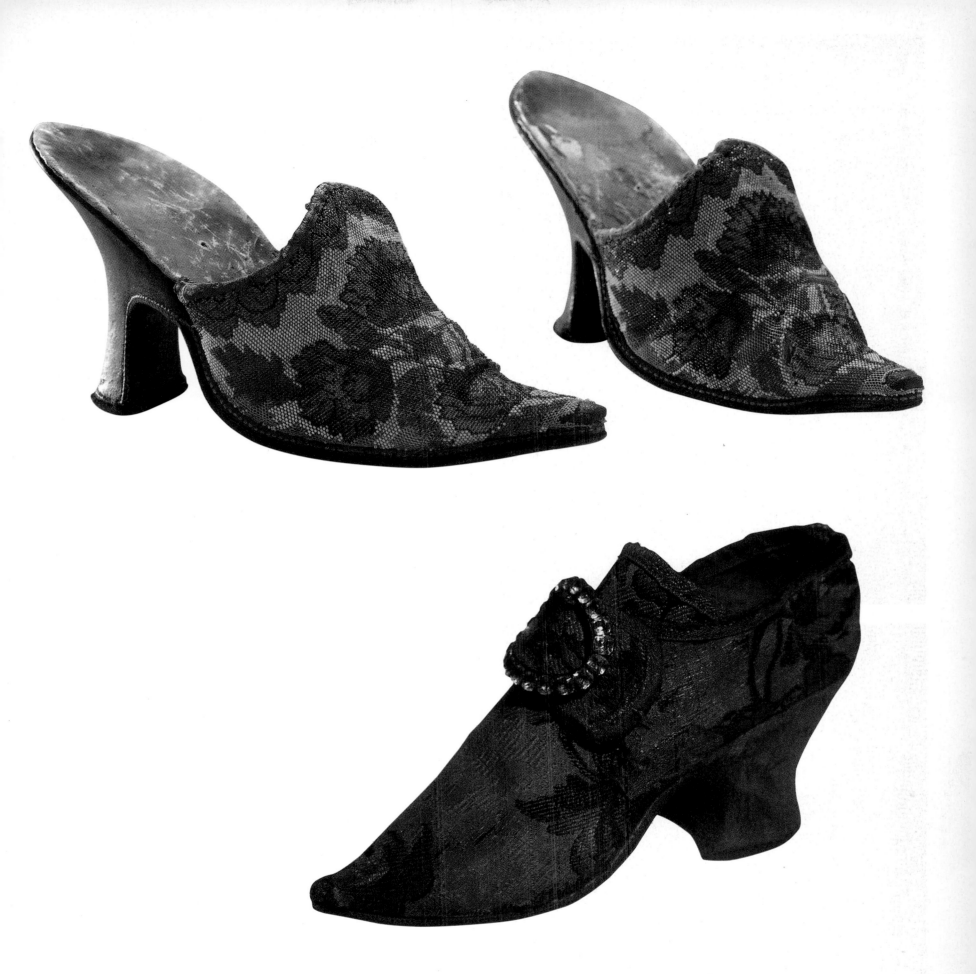

62. Embroided mules. France, early 18th century.

63. Woman's shoe. England, 18th century. International Shoe Museum, Romans.

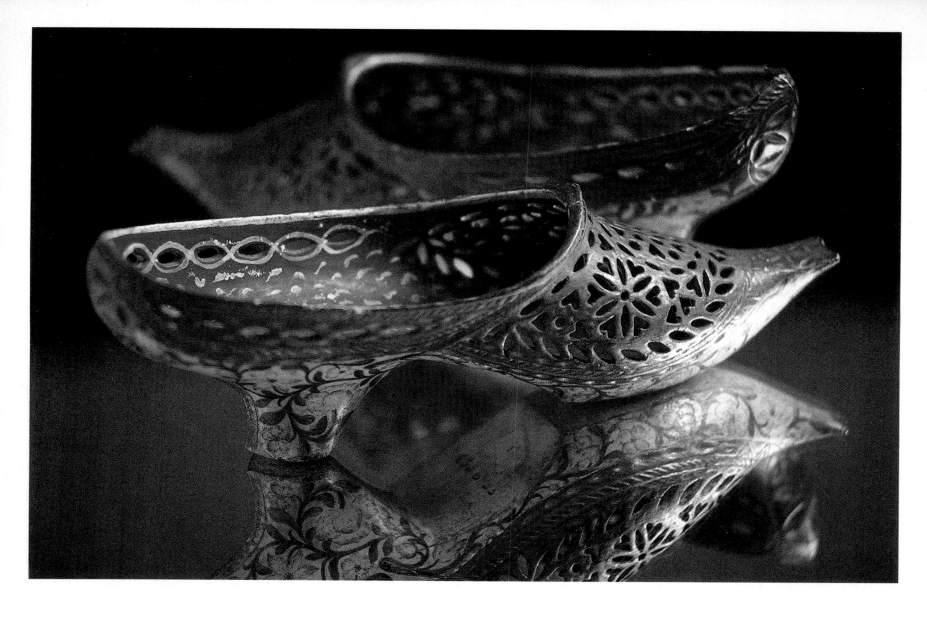

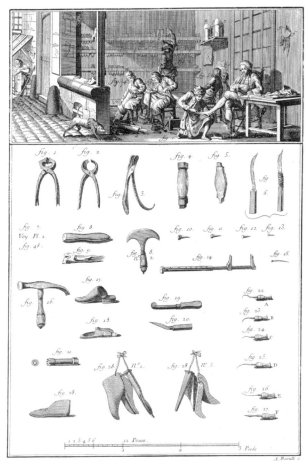

Cordonnier et Bottier.

64. Carved, lacquered and painted wooden clogs. Louis XVI period,

France, 18th century. International Shoe Museum, Romans.

65. Plates from Diderot and Alembert's Encyclodedia.

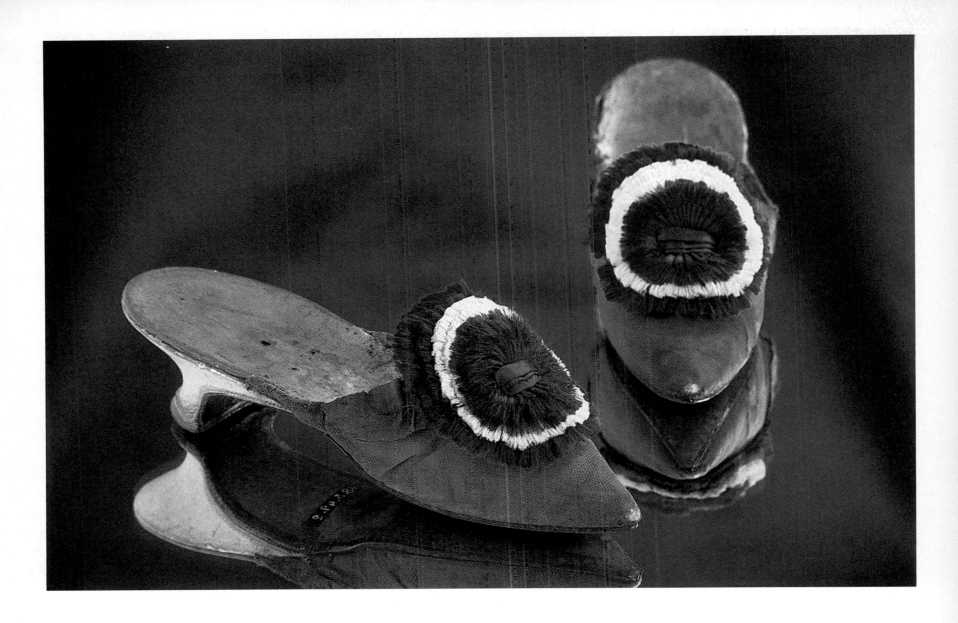

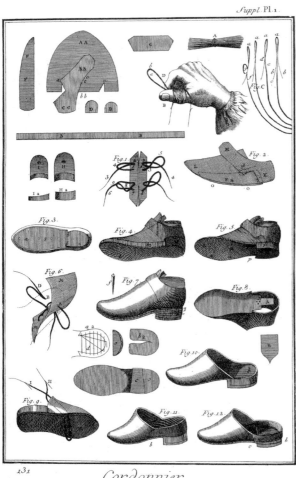

Cordonnier

66. Woman's mule. France, around 1789. Guillen Collection, International Shoe Museum, Romans.

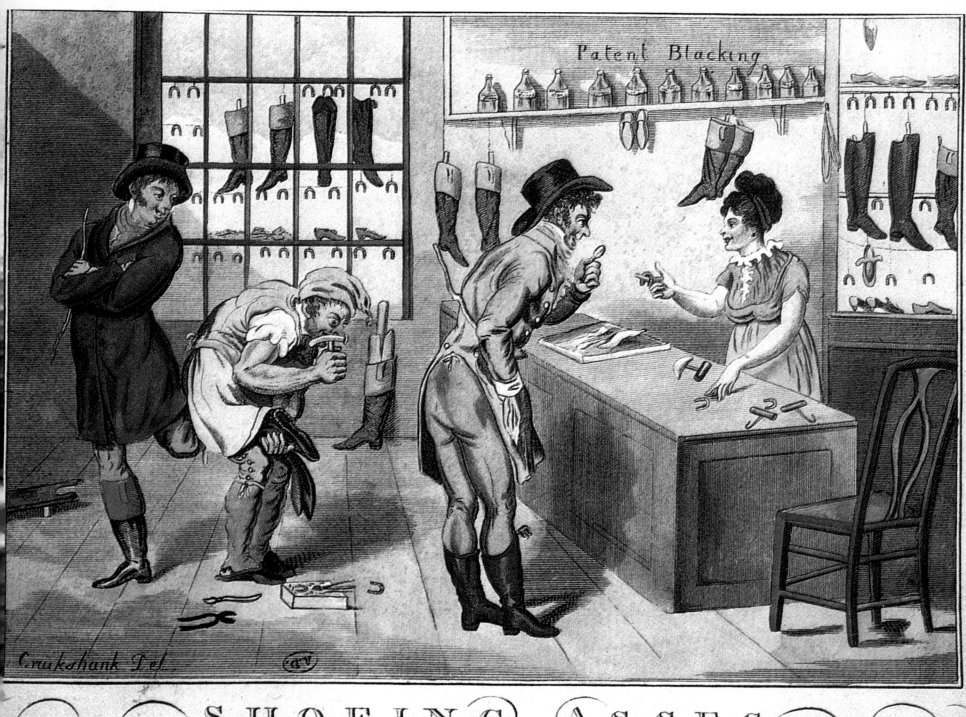

SHOEING ASSES.

The Present Fashion of Making Boots Everlasting.

Publish'd Apr. 20. 1807. by LAURIE & WHITTLE. 53, Fleet Street, London.

166

67. Cruikshank. "Shoeing Asses". International Shoe Museum, Romans.

19th century

19th-century women wore woolen ankle boots, but were especially known for their ballet shoes of fine glazed leather, satin, or silk. Ballet shoes fit a woman's foot closely like a glove and were held by ribbons crossed around the ankle. Very fragile, these ephemeral shoes scarcely lasted the duration of one ball.

An 1809 inventory of the wardrobe of Empress Josephine (1763-1814) listed seven hundred and eighty-five pairs of ballerinas made by the shoemaker Lalement. Dancing took place frequently during the Empire period, at court and elsewhere, during interludes between battles.

As for men's footwear, knee pants and silk stockings reintroduced by Napoleon showed off Empire-style escarpins, flat pumps made of patent leather and decorated with a buckle. The military-style boot was standard footwear for soldiers; it could be short or tall, with or without cuffs.

The Emperor, a shrewd strategist declared: "A well-equipped soldier requires three things: a good rifle, a military coat, and good shoes." Yet Napoleonic military shoes could be the subjects of humor, as in this story from the memoirs of an officer in the Great Army: "One day I went with General P… into an uninhabited house; it was pouring down and our clothes were soaking wet, so we lit a fire and warmed ourselves.

— Sit down, the General said to me.

— Why?

— I want to take your boots off.

— You're kidding me!

— No, I am not. Give me your foot.

— General, I can't allow it.

— Your boots are soaked and your feet are in water. You're going to catch cold.

— But I can take them off myself.

— I want to take them off for you.

Against my wishes, the General would remove my boots, to my extreme astonishment. When he was finished: Now my turn, he said. One good turn deserves another. Take off my boots.

— I'd be delighted.

— It was in order to get you to do this that I acted as I did

During the Restoration and the reign of Louis-Philippe, men wore boots and escarpins made of black leather. Only soft half boots were allowed to be beige, tawny, or brown.

The British dandy George Brummell (1778-1840), better known as Beau Brummell, wore laced ankle boots with narrow pants. Nicknamed the "fashion king," his clothes become a standard of elegance that knew no boundaries. The Prince of Wales and King Georges IV of England (1762-1830) were among his admirers.

Women also wore flat ankle boots made of cloth and laced on the side. A taste for satin and silk escarpins tied with ribbons lasted until 1830.

The heel returned under Louis-Philippe (1773-1850), but it was not until 1829 that news of its astonishing reappearance was published in the fashion periodical Le Petit Courrier de Dames: "We dare risk reporting shoes with a high heel positioned mid-sole, raising the in-step and thereby lending grace to walking. At least if our heels are constructed this way, they will not be ridiculous like our grandmother's heels."

Another fashion publication, *Les Modes Parisiennes*, in 1850 reported: "Some women are wearing heeled shoes according to their whim; this shows a desire to succumb to fashion, because they are very uncomfortable for dancing; ankle-boots have also begun to have little heels; these can only be suitable for women who do not have to wear rubber overshoes." The Second Empire preferred luxury and had an appetite for parties.

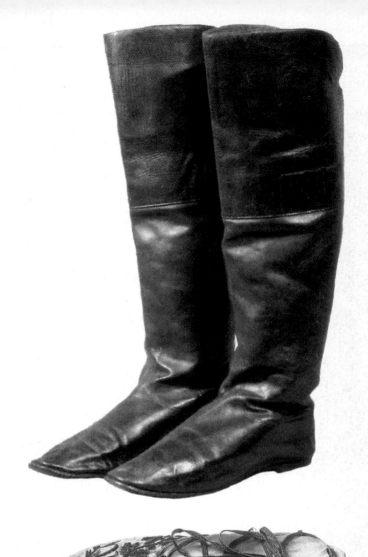

68. Emperor's boots. Private collection.

69. Flat court shoes of Napoleon I for his coronation in 1804. Lost during World War II.

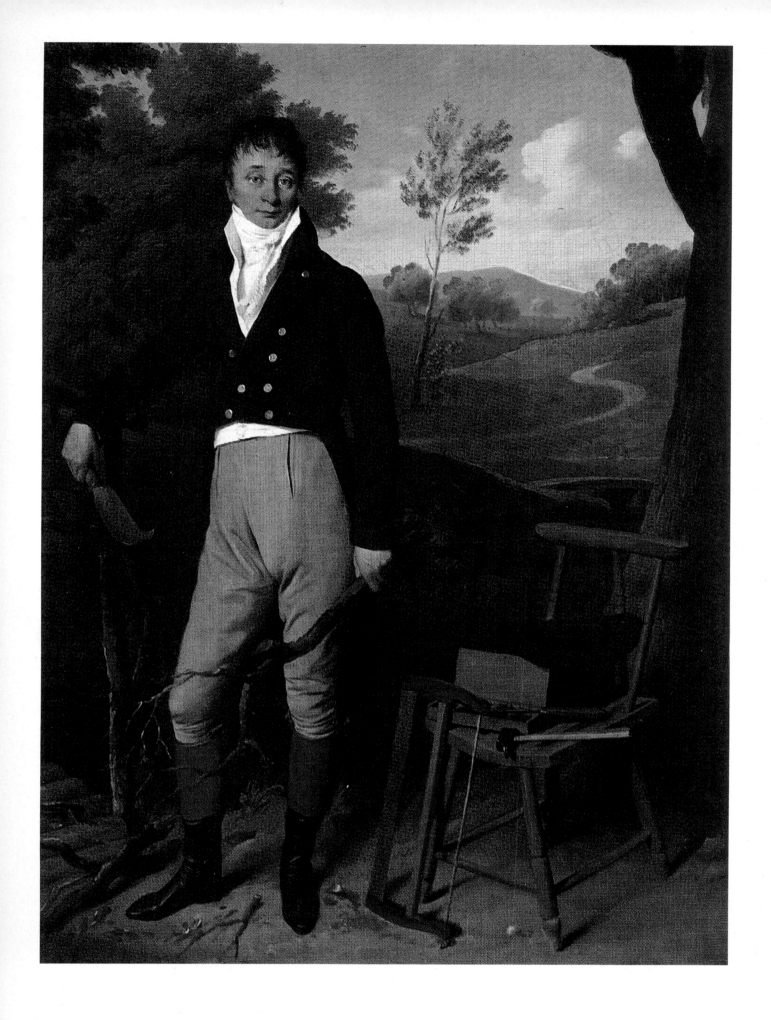

70. Louis Boilly. *Portrait of a Man*, 1805. Museum of Fine Arts, Lille.

71. Boots of Imperial Prince Jean-Joseph-Eugene-Louis Napoleon, only son

of Napoleon III and Eugenie de Montijo. International Shoe Museum, Romans.

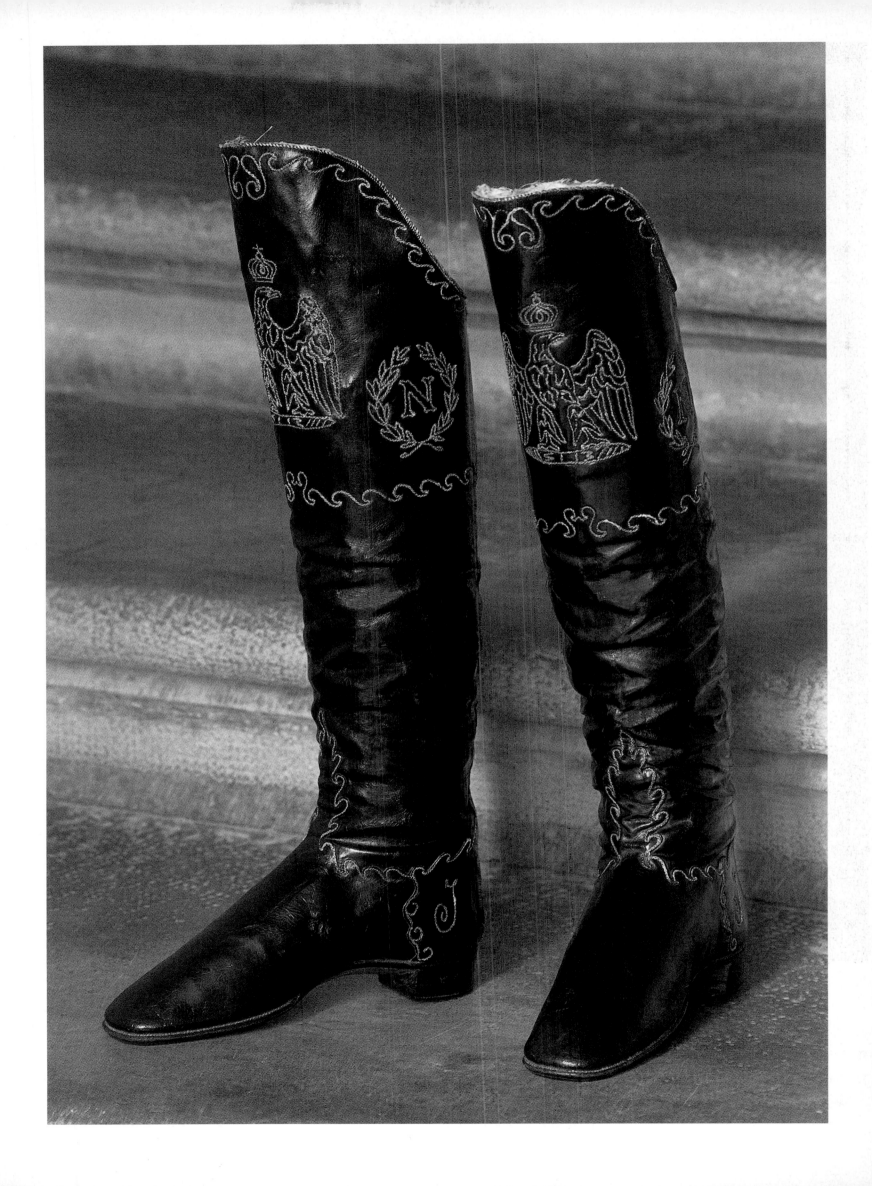

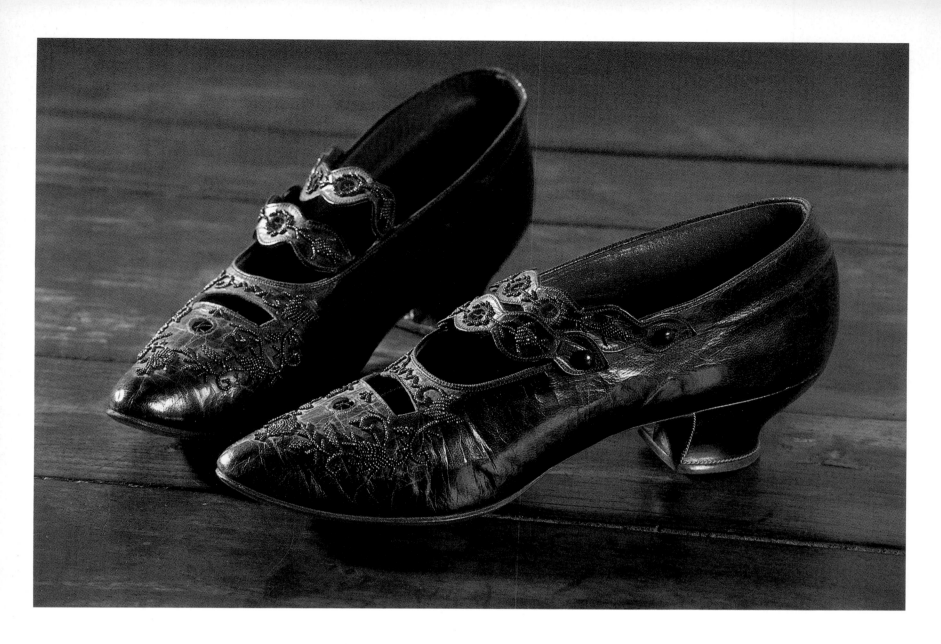

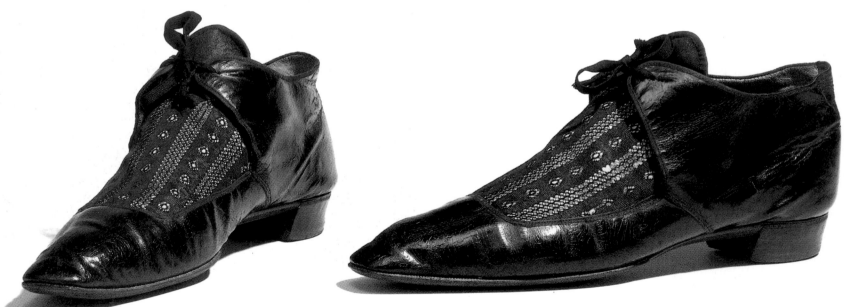

72. Woman's shoe in bronze kidskin, double attachment. Charles IX.

Buttoned on the side, embroidery with gilded metal beads, leather sole, reel heel.

19th century. International Shoe Museum, Romans.

73. Pair of men's shoes in black leather and openworked black silk.

Around 1830. Galliera Museum, Fashion Museum of the City of Paris.

Photo by Pierrain, PMVP.

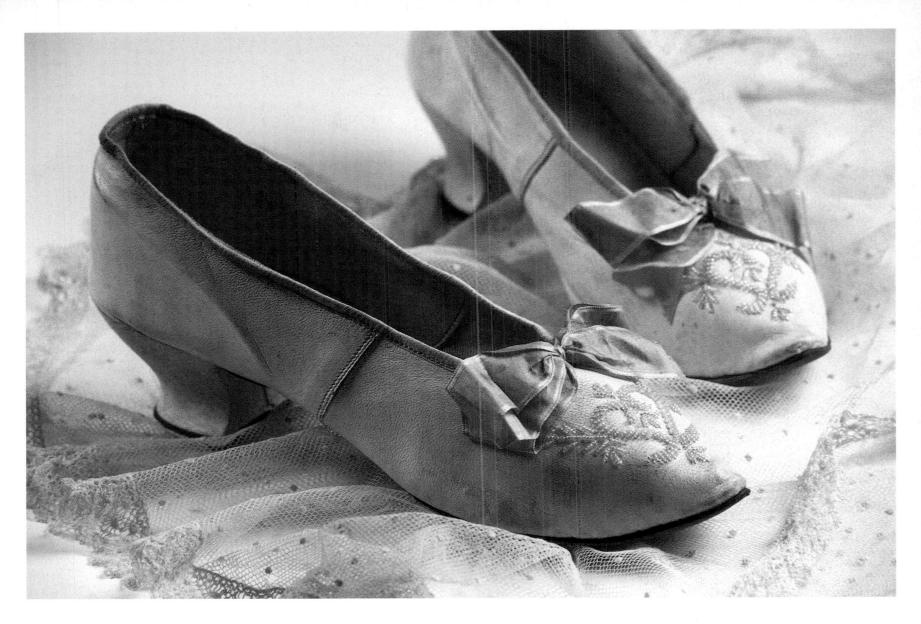

In contrast to the bourgeois court of Louis-Philippe, that of Napoleon III (1808-1873) proved to be extremely brilliant. Its salons and boulevards became a theater of society life, while the operettas of Jacques Offenbach, in particular *La Vie Parisienne*, mirrored the period's joie de vivre with a sense of humor. The passion for crinoline born around 1850 led to a revitalization of couture. The Empress Eugenie (1826-1920) brought fame to her couturier, Charles-Frederic Worth, who opened his salon in 1858, clothing the actresses and courtesans of the period, in addition to his imperial client. The bourgeoisie meanwhile accelerated their rise and pursued financial gain. The ankle boot reigned supreme, made of leather or cloth and very narrowly shaped. Decorated with embroidery and braids, it was either laced up or buttoned via a row of little buttons, whence the invention of the tire-bouton or buttonhook. The Second Empire also marks a decisive stage in the history of footwear, characterized by advances in mechanization and large-scale industry. Traditional shoemaking, which changed in 1809 when a machine for tacking soles appeared in England, was transformed by the industrial revolution. In 1819, another new machine made wooden pegs for tacking soles. But the biggest change came from Thimonnier's invention of the sewing machine, patented in 1830. A perfect invention, the sewing machine made it possible to stitch uppers of soft materials and began to spread among shoemakers in 1860. The technique improved their production yields, as machines positioned the heel, stitched the upper, and attached the upper to the sole. After 1870, it became common to use a form for each foot, which enabled shoes to correspond to anatomy. Industrial development began to overtake hand-made shoes as factories were established and expanded, in particular the Rousset Company in Blois in 1851. François Pinet's career is a classic example.

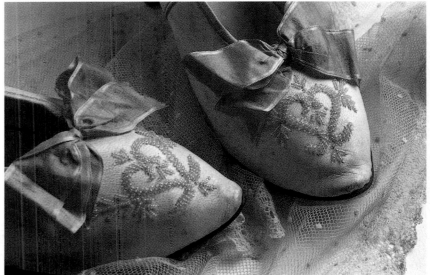

74. Bride's shoe, bead design in heart shape. Marriage the 10th of November 1896. International Shoe Museum, Romans.

75. Bride's shoe, detail, bead design in heart shape. Marriage the 10th of November 1896. International Shoe Museum, Romans.

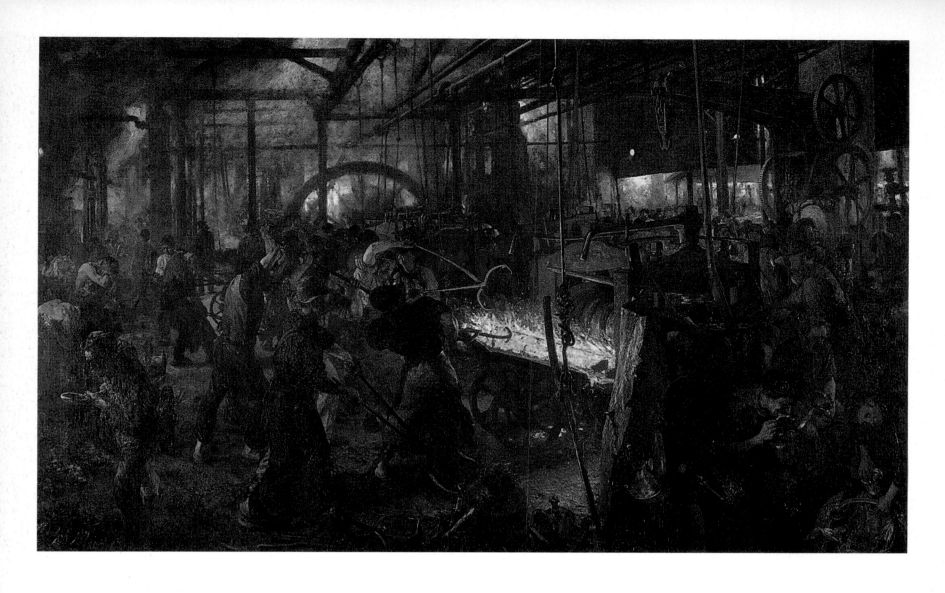

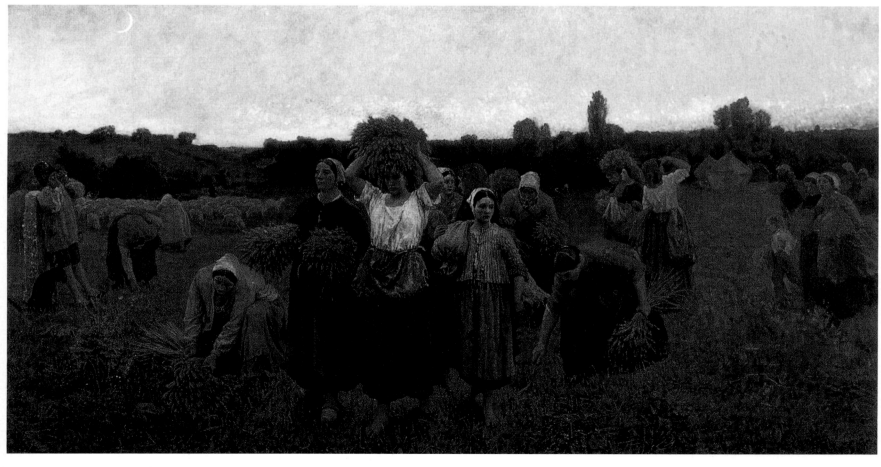

Shoes and Poverty

In the wake of the Second Empire's Fête Impériale or Imperial Celebration, the taste for magnificent clothing was matched with opulence in the art of the shoe. Examples of these styles, worn by the aristocracy and the increasingly wealthy bourgeoisie, can be seen today in public and private collections. Evidence of the fashions of their times, they are proof of the traditional expertise handed down from one generation to the next, revealing the individuality and the craftsmanship of their creators, whether famous or anonymous. On the other hand, the less well-dressed lower classes wore their shoes until thoroughly deteriorated; so common was this reality, these shoes are rarely preserved today. Nevertheless, images of these shoes survive, thanks to the art of painting. The writer Pierre-Joseph Proudhon (1809-1865), a friend of Gustave Courbet (1819-1877), taught that art should serve society and extol social demands. Although Napoleon III cared about improving the workers' hard lot, social conflicts remained and shook the traditional value system despite his efforts. Artists responded to what was going on around them by depicting in their painting the economic and social transformation brought on by the machine and industrialization. German painter Adolph Menzel (1815-1905) first visited Paris in 1855. At the World Fair he discovered the pavilion devoted to Courbet's realism. Menzel was a court painter who commemorated ceremonies and celebrations, but he was also interested in factory labour, and looked at people with sincere and honest interest. This was important because an artist first had to consider the worker a worthy subject before the worker could become the painting's focal point. In *The Rolling Mill* (Nationalgalerie Staatliche Museum zu Berlin Preussischer Kulturbesitz), dated 1872-1875, labourers are depicted busy at work dressed in crude, old shoes with worn-down heels, worn without stockings. The writer and art critic Champfleury, author of a book on popular imagery and contributor to the socialist journal The People's Voice, inspired the painter Gustave Courbet. Courbet depicted the modest shoes worn by the working classes in his socialist paintings, such as *The Stone Breakers*, which disappeared from the Dresden Museum during the Second World War, and *The Burial at Ornans*. The Stone Breakers features a pair of clogs worn by the worker in right foreground, of which the left one is cracked inside. The worker moving rocks in the left foreground better protects his feet with rustic laced shoes of crude leather. *The Burial at Ornans* depicts poor and prominent villagers gathered for an indigent's burial in a communal plot. The sharp contrast between the different social classes is echoed by their shoes: the grave digger's simple laced shoes are worn out, whereas the elegant black shoes worn by the society figures look like new.

The son of a peasant, Jean-François Millet (1814-1875) painted scenes of rural life, each one a testament to the peasant's humble labour and the nobility of man on earth. Farm hands, who were day workers, are usually depicted in simple clogs, as seen in *The Angelus* (1857-1859), *The Wood Splitter*, and *The Gleaners* (Salon of 1857).

The painter Jules Breton was also interested in peasant life and painted lively scenes. In the *Call of the Gleaners* (Salon of 1859), he depicts young women in clogs or bare feet. A lack of shoes was a sign of abject poverty, symbolized by the French expression "va-nu-pieds," which literally means, "who goes barefoot." As Jean-Paul Roux explains: "During the middle ages wearing shoes became one of the primary indicators a person was well born. It was of such importance that for a long time the feudal lord sometimes carried peasant shoes alongside leather ones! This is but a survival. The man with shoes was everything, the shoeless person was nothing. Va-nu-pieds! This expression, now a fixed label, has no real meaning today and we rarely use it. Yet quite recently, hundreds of years or more, in the unequivocal testimony of nineteenth-century novelists, the phrase carried its full weight as a synonym of the word beggar, and signified a man so poor he could not even pay for a pair of shoes."

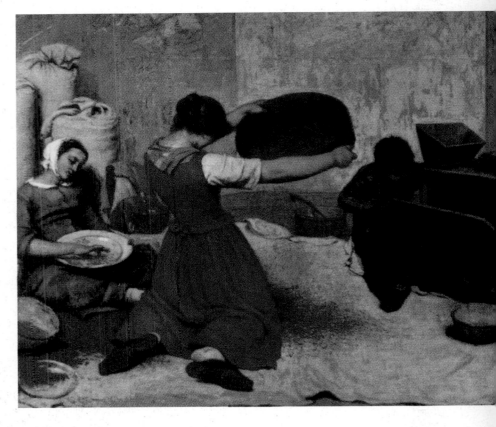

76. Adolph Menzel. *Rolling Mill*, 1872-1875. Oil on canvas.
Nationalgalerie, Staatliche Museen zu Berlin-Preussischer Kulturbesitz.

77. Jules Breton. *The Return of the Gleaners*, 1859. Oil on canvas.
90 x 176 cm. Orsay Museum, Paris.

78. Gustave Courbet, *The Sifters*, 1854-1855, oil on canvas,
Musée des Beaux-Arts, Nantes.

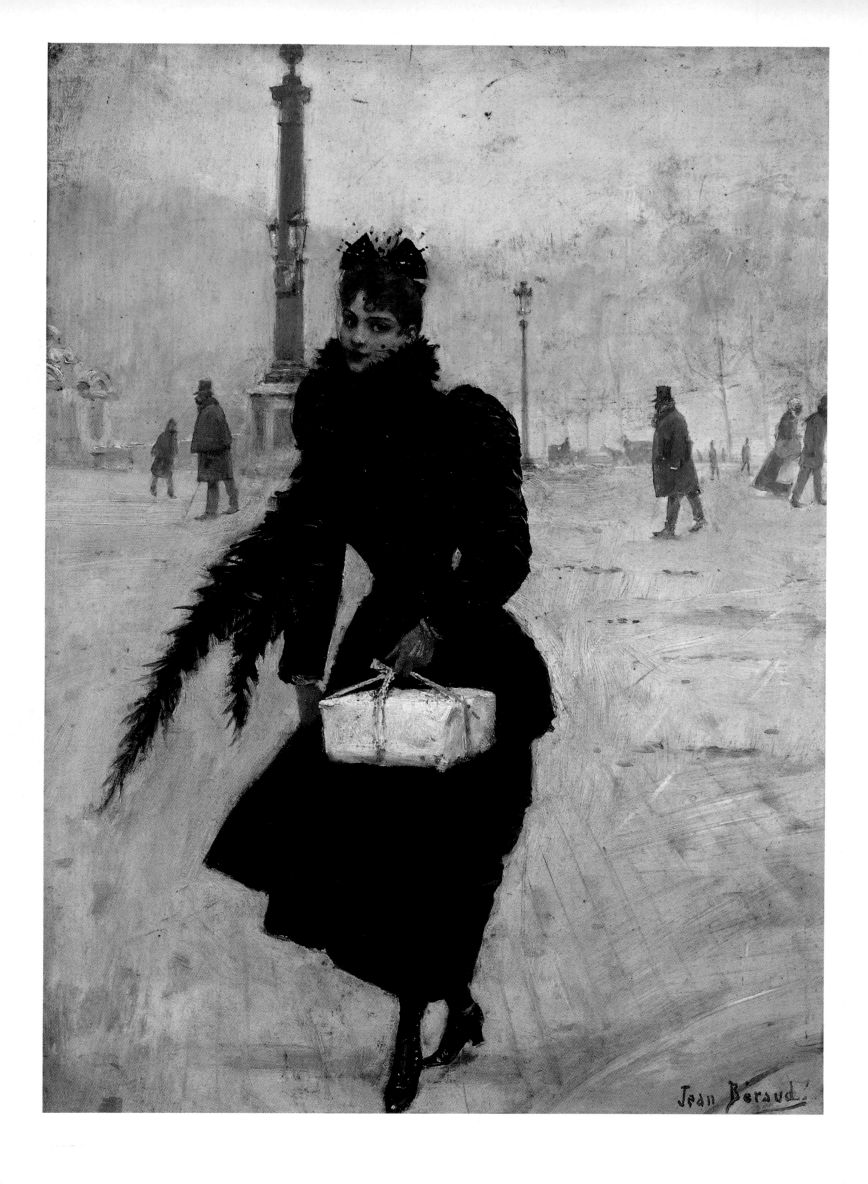

From shoemaker to head of a company

François Pinet was born in Château la Vallière (Indre and Loire) on July 19, 1817. The son of a shoemaker, he was introduced to the trade by his father. When his father died in 1830, Pinet was thirteen and was placed in the home of a master shoemaker to complete his professional education. He embarked on his Tour de France and in 1836 was declared a professionally accredited journeyman (Compagnon Cordonnier Bottier du Devoir, or Shoemaker-Boot maker Companion of Duty) under the name "Tourangeau la Rose d'Amour."

At age sixteen, with a total of twelve francs to his name, young François found work in Tours earning a weekly wage of five francs. Living on this modest salary, he saved to buy his own tools and to acquire his independence by working. He spent three years in Bordeaux, and then moved to Marseille, becoming the head of the Société des Compagnons Cordonniers (Workers' Association of Shoemaker Companions). In 1844, he went to Paris where he continued his training in large-scale manufacturing. An intelligent observer, Pinet was able to grasp the usefulness of manufacturing's division of labour and to see how its various components were combined to increase quality production.

In 1845, he became a traveling sales representative and started learning about business practices. In 1854, he took out a patent for a new heel manufacturing method that produced lighter and more solid heels than those composed of superimposed layers. In 1855, he opened a shoe factory to produce women's styles at 23 rue du Petit Lion Saint Sauvent. When the company grew, it moved to a larger spot (number 40) on the same street. Pinet married in 1858. His wife brought the qualities of heart, charm, grace, and vivacious spirit to the marriage. Quickly focusing her intelligence and sound education on the company, she became an enlightened collaborator.

François Pinet waited until 1863 to build new workshops and offices at 44 rue Paradis Poissonnière. The premises were constructed according to his own plans and under his management. In this new model establishment, functional for the era, workers felt appreciated and respected. Pinet employed 120 people in his workshops and 700 men and women who worked from home. The creations of François Pinet attracted a wealthy clientele in France and abroad. In Pinet's large shoe store on the boulevard de la Madeleine, elegant ladies rushed to buy ankle boots, escarpins, and derbies that encased the foot in the softest of leathers. Pinet's shoes came in shimming fabrics and in radiant colours, and were hand-embroidered and hand-painted. As a proprietor, Pinet also established in 1864 the first employers' association of federated shoe manufacturers and became its leader.

Pinet received many awards for his work, including a superb medal from the 1867 Paris World Fair that would thenceforth be engraved under the soles of his shoes as a sign of his talent. That same year, he invented a machine that could form Louis XV heels in one piece. Composed of a press and a dye, the machine's technology was awarded a new patent. Technological advancements of this kind marked the transition from craft industry to industrial manufacturing during the period. During the events of 1870-1871 that shook France, and especially Paris, Pinet provided financial assistance to the wounded and established a 20-bed mobile hospital unit at his own expense.

In 1892, during a traditional St. Crispin's banquet, he became a member of a new journeyman's society called the Union Compagnonnique. François Pinet died in 1897. A humble shoemaker from the provinces, he succeeded in dressing the feet of the world's most elegant women. In the process he made a valuable contribution to spreading haute couture's international influence. There were other 19th-century developments.

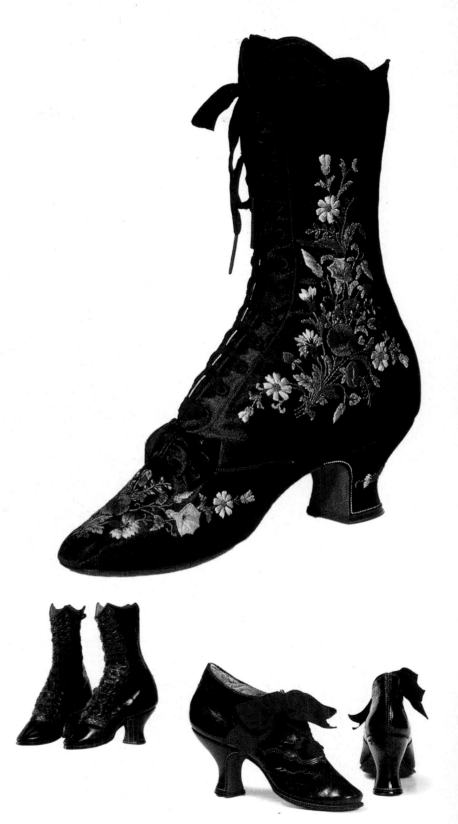

79. Jean Beraud. *Parisian, place de la Concorde*. Carnavalet Museum, Paris. Photo by Ladet, PMVP.

80. Miniature bottine in glossy kidskin, openworked upper, remarkable stitching producing the effect of leather lace, laced on the side; leather sole, reel heel. Executed by Rousselle. Second Empire. International Shoe Museum, Romans.

81. Hand embroidered woman's bottine in satin. Executed by Pinet. Paris, around 1875. International Shoe Museum, Romans.

82. Miniature woman's shoe in black kidskin, scalloped vamp, upper laced by a brown silk ribbon ending in a bow, leather sole, Louis XV heel. France, around 1880. International Shoe Mueum, Romans.

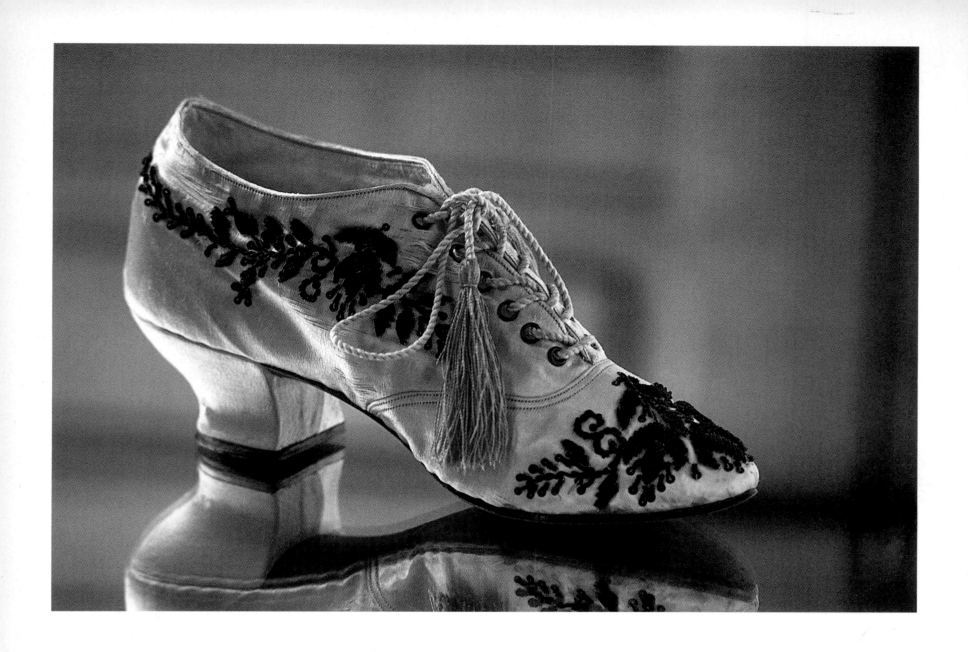

83. Woman's shoe. Oxford in white satin, embroidered patterns in silver, tasseled laces. Leather sole, covered reel heel. Executed by Pinet. Paris, around 1897. Guillen Collection, International Shoe Museum, Romans.

The advent of department stores in 1852 made a wide range of shoes readily available. The return of the heel, after being unsuccessfully revived under Louis-Philippe, become standard and took the demi-bobine or half-roll form. The arch of the foot being thenceforth supported by the shoe's shank, the heel could be positioned at the back edge of the sole. An aura of mystery surrounded the ankle boot hidden under crinoline. According to the notes and memoirs of Madame Jules Baroche, there came from England a more revealing fashion: "This year court ladies adopted a very English fashion: an ankle-revealing skirt of multi-coloured wool worn with a Louis XIII hat, a mischievous eye, a turned-up nose, and patent-leather ankle boots with heels. This outfit unfortunately requires a slender leg and a delicate foot. Otherwise it is smart, daring, casual, and better suited than any other for a walk in the woods."

But prince Napoleon found fault with the trend: "Women betray themselves in the morning with indiscrete skirts and in the evening with indiscrete blouses; what is to become of us?" The Empress wore tasseled boots to the races at Longchamp.

During this period, the female foot was much written about. Literature of the 19th century abounds with descriptions of feet dressed in mules d'appartement (slippers) and bottines (ankle boots).

Honoré de Balzac (1799-1850), Emile Zola (1840-1902), and Guy de Maupassant (1850-1893) were among the many writers who dwelled on this fashion accessory.

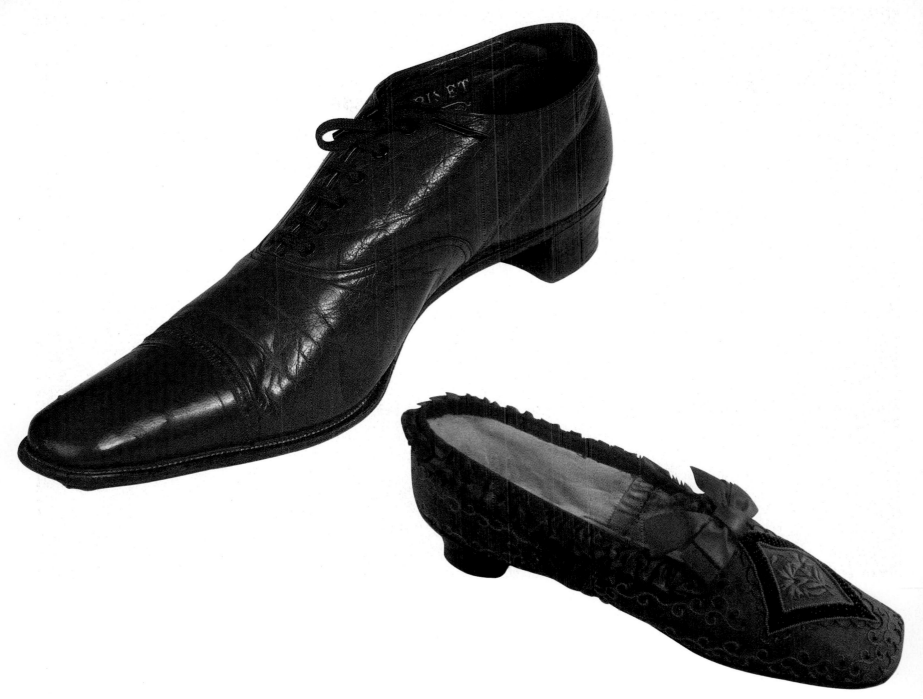

In *Madame Bovary*, Gustave Flaubert (1821-1880) describes more than one hundred pairs of shoes. Marc Constantin wrote the following description in the *The Almanac of Fine Manners* (1854): "The ankle boot has deposed the shoe and reigns victorious; nothing is prettier than a supple laced boot clasping the foot, which it makes look even smaller! It has a slimming effect on the lower leg and creates an elegant step."

For evenings or for a ball, women wore extremely sophisticated escarpins of tapestry or silk, which often matched their gowns. Gustave Flaubert refers to them in *Madame Bovary*: "Her beautiful outfit will be stored in the closet with pious respect, right down to her satin shoes whose soles were yellowed from the slippery wax on the floor." These styles were based on the open shoes with heels of the Louis XV and Louis XVI periods.

The mule d'appartement (slipper) in silk or velvet was another standard shoe. Men wore black boots or ankle boots. Children wore ankle boots that were smaller versions of the adult models.

From 1870 to 1900, shoes competed with ankle boots for in-town wear. The low-cut pump continued to be worn for evening. Round toes became pointed. Shapes were slowly changing, but the very recent revolution in dress caused by Paul Poiret, would have the foot in modern shoes thenceforth available for all to see.

84. Oxford style man's shoe by A. Biset in light brown kidskin. Elongated and upturned toe with perforated design. France, around 1890. International Shoe Museum, Romans.

85. Pump in embroidered calfskin. Paris, 1855. Guillen Collection, International Shoe Museum, Romans.

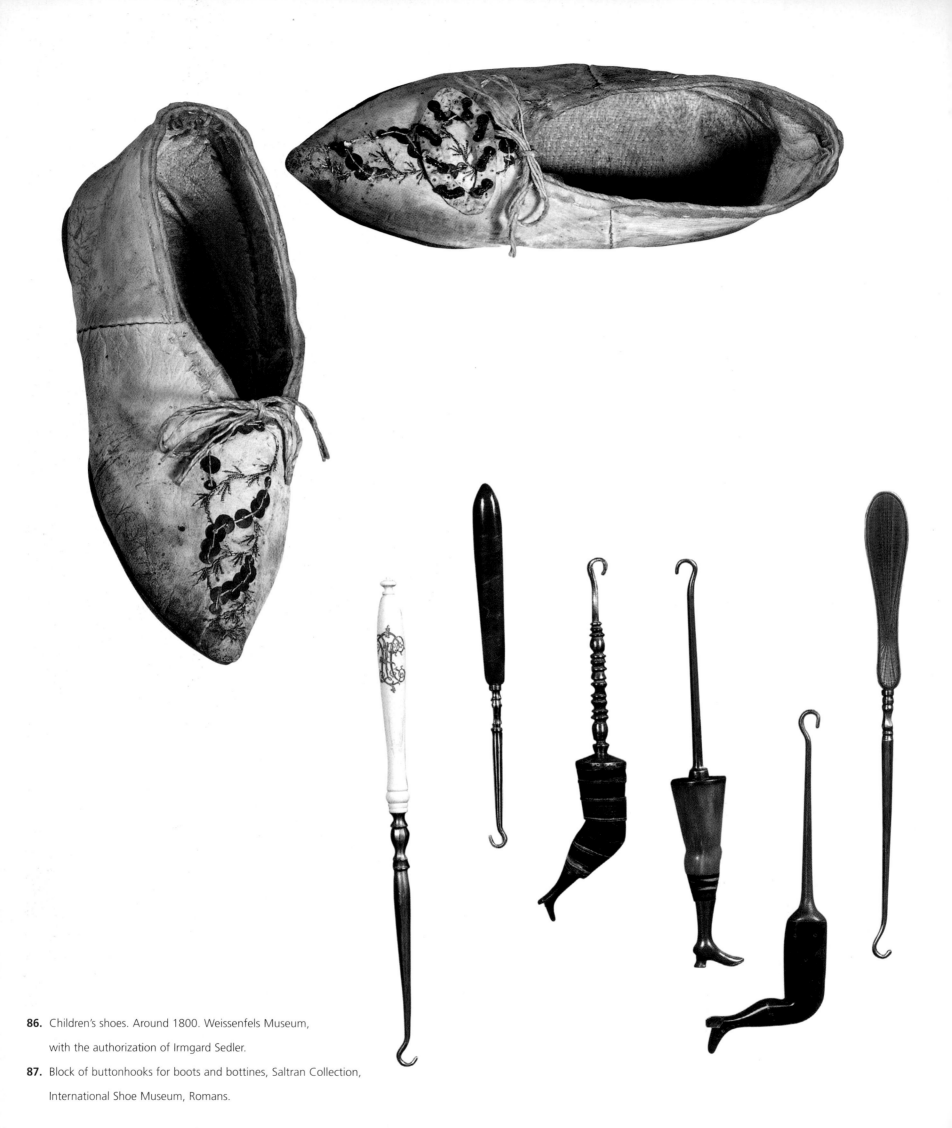

86. Children's shoes. Around 1800. Weissenfels Museum, with the authorization of Irmgard Sedler.

87. Block of buttonhooks for boots and bottines, Saltran Collection, International Shoe Museum, Romans.

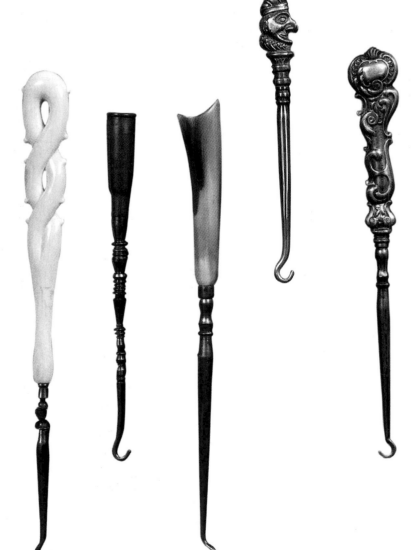

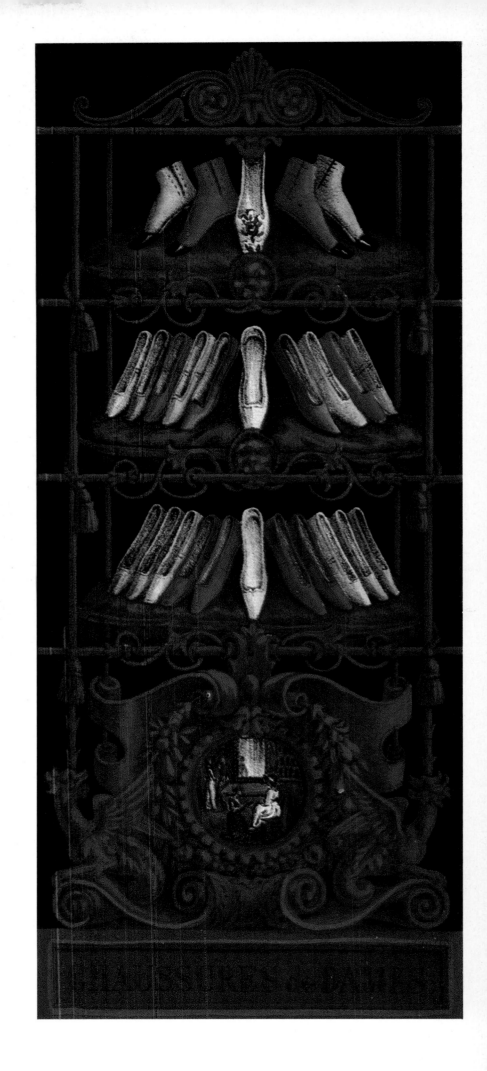

88. Painted shoe shop display. Around 1840. Lithograph.

Carnavalet Museum, Paris.

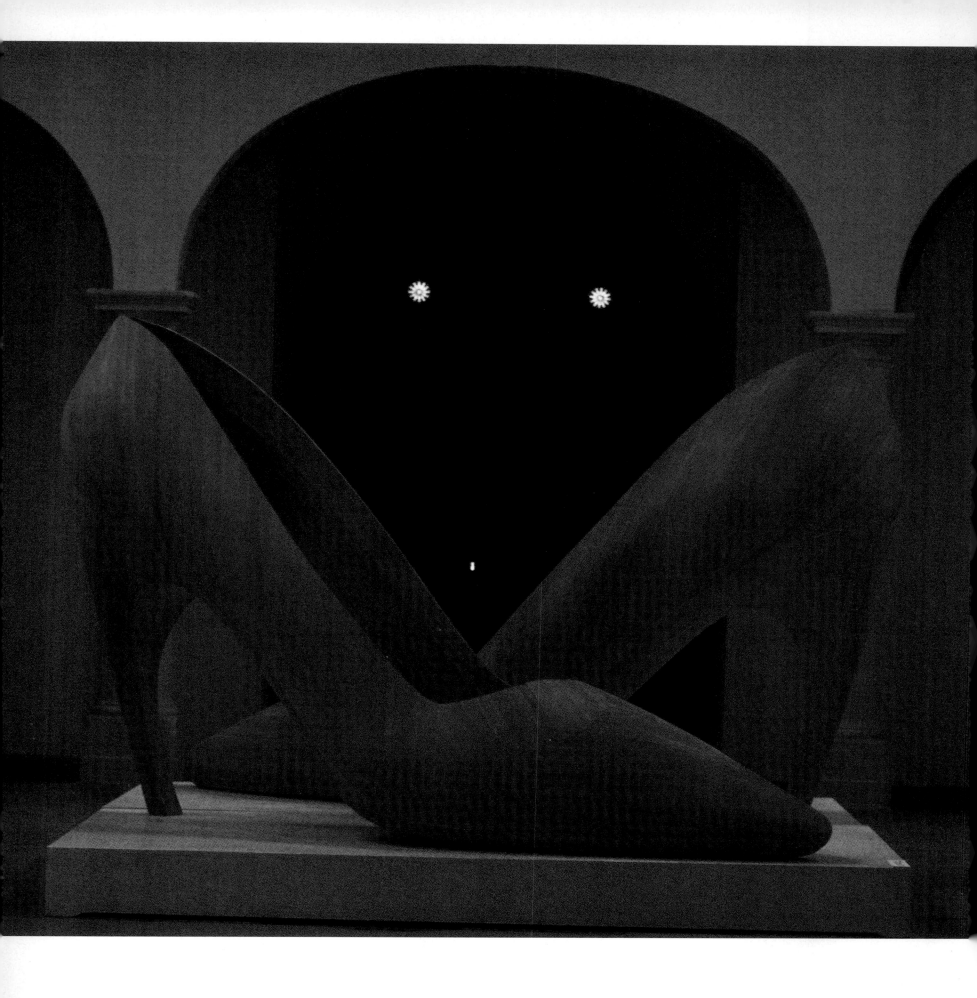

89. "Shock heel" shoes. Paris, 1987. Created by Roger Vivier,

International Shoe Museum, Romans.

The Shoe in the 20th century

The shoe's history and evolution in the 20th century can only be understood in relation to the personalities and the older firms that paved the way to our understanding of traditional and industrial fabrication. True "dynasties," some of these custom shoemakers and manufacturers are still growing into the 21st century. Many names are cited here taken from among the talented designers and prestigious firms, but many are absent, as this book cannot pretend to be exhaustive. All deserve greater recognition, not only for their contribution to the rise of fashion in France and the world, but also for passing their traditional know-how on to the next generation.

It is also impossible to understand 20th-century footwear in isolation from its closely related historical, economic, and artistic contexts. These underlying factors would lead to a revolution in clothing that would produce the versatile functionality of modern apparel. To fashion designers who deemed shoes a fashion accessory these factors were rich sources of inspiration.

Many historical factors contributed to the evolution of 20th-century shoes. First, the rise of international relations promoted foreign influences, while large world fairs, in which French couture participated, facilitated artistic exchange. Second, Haute Couture fashion shows and the informative role of fashion magazines, spread by photography and film, were among the principal agents of change. To these factors must be added the growth of sports and the introduction of the automobile. Additionally, a wealthy French and foreign clientele that only wore custom-made clothing and shoes continued to exist alongside the booming apparel industry, a phenomena that enabled mass production of Couture-inspired fashions accessible to the largest number of consumers at lower prices, which in turn promoted the growth of the shoe business. In this way names like André and even Bata became the pride of footwear's mass-market. The impact of the two world wars would also be considerable. Finally, the advent of Designer Fashion and technological innovations in footwear would carry shoes into the 21st century.

A number of events marked the years around 1900: the advent of the lady's suit revolutionized fashion; the English craze for sports and fresh air established itself in France; and a bathing suit that included cloth ankle boots with rubber soles was transported to Etretat and Trouville. Women who risked bicycle riding dared to wear baggy pants inspired by bloomers (also a rage on the other side of the Channel) and caused a sensation by showing their feet in shoes, as observed in the painting *The bicycle House in the Bois de Boulogne* (Carnavalet Museum, Paris), painted by Jean Béraud circa 1900. From 1900 to 1914, couturiers proliferated, riding the wave of la Belle époque and the house of Worth. There were Paquin, the Callot Sisters, Doucet, and Lanvin, among others. Ladies of society and courtesans sunk fortunes into their outfits. The nouveaux riches strutted about, arrayed in their most beautiful finery, trying to project an image of their newly acquired affluence. Until 1910, the button or lace-up ankle boot of "gold," beige, or black was standard for winter, whereas the covered shoe was worn in summer. Deep-cut shoes with Louis XV heels and a pointed toe box were the height of sophistication for evening, worn with matching dress and stockings. Elegance for men amounted to wearing button ankle boots, but low, top-laced shoes accompanied outfits for sports and casual wear. Most of these shoes were made by artisans scattered around Paris working in anonymity, making shoes rapidly, but skillfully, on demand, before the flowering of renown custom shoemakers became commonplace. The revolution in dress triggered by Paul Poiret eliminated corsets and shortened skirts. The wearing of straight skirts with soft, fluid lines inspired by the Orient cast a spotlight on shoes, which previously had enjoyed little visibility. The new style was reminiscent of the light clothes from the Directoire and Empire periods when shoes were worn exposed, revealing most of the foot.

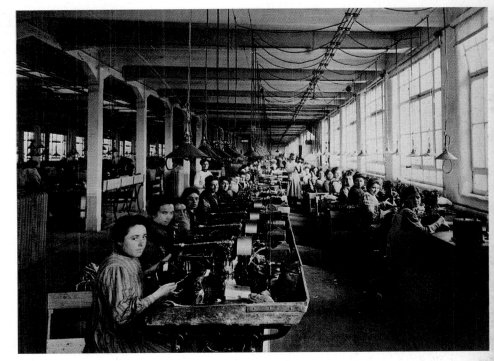

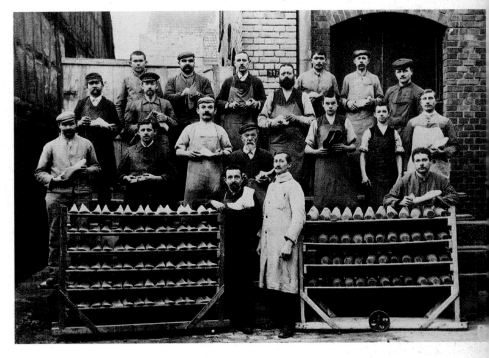

90. Stitching factory, "Sigle & Co" in Kornwestheim
(which will later be called "Salamander") around 1910.

91. Last factory, "Sigle & Co" in Kornwestheim
(which will later be called "Salamander") around 1910.

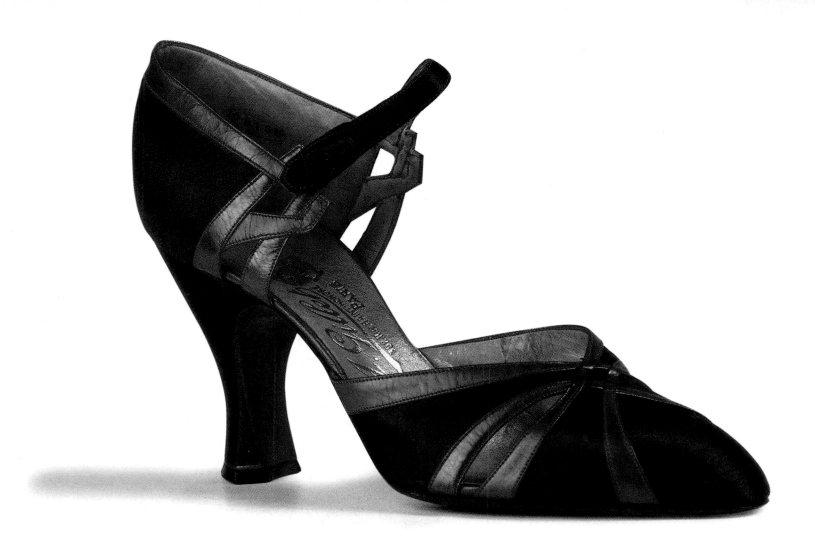

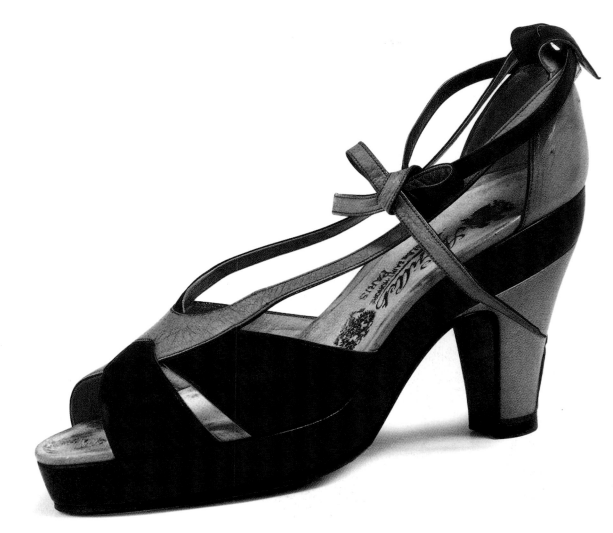

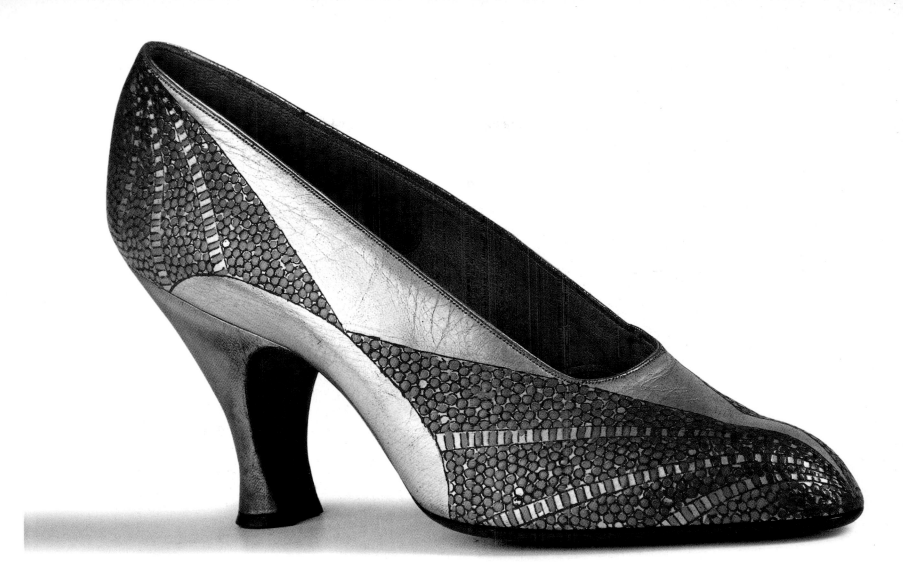

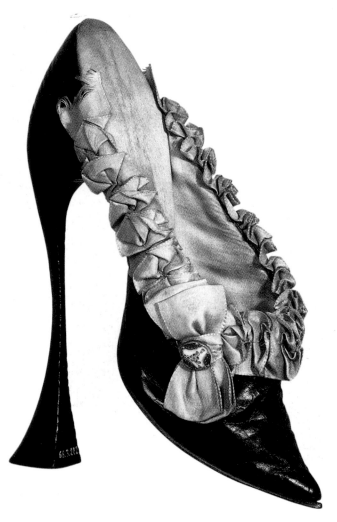

92. Woman's pump from shoemaker A. Gillet in the Charles IX style in garish green silk. Applications of gold kidskin. Louis XV costume heel. Paris, around 1928, 1930. International Shoe Museum, Romans.

93. Woman's town sandal in kidskin coloured cream and red by A. Gillet. Platform sole covered with red kidskin. Paris, Summer 1935. International Shoe Museum, Romans.

94. Woman's pump in silver kidskin. Design of pink dots and small green rectangles in geometrical spaces largely leaving visible the silver background. Covered Louis XV heel. Leather sole. Paris, around 1925. International Shoe Museum, Romans.

95. Mule, unsuitable for walking, in black kidskin and sky blue satin, small cabochon in porcelain. Height of the heel: 20 cm. Vienna, Austria, around 1900. Guillen Collection, International Shoe Museum, Romans.

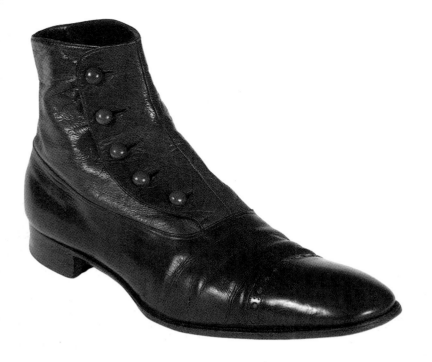

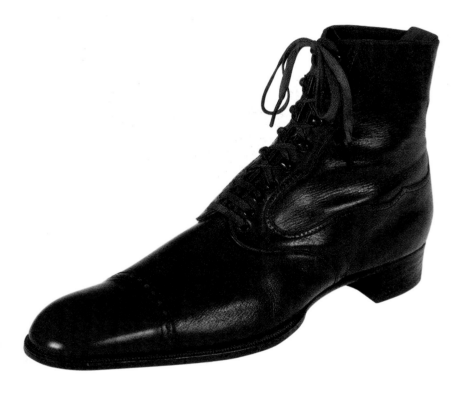

Paul Poiret's straight dresses also created a look that required a shoe with a more refined profile. World War I (1914-1918) disrupted the whole society's living conditions. Women, for example, found themselves having to cover for men in the most diverse jobs. In this way they experienced a need to dress more practically in a fashion that allowed their feet unrestricted movement. Now highlighted, the shoe quite naturally acquired a new elegance. The Roaring Twenties succeeded the terrible war years. Women cut their hair and the short skirt claimed a definitive victory. Long boots and black stockings gave way to light-coloured stockings to set off new shoes available in all the colours of the rainbow. The Charles IX style began its long reign. The low-cut shoe with the Louis XV heel came to be worn mainly in the afternoon. For evening, it was either of a matching fabric to go with the gown, or of gold lamé or silver.

Men's top-laced shoes, often covered with a small gaiter of black or gray wool, gave the illusion of an ankle boot. In the 1930s, Elsa Schiaparelli and Coco Chanel set the tone for fashion, and with the added influence from Madeleine Vionnet, evening gowns descended in length, emphasizing the figure's lines with a bias cut. In response, shoes became more slender, heels became higher, and shoe buttonholes tended to be hidden. Flats and crepe-sole shoes were worn with outfits for sport. At the same time, at the dawn of the Second World War, wedge soles appeared. Wartime leather restrictions imposed on the entire population turned wedge soles into a standard style. Unfortunately, wood (brightly painted or covered in fabric) and cork wedges were uncomfortable and ugly, although the innovation of the articulated wooden heel would provide some extra ease in walking. Designers also used substitute materials such as raffia and felt to make the uppers.

These heavy wedged shoes became pedestals for a straight silhouette with broad shoulders, until after the Liberation in 1947, when Christian Dior launched his "New Look." A very Parisian style, the New Look was characterized by a cinched waist and a large skirt that fell below the calf, worn with slender heels in perfect harmony with the silhouette. Henceforth, in the mind of designers, an elegant women's outfit would be unthinkable without high-heeled shoes. The stiletto heel was thus born in reaction to the heavy shoes associated with the war. A metal core guaranteed the heel's stability, but the stiletto left perforations in the floors of public places until a protective tip was invented. The heel survived until the 1960s, although its profile became slightly curved underneath the sole. The popularity of the mini-skirt led to its disappearance and shoes with round toes (succeeding pointed toes) replaced the stiletto. Two styles dominated store shelves: the Richelieu (the front upper sewn over the back upper) and the Derby (the back upper sewn over the front upper), while the moccasin, a shoe without laces, attracted a young clientele.

According to Sylvie Lefranc, head of the Bureau de Style de la Fédération de l'Industrie de la Chaussure de France (Fashion Office of the French Shoe Industry Federation) consumers lacked access to a wide range of shoe styles and products in the early 1960s. A malaise of sameness pervaded all the product lines, except for those of prestigious custom shoemakers, which were only available to the privileged few. Enter Roger Vivier, who had the innovative genius to pave the way to modern consumerism. In a manufacturing partnership with Société Charles Jourdan, Vivier launched a ready-to-wear line of fine shoes that were expensive but still affordable to a large number of consumers. Vivier was able to express his personal talent for bold silhouettes and the use of sophisticated materials in the line. The democratization of elegance gathered momentum as a trend and marked the advent of Designer Fashion footwear: new products were henceforth the subjects of aesthetic research, and contours and volumes were stylized to reflect the personality of their designer.

96. Man's bottine with buttons. France, from 1895 to 1910.

International Shoe Museum, Romans.

97. Man's bottine. Around 1912. International Shoe Museum, Romans.

Among the designers who had the ability to impart their own unique and identifiable look to their shoes were Roland Jourdan, following in the footsteps of Roger Vivier with his stylistic exercises focused on heels; Robert Clergerie, who lent his prestige to masculine and feminine style by creating new shapes; Stéphane Kélian, the inventor of the feminine braid and riding boot wizard; and finally, Walter Steiger, who handled line with a true designer's meticulousness. This new generation of fashion designers strongly influenced the 1970s and triggered a real craze among female consumers, who were passionate about shoes elevated to the full status of fashion object.

Alongside the phenomena of sophisticated urban fashion that had developed in reaction against the banality of standard shoes, there appeared a new trend generated by lifestyle. Originating in the United States and winning over Europe, the trend amounted to the advent of sportswear and jeans, or the casual look. Kicker's founder Daniel Raufast recognized the significance of the trend (it was especially marked in the youth and children's markets starting in the early 1970s) and developed a casual, playful product in response. During the same period, Mr. Helaine of Arche introduced a small, super-soft, and colorful boot that was distributed around the globe. The world of adventurers and nostalgia for pioneers and soldiers attracted a new generation of young men, as footwear with a history – Clark's Desert Boots, Pataugas, and Palladium's Pallabrousse – was adopted for leisure and weekend wear. New milestones in technical performance were reached in the 1970s with the successful introduction of rubber soles molded on fabric uppers; once the movement was launched, there was no turning back.

Beginning in the 1980s, sportswear ceased to be the only source of inspiration for new styles, as the active sports themselves dictated the rules. The Girbauds were among the pioneers in this area, co-opting specific items from various sports contexts and giving them the right to be cited. The major specialized brands followed suit by going after the youth market: Adidas, Reebok, Converse, Puma, and Superga became fashion players in their own right. Events happened quickly in this industry segment, but it should be noted that Nike played an important role in developing new lines featuring modernist design.

Other fashion trends arose from an openly ecological approach – before anyone had ever heard of the Greens. These currents persisted over the decades, ever faithful to the cult of the natural, ergonomics, and authenticity. Bama, Birkenstock, and even Scholl were among the leaders to whom the contemporary Camper is heir.

Fashion's 360-degree turn toward more intimate and primary values privileged the person over appearances and is especially evident in footwear, which is an accurate reflection of contemporary lifestyles.

Sportswear now "contaminates" the world of elegance as well. What couture house does not have running shoes and high-tops in their collection? Even men have been seduced by the casual chic of Tods and Hogan, after experiencing the sturdy comfort of Paraboots.

But Cinderella's slipper still inspires fantasy, and elegance and glamour exist now more than ever. Sophisticated women's shoes today have new defenders. New designers carry the torch of the great artists of seduction, redesigning new contours and original heels, playing with materials and decoration: Rodolphe Ménudier, Michel Perry, Manolo Blahnik, Pierre Hardy, and Benoît Méléard are among the most visible.

The rapid change in footwear, from both a design and manufacturing perspective, is perfectly illustrated by the careers of the most illustrious custom shoemakers: Andrea Pfister, Berluti, Ferragamo, Massaro, and Yantorny. Each name represents a different trajectory, but all stand for devotion to excellence. Here are their biographies, which offer a behind-the-scenes look at the art of the shoe.

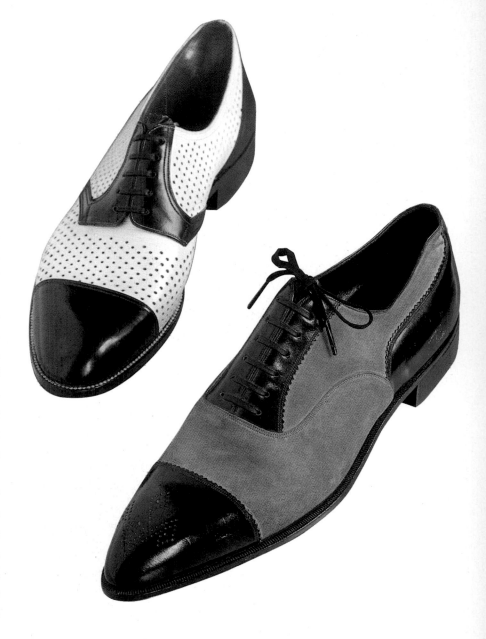

98. Man's shoe. Black suede and black veneer. UNIC Romans, around 1923.

Man's shoe in white perforated calfskin and black calfskin.

UNIC Romans, around 1938. International Shoe Museum, Romans.

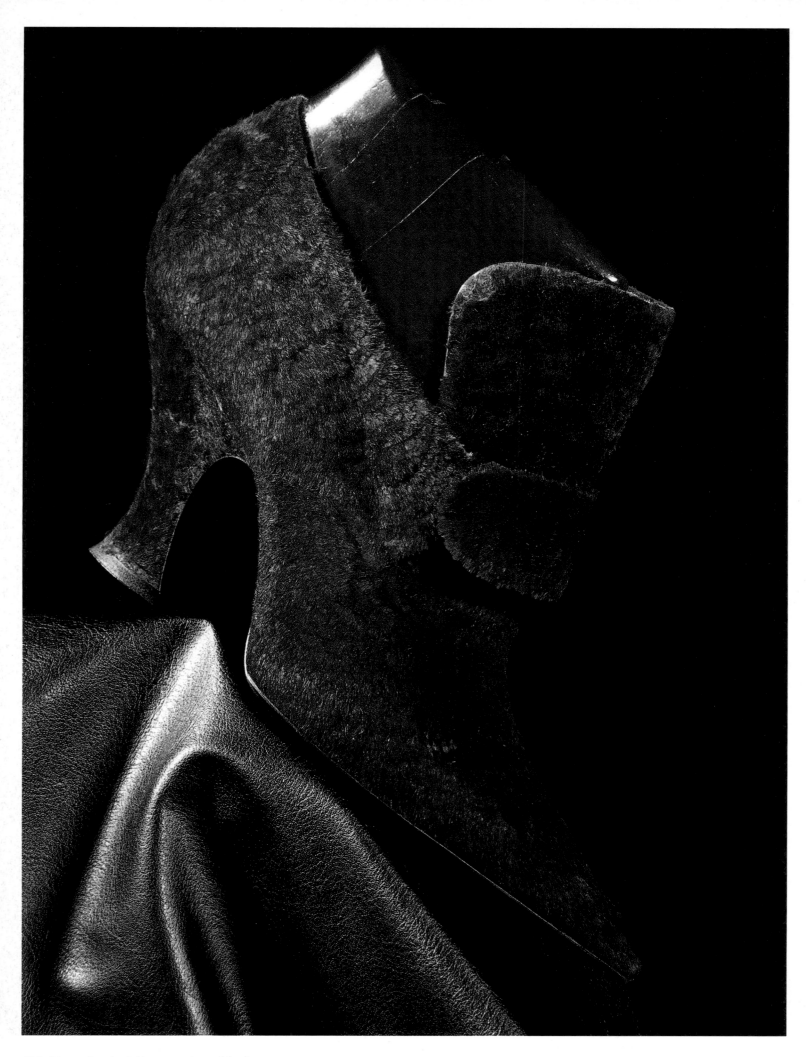

102. Masterpiece by P. Yantorny: shoe of feathers.

International Shoe Museum, Romans.

Pierre Yantorny
The Most Expensive Shoes in the World

The veil of mystery around Pierre Yantorny, who called himself the "most expensive shoemaker in the world," has finally lifted, thanks to the release of his personal journal, photographs, papers, and shoes left to the International Shoe Museum, Romans, by the artist's nephew. These records will allow us to revise his biography and to dispel the myths about his Indonesian origins and his role as Conservator at the Cluny Museum in Paris.

Pierre Yantorny was an Italian, born on May 28, 1874, in Marasso Marchesato, Calabria. He only attended school from age eight to eight and a half, at which time he began his working life in a macaroni factory where he earned twenty cents a day, working from six in the morning until six in the evening. He subsequently went to work for an individual as the caretaker and exerciser of a horse. When his father settled in Chicago, the twelve year old went to Naples and apprenticed with another apprentice shoemaker; his only payment consisted of the knowledge he acquired.

Six months later, hired by a real boss, he was able to save some money, enabling him to set off for Genoa. After a short stay, he went to Nice where he perfected his craft, but already he was dreaming of Paris. To finance his trip and save forty-two francs to pay for a train ticket, another shoemaker suggested that Yantorny apply to the Marseille slaughterhouse to work with sheep.

As Yantorny writes in his journal:

"And so I arrived in Paris on June 13, 1891, after traveling three days, because it was not a fast train; at four in the morning I made my triumphant entry into the French capital. I had been given the address of a shoemaker's workshop on the rue Saint-Honoré where I might be able to find tradesmen who could help me get work. But damn! The workshop had disappeared five years ago."

Thanks to the kindness of an Italian restaurant owner on the rue Traversière, Yantorny found a tradesman who worked for the major Paris houses and who agreed to take him on. The workday began at four in the morning and lasted until ten in the evening. Hard work and talent quickly led to his wielding the knife and the awl like a pro. But, alas, his benefactor disappeared without leaving an address.

Yantorny took a job washing dishes in a restaurant for three months so he could afford to buy his own tools.

However, unable to find work, he returned first to Genoa and then to Nice on January 17, 1892, with twenty cents in his pocket. He spent the winter there further perfecting his craft then returned to Paris where he stayed until 1898, presenting himself as a tradesman worthy of the top firms – a designation that pops up constantly in his journal.

Two years in London would introduce him to a new aspect of shoemaking, for it was there he learned the art of making shoe trees, which he deemed an indispensable complement to that of shoemaking and form making. This experience moreover presented an opportunity for Yantorny to learn English, a considerable asset in terms of his future American clientele.

Upon returning to Paris for the World Fair, he temporarily abandoned his shoemaker's craft in order to learn form making. His small room on the rue Saint-Dominique became the scene of his personal investigations. As he notes in his journal:

"This is where I began my study of form making, all by myself; I worked long hours, going days without eating; experience itself feed me, because I saw that I was making progress in what I was trying to do."

Four years later, he rented an old bakery at 109 faubourg Saint-Honoré, and established himself as a maker of forms for shoemakers. The perfecting of four different models with, in his own words, "all the necessary lines to charm the eye" brought him a tremendous amount of work. But he continued to entertain the idea of acquiring a wealthy clientele:

"I wanted to make shoes for people who wore shoes to coordinate their outfits and naturally many more sacrifices had to be made to acquire this clientele…"

A few years later, he set up shop above 26 place Vendôme, where the jeweler Boucheron is currently located. When he failed to receive orders and fell under criticism from the shoemakers' corporation, he said: "actions speak louder than words and time will be the judge of the rest."

To attract customers, Yantorny placed a sign in his window that read, "the most expensive shoes in the world." The expression served as a trade name. A master of his craft, he sought the wealthiest of clients who had the taste, the time, and above all the means to put down a deposit of three thousand francs and submit to the six to eight fittings required to produce the perfect shoe.

In his journal, Yantorny stresses the art of fitting a pair of ankle boots: the process had to result in a perfect correspondence between form, foot, and shoe. According to Yantorny, negligence on the part of the shoemaker could lead to ingrown toenails, calluses, corns, and even enlarged toes, which leads him to conclude:

"If the client purchases from the shoemaker all these ailments, he will have them for the rest of his life and no doctor or surgeon on Earth will be able to heal him. This is why individuals who care about their health and well-being must take care and not entrust their feet to the first shoemaker that comes along."

Yantorny goes on to humorously survey the effects of wearing ill-fitting shoes in various circumstances:

"If you have poorly made shoes and they get wet, you'll catch a cold and other illnesses" (which is confirmed by Pasteur);

"If you are in business negotiations and your feet hurt because of your shoes, you'll be in a bad mood and you'll be unable to rise to the occasion of properly conducting your business";

"If you go to the theater to see a production you like and you wear shoes that hurt your feet, you won't have any fun"; and finally,

"If you go out to dinner, no matter how fine the food and no matter how pleasant the company, if you feet hurt you won't enjoy yourself at all."

This is why Yantorny insists the foot be dressed in the perfect comfort produced from a quality shaped shoe and foot mold.

Packed with technical advice, Yantorny's journal provides information about the perfection of his craft. The shoemaker shares with us his love for his trade, which extends to the smallest details:

"For women's shoes, eyelets must be handmade like we do for button holes; but to be pretty, the eyelet must be very round and the points flat enough that they don't damage the grain of the leather, and so that they can be very close together."

As for aesthetics, just open his journal and see how much it concerns him:

"My only concern is to constantly combine tradition with artistic creativity.

1°/ The traditional side is doing no harm to the foot.

2°/ The artistic side involves giving the foot an illusion of being as small and as thin as possible and even correcting natural defects.

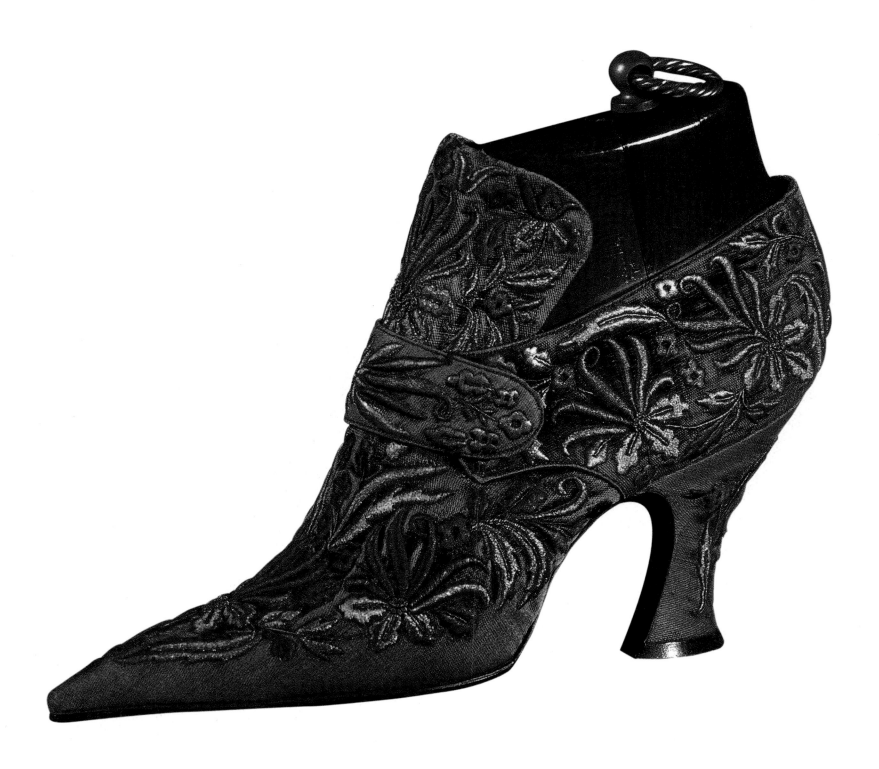

103. Duke of Guise by P. Yantorny. Crimson silk velvet embroidered with gold

and silver thread. Inspired by liturgical cloths of the 17th century;

Louis XV heel. Paris, around 1912. International Shoe Museum, Romans.

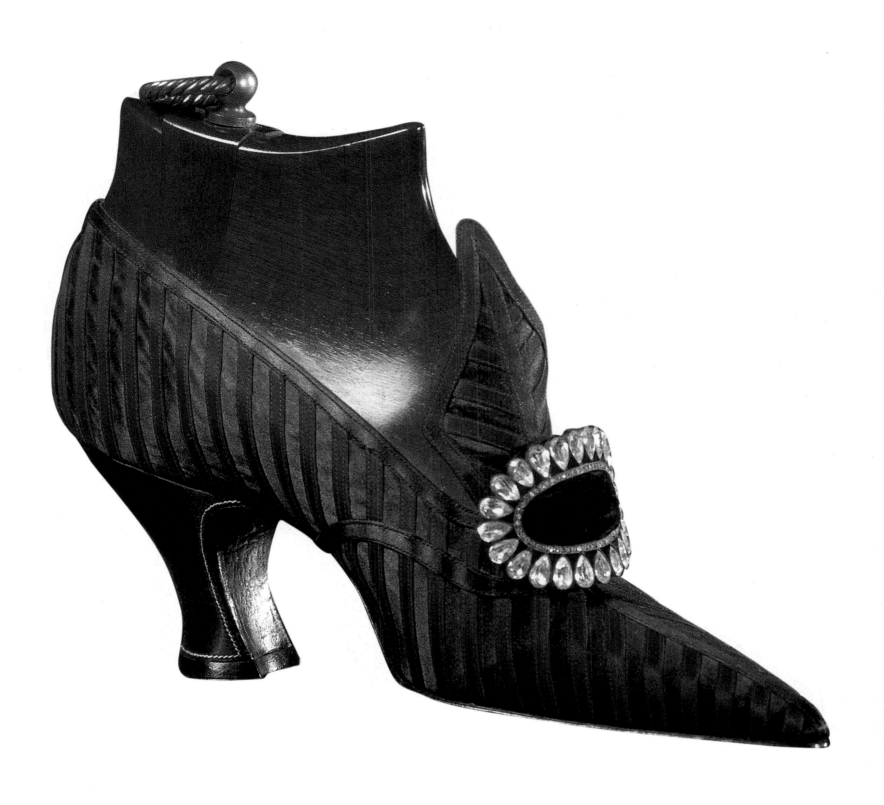

104. Duke of Guise by P. Yantorny. Background in black satin and applications of red satin bands, buckle adorned with strass and Louis XV heel. Paris, around 1912. International Shoe Museum, Romans.

pour avoir des clients dans ces conditions il a fallu la transformation complète de toute la cordonnerie du monde. C'est donc pour vous donner une idée de ma nouvelle école.

Le Soulier en Plumes

Le chef d'œuvre que j'ai voulu soumettre aux yeux du public c'est le soulier de plumes qui est fait avec de petites plumes d'oiseaux venant du Japon mesurant chacune à peu près 1 millimètre et demi. Il a fallu 6 mois pour pouvoir en achever une paire. Je n'ai pas fait cela pour une spéculation de vente mais seulement pour un objet artistique et faire voir jusqu'où je pouvais pousser le degré de la cordonnerie.

·LE·BOTTIER·LE·PLUS·CHER·DU·MONDE·

P. YANTORNY

N°   26, Place Vendôme

Paris, le   19

Reçu de

la somme de   dix mille francs   à valoir sur l'ensemble de sa commande conformément au règlement de la maison.

105. Extract from the journal of shoemaker P. Yantorny.
International Shoe Museum, Romans.

106. Receipt from P. Yantorny, "the most expensive shoemaker in the world".
International Shoe Museum, Romans.

107. Trunk from P. Yantorny, made for Rita Acosta Lydig. Leather and silk.
The Metropolitan Museum of Art, New York.

Example: for a shapeless foot, make shoes that give the foot all the lines and balance needed to be eye-catching."

The expression "to be eye-catching" punctuates the journal in which he also comments on industrialization:

"Industrial shoe manufacturing has poor shoe forms and makes little boxes for feet that one calls shoes. Handcrafted shoes must be made according to the client's aesthetics" and

"It is very difficult to make shoes that conform to a person's feet and individual aesthetics";

"If there is a seam behind the vamp, very often it is done badly and throws the heel off, as well as the leg, when you look at a person from behind."

Although Yantorny says in his journal that getting rich was not his goal, his creations were pricey. Before 1914, the first order came to thirty-five thousand francs, probably in recognition of his talent and strong personality. A sumptuous leather-bound order book with parchment pages confirms the high price of this first order, which comprised the creation of several different shoe forms, a traditional and artistic study of the foot, fifty pairs of shoes without trimming at the price of one hundred and twenty-five francs each, fifty shoetrees, two trunks for boots and shoes, six pairs of stockings for each pair of shoes (amounting to three hundred pairs of stockings), and finally buckles, shoe horns, button hooks, and all the accessories needed for upkeep.

Who were his clients? Few in number and seen by appointment only, they were Russian and French, but above all American women, like the wealthy Rita de Acosta Lydig. One of the most elegant and prominent woman in New York, Lydig ordered over three hundred pairs of shoes. True works of art, they were kept in Russian leather trunks with velvet panne interiors that could hold twelve pairs. The Metropolitan Museum in New York has an example of one of these extraordinary trunks. Each shoe came with its own shoetree engraved with the name Rita. Some of these shoes were made in vintage fabrics: Yantorny was a connoisseur of textiles and obtained velvets, brocart, satin, and lace from collectors in order to produce his creations.

This tireless worker eventually felt the need to step back and gave himself a two-year sabbatical in India around 1930. Those closest to him remember the story well:

"One day I realized that I was starting to notice the things that I had never done.

So I took the train to Marseille and the boat to Bombay. I didn't stop until I reached Darjeeling. There I walked until I reached a spot where I could contemplate Mount Everest without anyone bothering me; and I stayed there for five days, just staring at the Himalayas in their tranquility. This is what most people need to do: to stop and look at something outside their ordinary experience."

He returned from this lengthy Asian interlude a vegetarian and devotee of silence and meditation. Nevertheless, his Italian temperament quickly re-asserted itself and at his home in the Valley of Chevreuse, the shoemaker became a farmer. He sowed seed behind a plow drawn by two oxen, harvested his own wheat, and made his own bread.

When going to work, Yantorny always got upset at the sight of passers-by in the street wearing imperfect shoes. From his meditations, he came up with the idea of establishing a new school for shoemaking. His dream of leaving behind a complete codification of his craft, for instructional purposes, held an important place in his journal:

"We need a school and the students in this school need to pass examinations and to be awarded the prizes based on their level of intelligence; in other words,

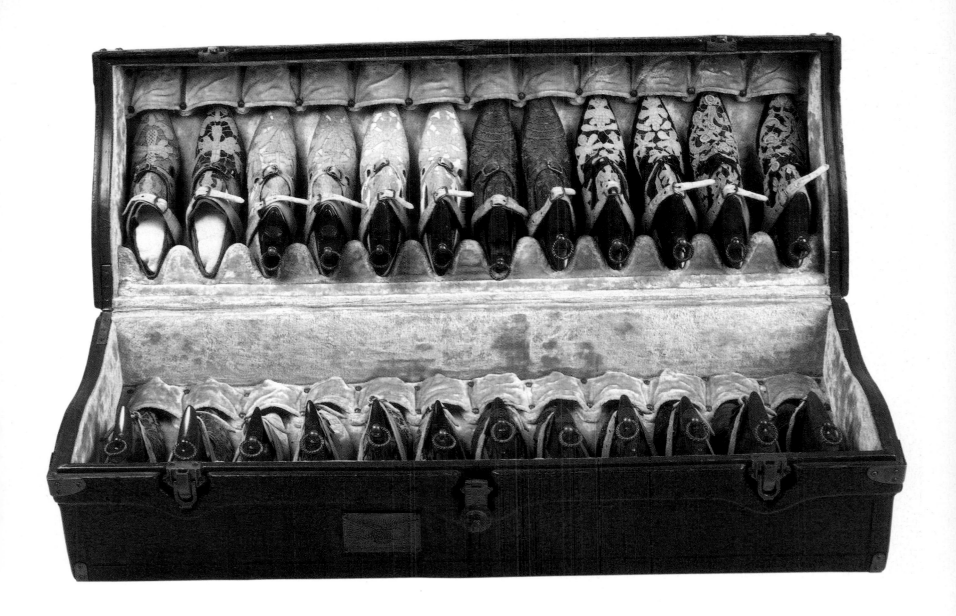

first-place shoemaker; second-place shoemaker, and third-place" and "The young people selected must be taken to the mountains, far away from large towns, so they can learn well without big-city distractions."

Yantorny recommended admitting students at age fourteen, he believed mastery of the craft required eight years, five of which were devoted to forms and shoetrees. The examination would consist of measuring the feet of three different people and making forms, shoes, and shoetrees for each person. The successful candidate would receive the title master shoemaker and as Yantorny adds:

"If he gets first prize, he will have the right to make shoes for the most elegant and richest people on earth and will garner high prices for his shoes."

Yantorny's school was never created. On the other hand, his own research was awarded. In 1924, he registered a shoe-lacing patent in the United States. Eleven years later, Cardinal Pacelli, the future Pious XII, thanked him in the name of Saint Peter for his generous offering to the works and needs of the Holy See, with a special apostolic benediction from the Pope for Yantorny and his family.

This man who was fluent in three languages (his maternal Italian, French, and English) could neither read nor write. His companion therefore had to lend a hand and record his journal as he dictated. The journal ends with Yantorny's description of his feathered shoe, now preserved in the International Shoe Museum, Romans:

"The masterpiece I wanted to present to the public was the feathered shoe made with small Japanese bird feathers each measuring around one and one-half millimeters. It took six months to make one pair. I didn't make it with the intention of selling it, only as an art object and to show just how far I could push the envelope of shoemaking."

Then he concludes:

"My only aim is to leave something to a museum of the shoe that future generations could admire, not a financial legacy, but the artistry found in shoes."

The most significant creations of this atypical shoemaker, who died on December 12, 1936, are divided between the Metropolitan Museum of Art, New York, and the International Shoe Museum, Romans.

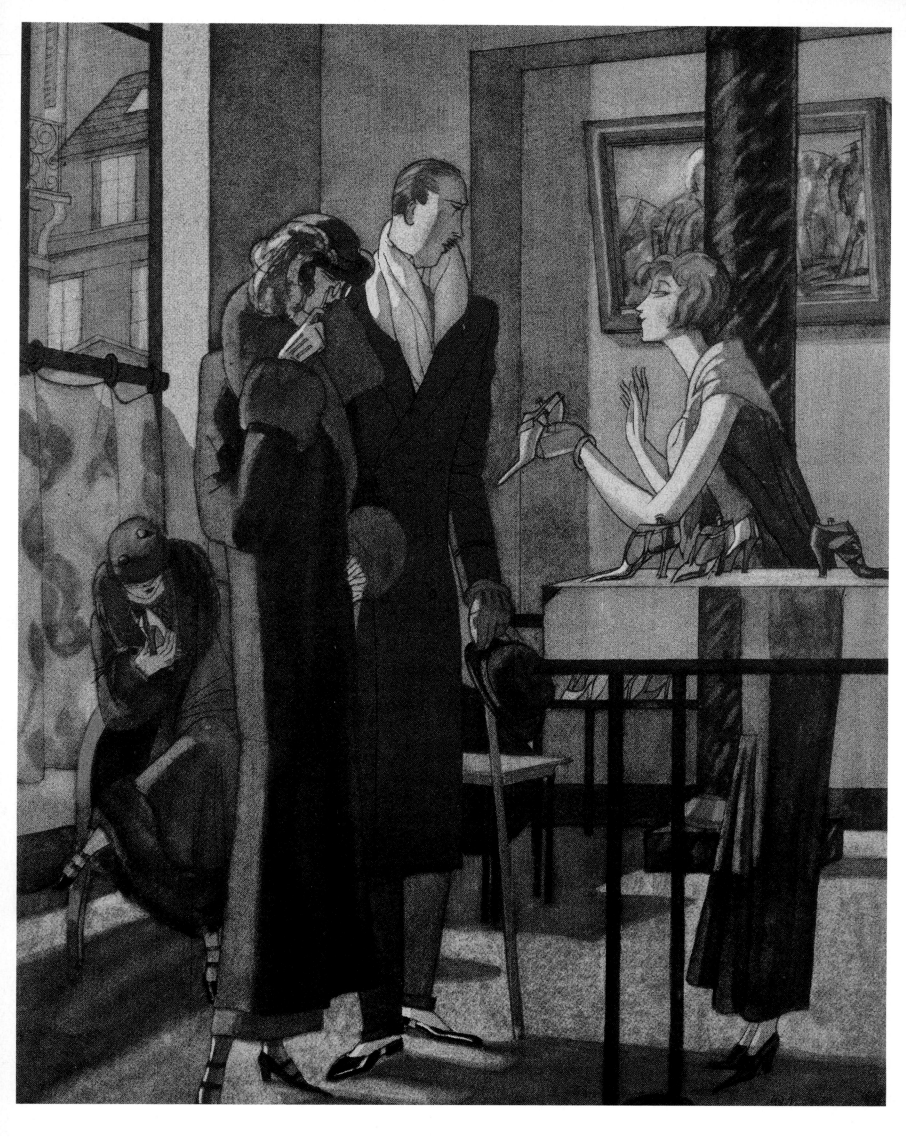

André Perugia,

Last of the Great Renaissance Artists, First of the Moderns

Considered one of the 20th-century's greatest custom shoemakers, André Perugia was born in 1893 in Tuscany, the son of a shoe repairman. The family fled poverty by emigrating to Nice, where the father set up shop as a shoemaker.

His apprenticeship began in his father's workshop and continued with a boot maker in Nice when he was sixteen. Perugia quickly realized that he knew as much as his boss and decided to take over his father's shop. There he felt the limitations of the shoemaker's trade, already demonstrating a strong inclination towards invention.

Perugia's shoe styles attracted the interest of the wife of the head of the Negresco hotel, who offered him a window to display his shoes to hotel patrons. Paul Poiret came upon them during a trip to Nice, where he had gone to show his collections to Hindu princesses and to a wealthy clientele vacationing on the Riviera. Poiret wanted to enhance the splendor of this fashion show with colorful accessories and only André Perugia agreed on such short notice to produce the models sought by the couturier. After a triumphant showing, Poiret offered to set up Perugia in Paris, but the war disrupted the plans, which did not come off until 1920.

Poiret effectively introduced Perugia to his elegant clientele at his fashion show. Perugia did not have to wait for success and he returned home with a full order book. But he was still in his small family shop, and he dreamed of making shoes for the glittering world of Parisian high society.

One year later, the dream became a reality with the opening of a boutique at 11 faubourg Saint-Honoré. The shoes of famous customers displayed along with their names and a few extravagant styles captured journalists' attention. It was easy for Poiret to promote the young man; Perugia's talent did the rest.

The shoemaker created a number of models for the couturier, including the "Arlequinade" and "Folie," which corresponded to names of Poiret perfumes. Meanwhile, a top-drawer clientele filed into the house of Perugia, including Mistinguett (French music-hall idol), Josephine Baker (exotic dancer of the Roaring Twenties), queens, princesses, stars of stage and screen, and aristocrats. Perugia only made women's shoes, although he would good-naturedly make masculine models as an exception, for Maurice Chevalier, for example.

Beginning in 1927, Perugia crossed the Atlantic to capture a wealthy American clientele. Success in America was also by appointment only to "Monsieur Perugia," which became "Mister Perugia." In 1933, established at 4 rue de la Paix, he introduced the "Padova" brand distributed in the United States by Saks Fifth Avenue.

His foreign sales network grew with RAYNE in England. Additionally, in 1936, the Queen of England paid him the honor of an order during a visit to Paris. In 1937 he would establish himself once and for all at 2 rue de la Paix until the end of his career.

Perugia left a vast body of work. To interpret and understand his oeuvre the observer must consider its technical aspects, its themes of inspiration, and Perugia's collaboration with couturiers. The work of a custom shoemaker is similar to that of a haut couturier. The shoemaker takes an impression of the foot (by making a plaster cast or a drawing) and takes measurements. The style and the height of the heel determine the form. From these elements an initial frame without ornament is made, which the shoemaker can open at the top, on the side, and at the heel during the fitting. When the frame was perfectly adjusted to the customer's foot, the shoe was ready for fabrication. A portion of Perugia's orders was executed in his workshops; the remainder was made by shoemakers working at home.

For Perugia, difficulty in execution and expense mattered little, whereas the shoe's suitability for walking and its proper fit were paramount.

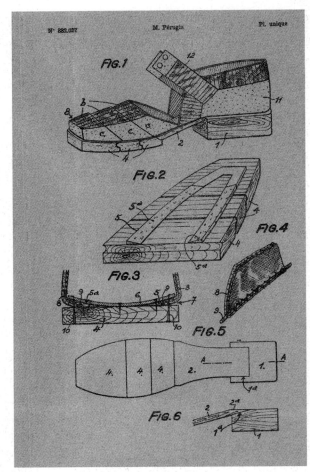

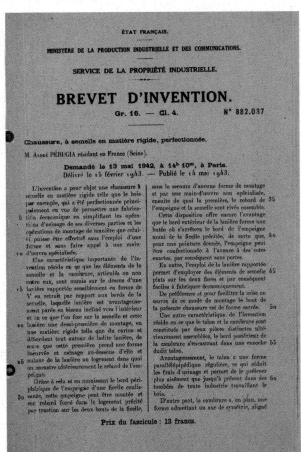

108. Print: The House of Pérugia or the Fashionable Shoemaker. Guilen Collection, International Shoe Museum, Romans.

109. Patent awarded to Pérugia in 1942. International Shoe Museum, Romans.

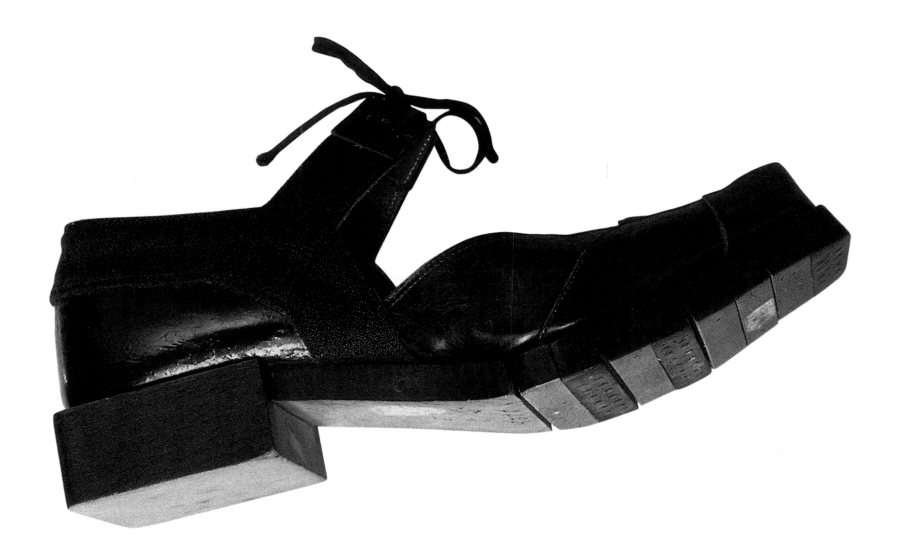

110. War shoe: vamp made up of strips of cloth and skins, fitting of boiled hide, square heel, wooden sole of blades attached to canvas. 1942.

111. Print: *Consultation-Pérugia Shoes.* International Shoe Museum, Romans. Photo by Joël Garnier.

112. Display window of Pérugia shop, Faubourg Saint Honoré, Paris.

Perugia's customers ordered nearly forty pairs per season at an approximate unit price of fifty thousand francs, which amounted to a significant annual sales figure in the 1920s. Perugia's oeuvre shows the use of an extraordinary diversity of materials: exotic and often surprising leathers (including lama stomach skin and antelope skin, which was painted and embroidered with purl), fabrics, laces, vegetable fibers, and horsehair, among others.

He did not hesitate to completely transform traditional leathers: snakeskin became gold and alligator skin sported cheerful colours. To this was added the opulence of embroidered and enameled ornamentation, which transformed the shoe into an exclusive design. Perugia was a perfect master of his craft.

Perugia was also perfectly aware of his limitations, which motivated him to keep raising the bar through technical research. He never stopped devising new processes, forty of which bear registered and meticulously illustrated patents. These patents punctuate his entire career from 1921-1958. To Perugia we owe in particular not only the 1942 invention of the articulated wooden heel, which thrived during the Second World War, but also the 1956 invention of the clever interchangeable heel system. Additionally, Perugia invented a metal instep; iron craftsmen made his heels for him. Perugia shoes defied the laws of balance by changing the established structure of the heel.

His interest in bare footedness led him to launch a sandal for evening. Without making the shoe inappropriate for walking, he eliminated as much of the upper as possible and used a transparent vinyl to create the illusion of a bare foot. Mindful of improving the fit of shoes, he thought of the foot in movement rather than in repose as was customary.

For Charles Jourdan, to whom he was a technical advisor from 1962 to 1966, Perugia adapted his patented inventions and his know-how to an industrial scale, but he was not involved in the creative process strictly speaking.

Perugia displayed originality in the art of the shoe from his very first creations. Times changed and different cultures nourished his design themes. The oriental theme appears throughout his oeuvre and is seen in shoes for evening, town, apartment, and even the beach. Perugia's oriental style was part of a fashion movement generated by the craze for the Ballets Russes. From 1909, Diaghilev's company performed in Paris. The ballet Shehezerade flaunted the sensuality of harem women in a commotion and explosion of colours and pleasantly distracted the public with the charms of the Orient. On June 24, 1911, Poiret organized a Persian celebration called "The Thousand and One Nights" and met his guests dressed as a sultan. His trip to Morocco in 1918 also enriched his imagination. It was surely under Poiret's influence that Perugia immersed himself in orientalism, which became a favorite theme. The effect is seen in Perugia's Chinese-inspired motifs, such as the apartment mule with raised heels. Perugia then looked towards Japan and made notched soles in imitation of the gaiter spat; closer to home, he found inspiration in Venetian mules that displayed masks.

Turning to history for inspiration, Perugia took the Greek cothurne and Roman campagus as models. The medieval period inspired his taste for the rustic shoes of the 10th and 11th centuries, made of a tall upper held by a thin cord. He succeeded in making an elegant version of this type: the "Dagobert." In addition to an evocative name, the Dagobert had an upper held by a thin cord hidden by a small cuff. The Charles IX, the Salomé, and the court pump known as the escarpin followed. Some of these shoes, with their tall uppers of beige antelope skin printed in gold and with openwork diamond patterns, were reminiscent of the cut windows of gothic churches.

But the shoemaker's own artistic milieu had a considerable impact on him. Poiret, who was a patron of painters, writers, and designers, turned Perugia into a connoisseur and enlightened art collector. The geometric ornaments of his shoes express a cubist aesthetic. Between 1925 and 1930 Art Deco motifs were everywhere. Perugia's wood heels, first sculpted and then gilded with gold leaf, reveal true artistic labour. This exclusive shoemaker was the first to exhibit in the Salon's Decorative Arts.

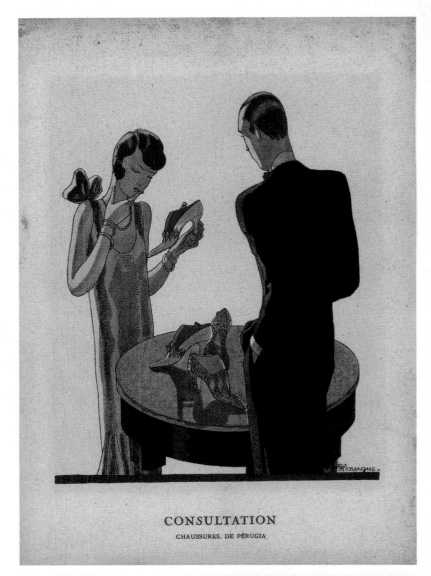

CONSULTATION

CHAUSSURES, DE PÉRUGIA

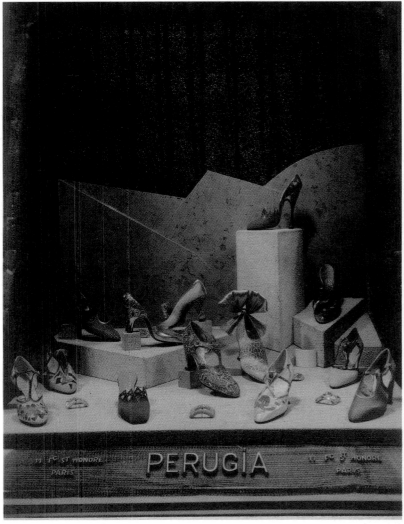

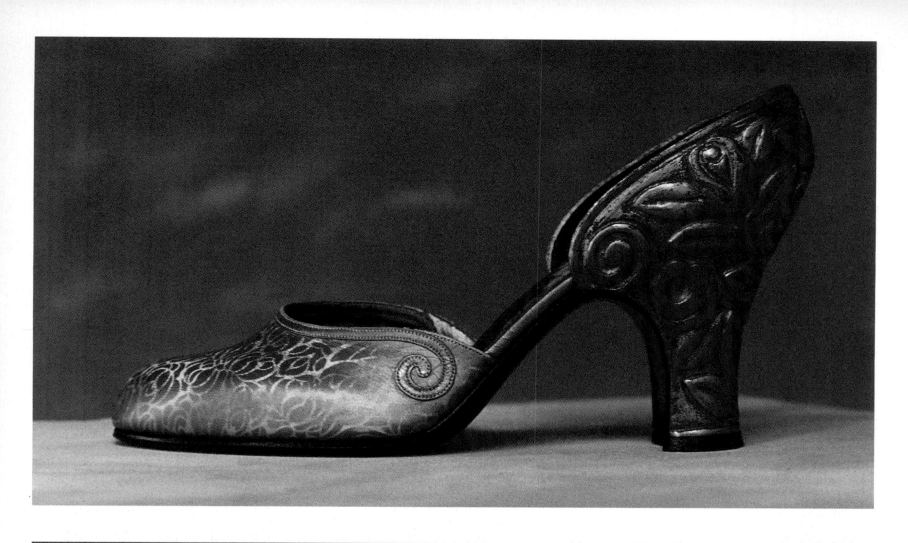

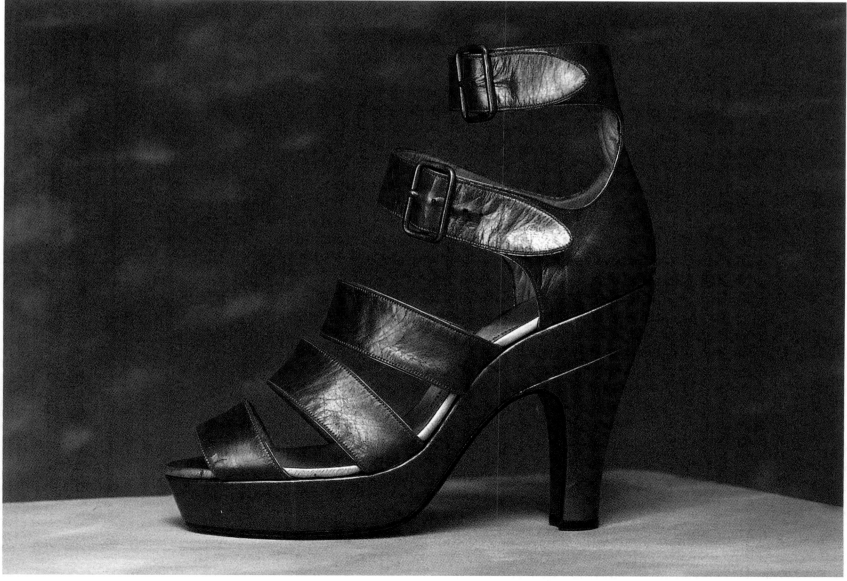

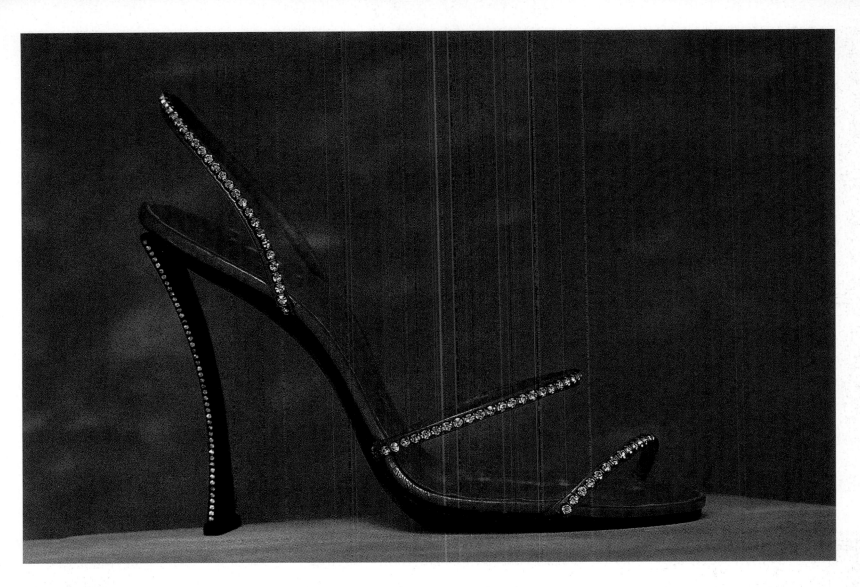

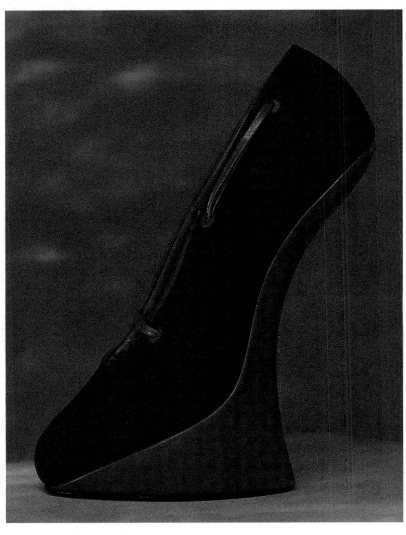

113. Perugia. Pump in blue kidskin printed with gold, heel and quarter from a single piece of wood carved and gold leaved. Around 1950 (copy of a style created in 1923). International Shoe Museum, Romans.

114. Perugia. Style created for Arletty. Evening sandal in gold kidskin, cork platform sole covered with gold. 1938. International Shoe Museum, Romans.

115. Perugia sandal in gold kidskin and strass, metal heel inlayed with strass. 1952. International Shoe Museum, Romans.

116. Perugia. Heelless shoe in purple velvet calfskin, lace of gold kidskin, base of polished cork coloured gold. 1950. International Shoe Museum, Romans.

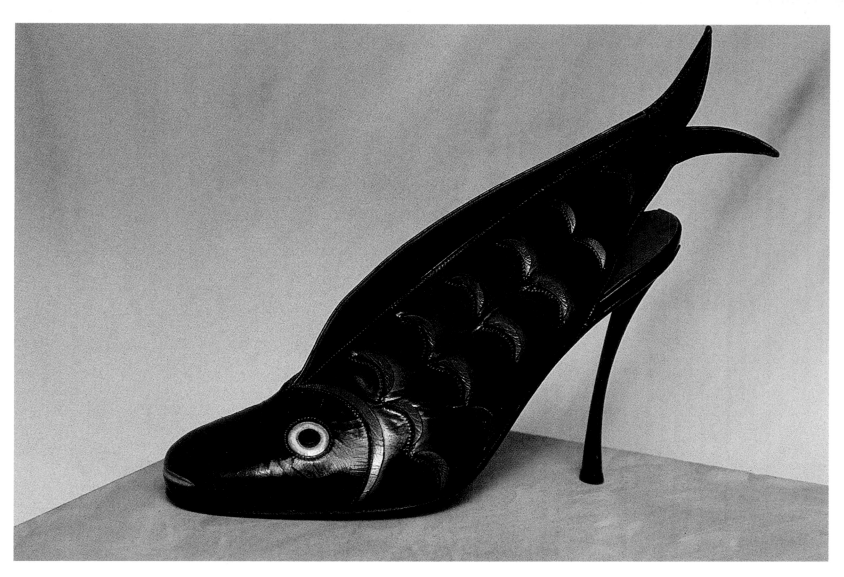

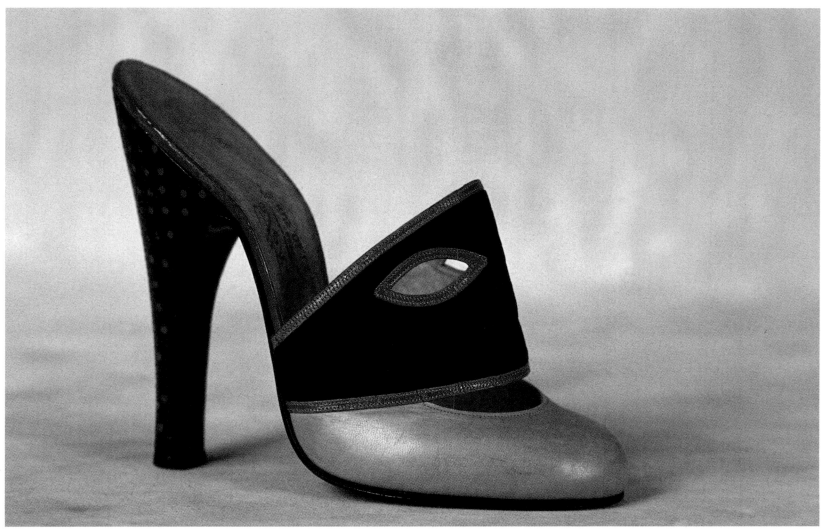

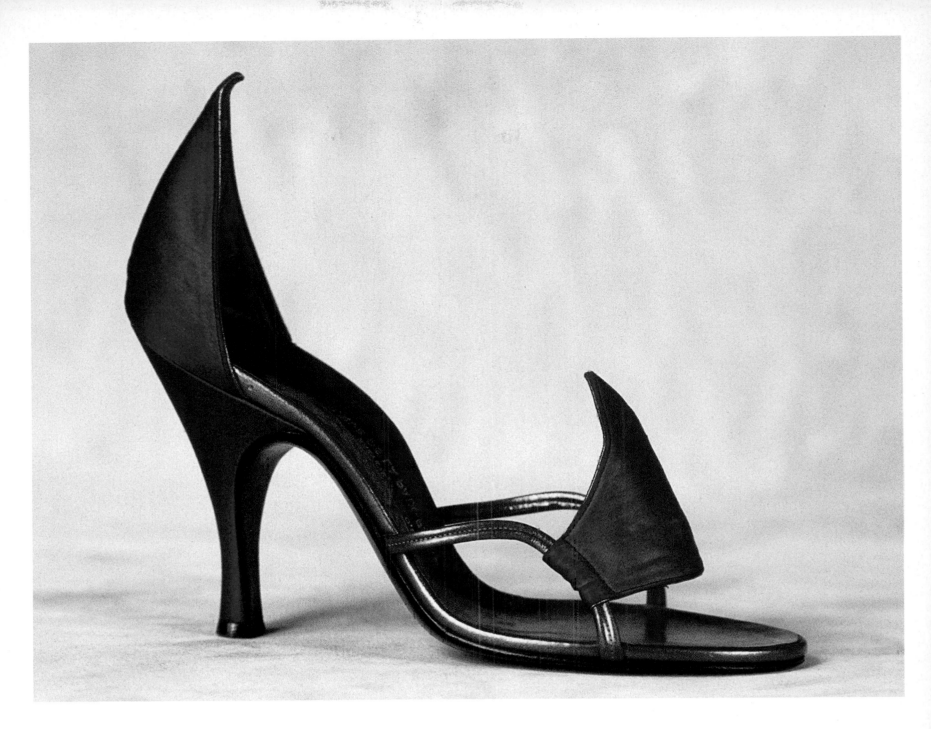

Around 1955, he reached the pinnacle of his career with a collection created in the United States. Each shoe was meant to be a homage to a 20th-century painter: Picasso, Braque, Matisse, Fernand Léger, Mondrian, et cetera. But Perugia's shoe as an art object still fulfills its primary function for walking. In addition to these bold creations, Perugia made many models for couturiers. As Paul Poiret's official shoemaker, he created pointed shoes with rich ornamentation and in various bright colours, that perfectly harmonized the couturier's long, straight silhouettes.

A long collaboration from 1930 to 1950 with Elsa Schiaparelli, with whom he shared a complementary competence, gave birth to new and original forms that were especially remarkable in their extraordinary modernity. After the Second World War, Perugia placed his talent in the services of Dior, Jacques Fath, Balmain, and Hubert de Givenchy. During this period he continued to divide his time between France and the United States, where he collaborated with I. Miller, one of America's most famous custom shoemakers. His superb career came to an end with Charles Jourdan, to whom he left his extraordinary personal collection. An inspiring artistic resource, it is on view today at the International Shoe Museum, Romans. André Perugia died in Nice on November 22, 1977. Even though some of his designs were drawn from the past and mined orientalism for inspiration, this exclusive shoemaker's status as an innovator is confirmed by the results of his technical and aesthetic research.

Perugia's place in the world of fashion elevates the beauty of the shoe and affirms its modernity. His perfection of new materials, new forms, and new fabrication processes remain valid today. "Last of the great Renaissance artists and first of the moderns," Baudelaire's apt description of Delacroix can also be applied to this shoemaker for the excellence of his art of the shoe.

117. Perugia. Pump in kidskin, black glaze, upper shaped as a fish, heel composed of a metal blade enameled black, style modeled after a painting by Braque. Around 1955. International Shoe Museum, Romans.

118. Perugia. Mule in cream coloured kidskin and brown velvet with gold embroidery, heel covered with black and gold discs. 1949. International Shoe Museum, Romans.

119. Perugia. Evening sandal in red satin and gold kidskin, style created for Jacques Fath. Around 1953. International Shoe Museum, Romans.

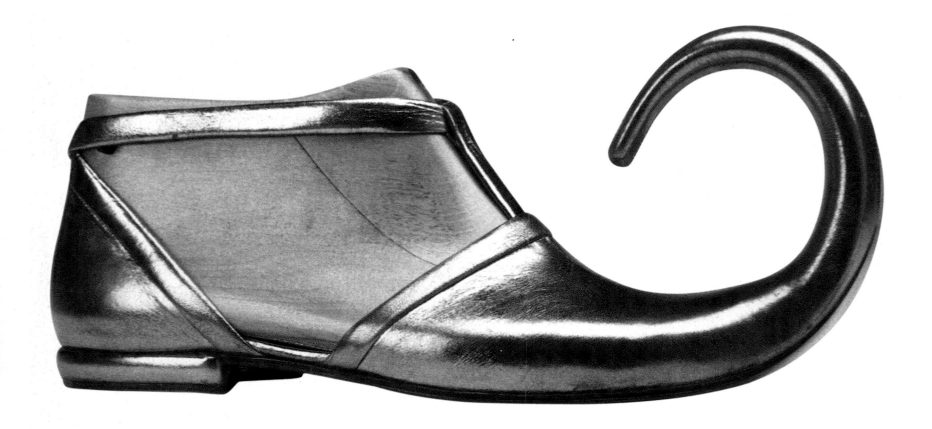

120. Bronze leather replica, 1985, after a style created in 1923 by Salvatore
  Ferragamo in Hollywood for the film *The Ten Commandments*,
  directed by Cecil B. DeMille. Ferragamo Museum, Florence.

121. Salvatore Ferragamo and Emilio Schubert during the first exhibition of fashion in
  Florence in 1951. They presented their latest invention, "The Kino".

122. The Ferragamo workshop in Florence, after the return of Salvatore Ferragamo in
  1927. These photos were taken for the magazine *Gran Bazar* and published in
  the end of the 1920s. Ferragamo Museum, Florence.

Ferragamo

Salvatore Ferragamo was born in 1898 in Bonito, a poor little village in southern Italy. The son of a peasant, he made his first pair of shoes at age nine. Salvatore made these shoes as a gift to his sister in honor of her first communion, because he did not want her going to church on that day wearing clogs. Encouraged by this initial experience, he embarked on an apprenticeship with a shoemaker in Naples. In 1914 he immigrated to the United States, where he lived for thirteen years, working primarily for the motion picture industry and making shoes for the biggest names in cinema to wear on screen and in town. Concerned about comfort and elegance, he studied anatomy at the University of California. This education taught him the fundamental role the arch of the foot played in distributing the weight of the body. He then perfected a steel arch support that he thenceforth included in all his designs. Returning to Italy in 1927, he established himself definitively in Florence in 1935 near the district where traditional craftsmen had their shops. He then purchased the Palais Spini-Feroni, which remains the home of the internationally known family business today. Economic problems in Italy during this period, followed by the war, prompted Salvatore Ferragamo not only to use inexpensive materials, such as braided paper, straw, and hemp, but also to replace his famous shank with cork. These difficulties did not hinder his remarkable creative imagination. Quite the contrary, because it was then that he made his most famous creation: the wedge sole, which was wildly successful and glorified the shoemaker's genius. New inventions marked the 1940s, such as the invisible sandal with upper made of nylon thread and heels sculpted in the form of an "F."

The exhilarating atmosphere of Italy in the 1950s made Rome, Amalfi, and Portofino tourist destinations for the wealthy, who never failed to make a stop in Florence to buy the famous shoemaker's latest creations. One day Greta Garbo bought seventy pairs in one fell swoop. The Duchess of Windsor stocked up on bi-coloured shoes each spring. Ferragamo's creativity, originality, and imaginativeness combine harmoniously with extraordinary technical knowledge. These qualities won him the 1947 Neiman Marcus Award. Twenty years later, his daughter Fiamma repeated this achievement. Salvatore Ferragamo died in 1960. He still speaks to us through his most beautiful creations exhibited in the museum that bears his name, which is established in the Spini-Feroni palace for the delight of all visitors.

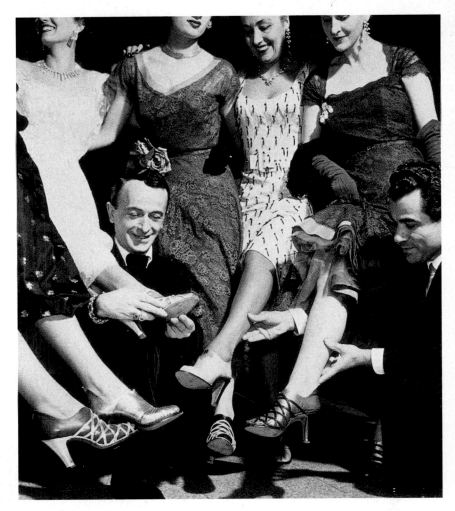

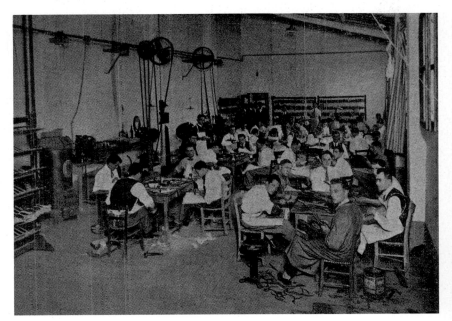

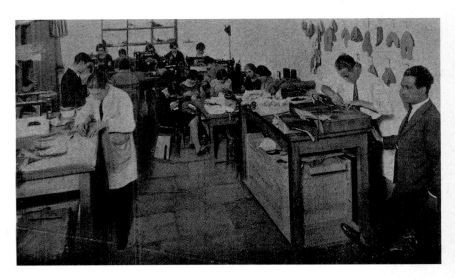

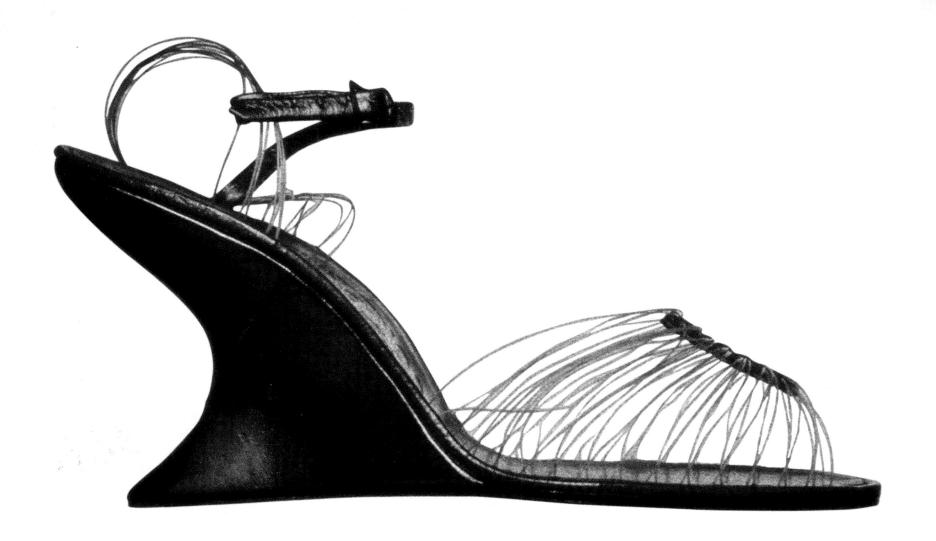

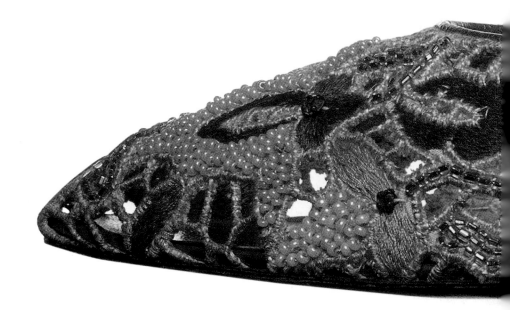

123. Ferragamo. Sandal in nylon and gilded leather. Ferragamo Museum, Florence.

124. Ferragamo. Style created for Sophia Loren, beads and motifs embroidered in satin. Ferragamo Museum, Florence.

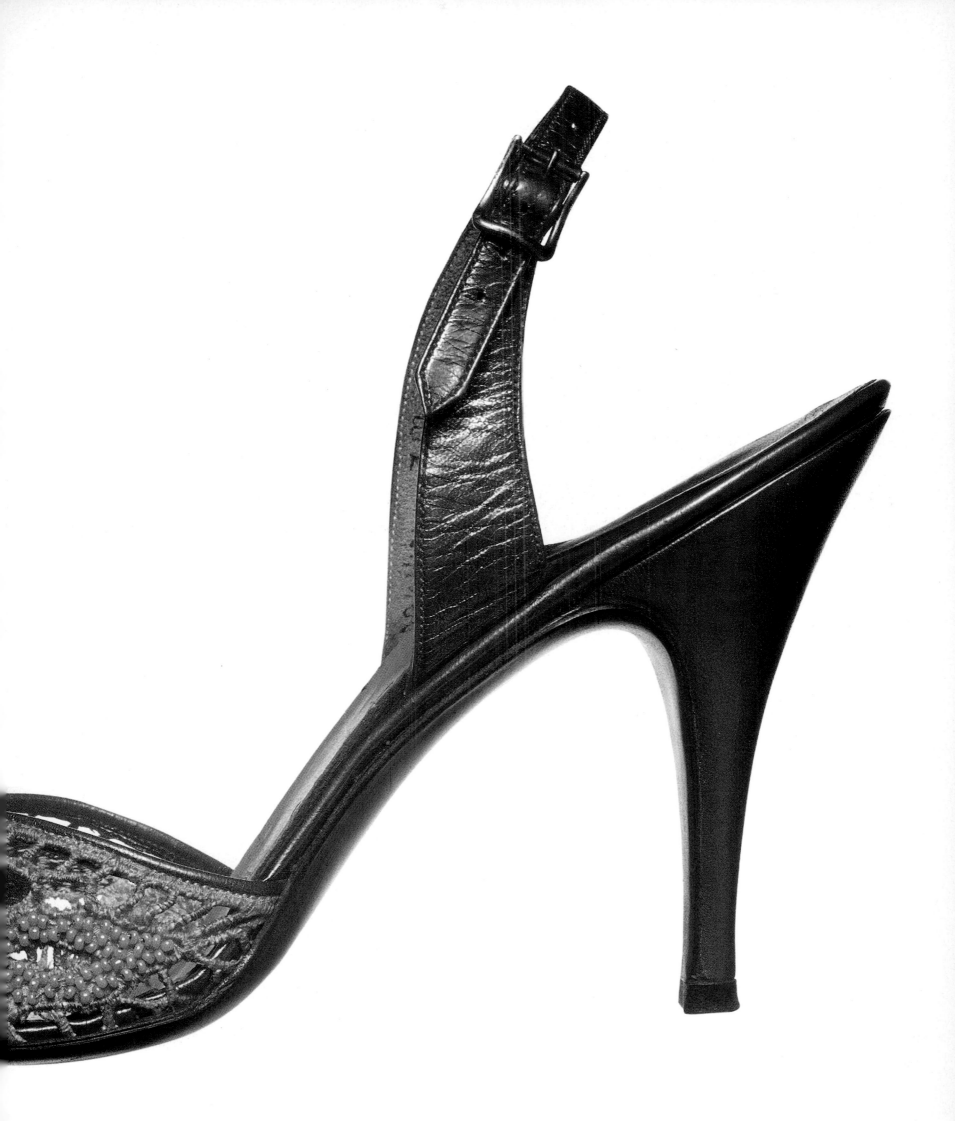

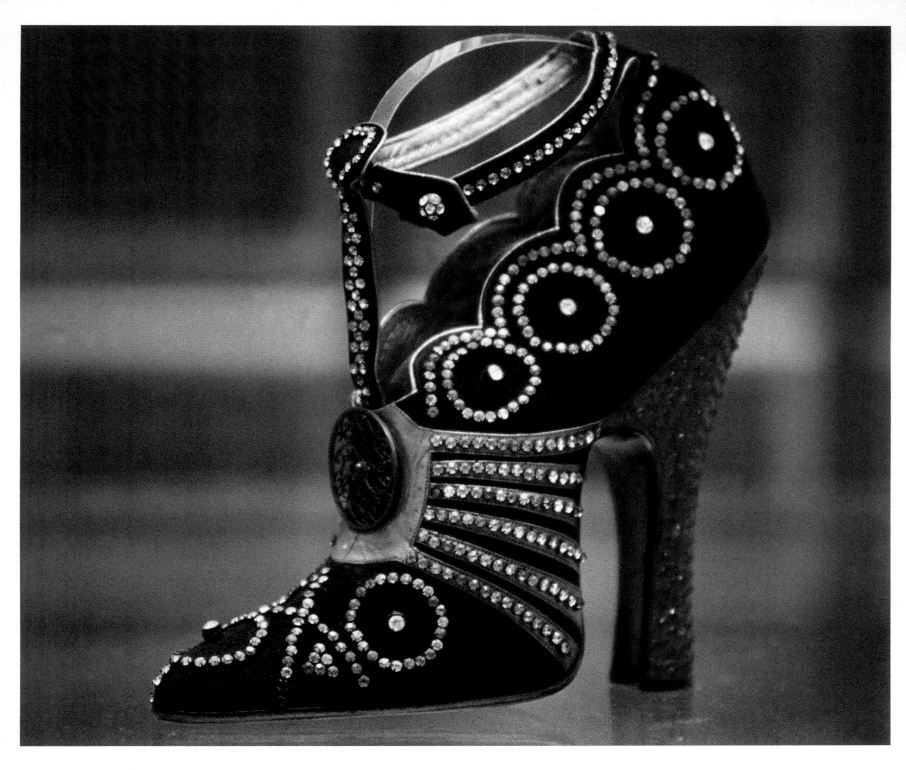

Alfred Argence

Established in 1900, Argence first opened its doors in Paris at 89 rue du faubourg Saint-Honoré, before moving to the rue des Pyramides, where it remained until closing. This prestigious firm, which focused on elegant women's shoes, was a member of the Syndicat des Bottiers de Paris, and attracted an elegant and famous clientele, including Sarah Bernhardt and Cléo de Sérode. Argence received many awards in the context of international exhibitions, such as the 1908 general labour exhibition in Florence and the 1908 international exhibition of modern industry and decorative and commercial arts in Rome. Alfred Victor Argence succeeded his father and worked in collaboration with Haute Couture. He was awarded many prizes at various exhibitions, such as "Artisans of Paris" in October 1942 and the "Exhibition of Shoemaking Firms" organized by the National Federation of French Shoemakers and the Union of France in the framework of the Congress of the International Leather Bureau in Paris in September 1948. The firm's business gradually declined before closing down in the early 1980s.

125. Evening shoe. Mary Jane in black suede, applications of gold kidskin, stass embroidery, silver filigree buckle. Louis XV heel covered with gold celluloid and strass. Pump realized by Julienne. International Shoe Museum, Romans.

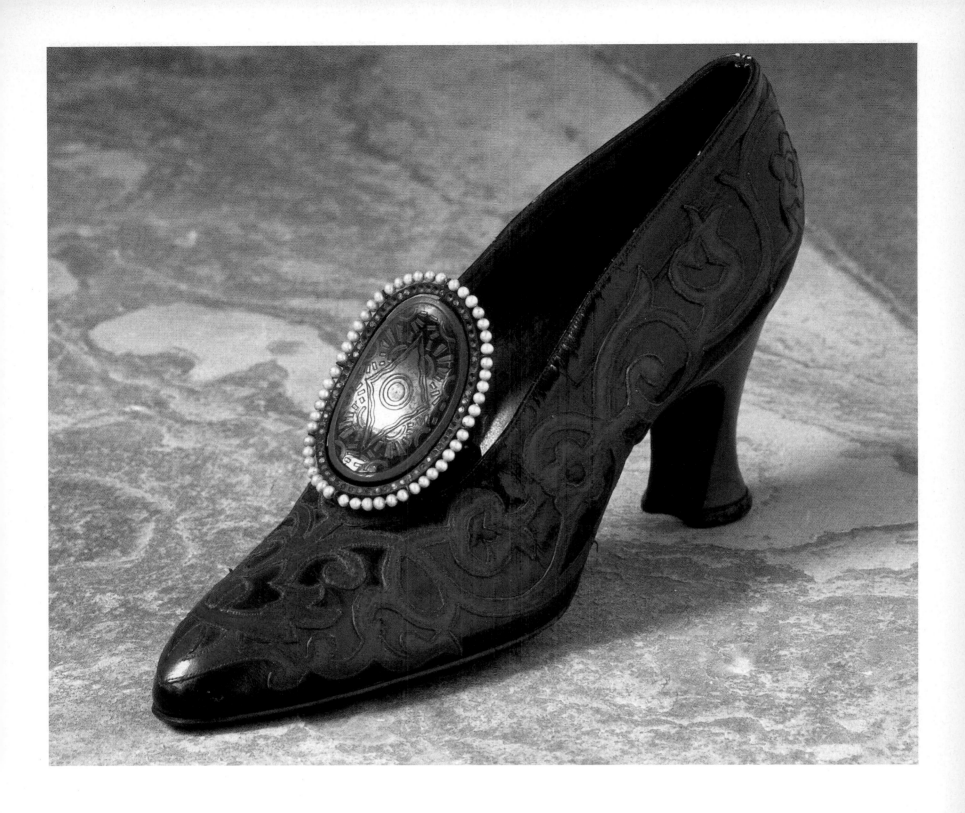

Julienne, Female Shoemaker

The daughter of a master shoemaker, Julienne started learning the secrets of the trade at a very young age.

In 1919, she set up shop in Paris at 235, rue Saint-Honoré; a boutique in Biarritz followed later. Her imaginative skill as a model-maker and her technical knowledge of traditional French craftsmanship positioned her at the forefront among the best.

Julienne specialized in fine shoes for distribution, attracting a clientele of elegant women with limited budgets who could not afford custom shoes.

Julienne's shoes were pretty replicas of custom-made styles; the excellence of their materials and forms sharply distinguished Julienne's shoes from banal, mass-produced brands. Always ahead of new trends, Julienne assimilated the exotic influences of the colonial exhibition and adapted them for Parisian taste. Julienne stopped working before the Second World War.

126. Pump realized by Julienne. Large bakelite buckle decorated with white beads, application in red kidskin. International Shoe Museum, Romans.

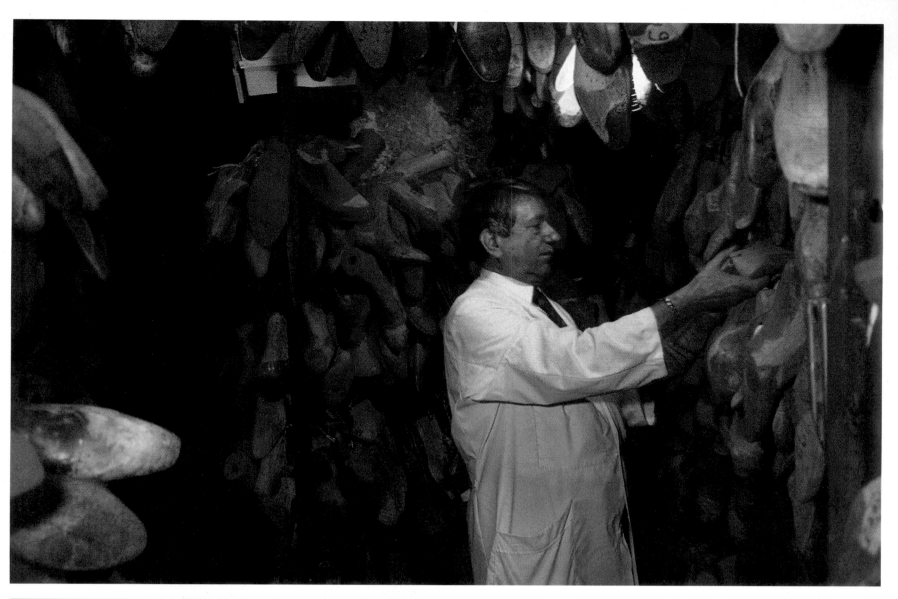

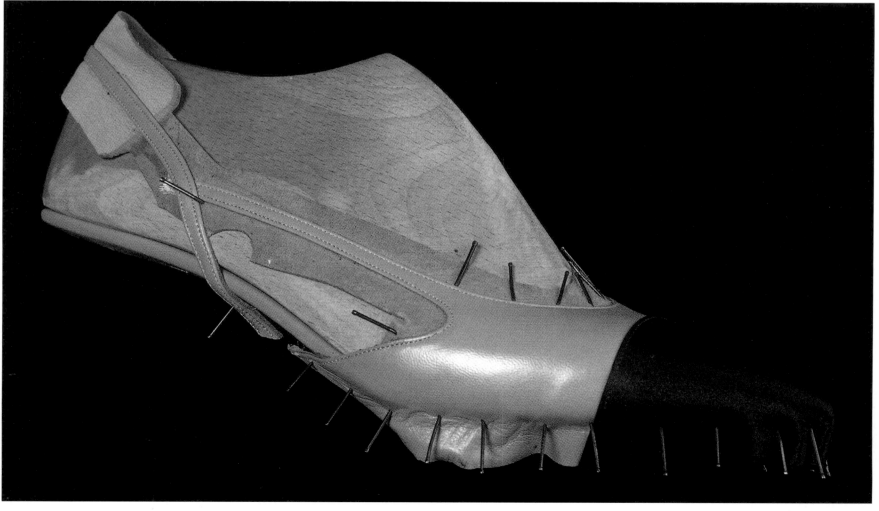

La Maison Massaro
A Shoemaking Dynasty

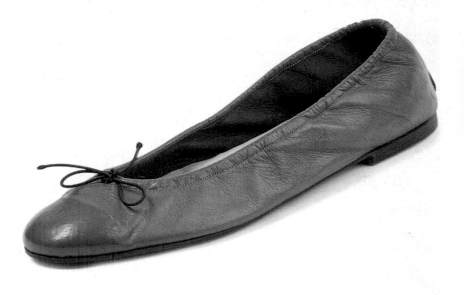

Sébastien Massaro founded the firm that bears his name in 1894, setting up shop at 2 rue de la Paix in Paris. His four sons, François, Xavier, Donat, and Lazare learned the trade under their father's supervision.

Lazare's son, Raymond Joseph Massaro, was born on March 19, 1929. His career lead him to the Ecole des métiers de la chaussure (a French trade school for shoemakers) on the rue de Turbigo in Paris, where he obtained vocational training qualification (C.A.P) in Louis XV women's shoes in 1947. The young Raymond finished his training in the family workshop. He remembers his father at the time making shoes for Elsa Schiaparelli, the Duchess of Windsor, Countess Von Bismarck, the millionaire Barbara Hutton, Shirley MacLaine, and Elizabeth Taylor, all of whom were regulars of the boutique on the rue de la Paix, along with other celebrities.

The Massaro family designed mainly for individuals, but it was developing closer ties with Parisian Haute Couture firms. In 1954, Lazare Massaro created a ballerina shoe for Madame Grès that would influence the entire period. This was followed by his invention of the famous bi-coloured sandal in beige and black for Coco Chanel in 1958.

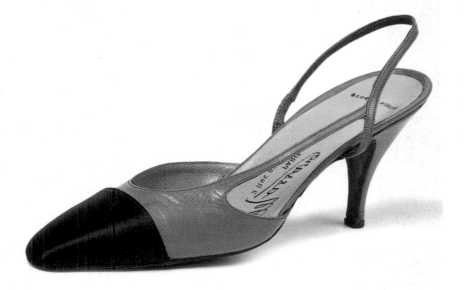

Raymond Massaro took over the firm's management and continued his the work of his father and grandfather. Many celebrities called upon his talent, including King Hassan II, to whom he became shoemaker, the actress Romy Schneider, and more recently the private Haute Couture collector Mouna Ayoub.

Raymond Massaro also filled some unusual requests for shoes that were quite humorous. Once there was a maharajah, a regular resident at a luxury hotel in Paris, who came to the capital with his personal secretary. The Asian secretary was so used to his country's ancestral tradition of going barefoot inside the palace, that he was unable to walk in shoes inside the expensive hotel without great difficulty. The Indian vassal prince wanted to respect French customs out of courtesy. So he asked his shoemaker to make a pair of shoes without soles that would allow his secretary's feet to come into direct contact with the ground. The clever shoes allowed the secretary to bow to both French and Indian traditions.

Major couture firms also came calling to Raymond Massaro, including: Emmanuel Ungaro, Guy Laroche, Gianfranco-Ferré, Christian Dior, Thierry Mugler, Ocimar Versolato, Christophe Rouxel, Olivier Lapidus, Jean-Paul Gaultier, and Dominique Sirop. He produced various styles for Karl Lagarfeld at Chanel, and made resin heels that looked like women's legs for Azzedine Alaïa. Constantly innovating, this designer is totally committed to originality.

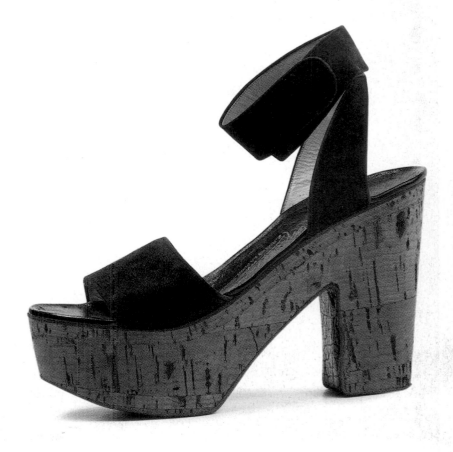

In 1994, the French Minister of Culture exclusively awarded Raymond Massaro the title Master of Art for combining consummate craftsmanship with a creative spirit. The shoemaker also belongs to the "Committee Signé Paris," established in 1997 to promote in France and abroad firms dedicated to excellence that represent Paris fashion through the quality of their artistic know-how. In 1999, Raymond Massaro exhibited his shoes in Tokyo as part of Japan's Year of France.

Raymond Massaro is also devoted to the science of foot orthopedics.

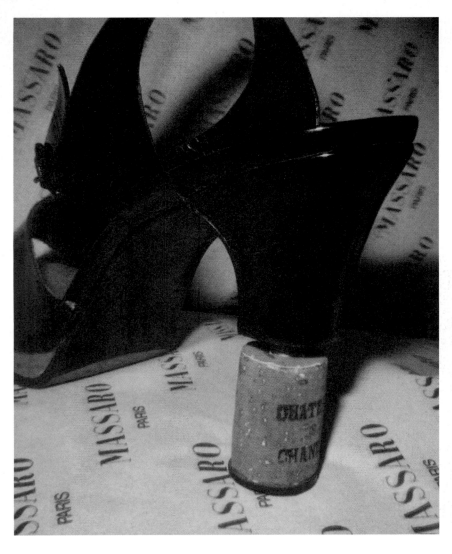

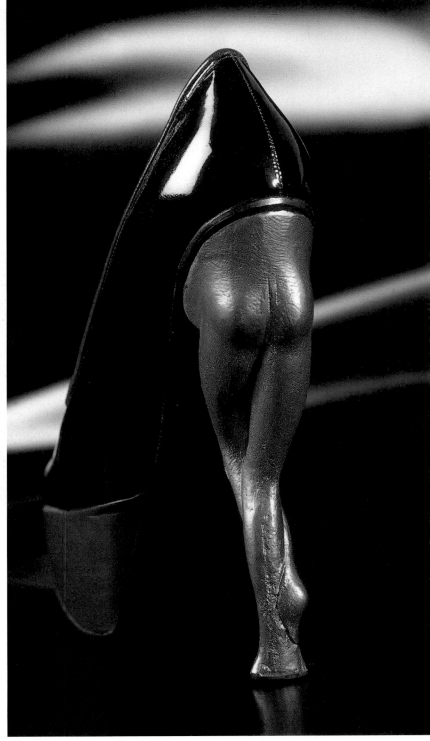

Previous pages:

127. Massaro in his workshop.

128. Shoe in production for Chanel by Massaro.

129. Elastic pump created for Madame Grès (beachwear) by Massaro. 1955.

130. Shoe created by Massaro for Chanel, 1958.

131. Shoe created by Massaro, 1992.

132. Black-varnished sandal with platform sole in cork created by Massaro for Chanel in summer 2001. On the cork heels, the inscription "Château Chanel" can be read.

133. Massaro. "Legs" platform shoes for Azzedine Alaïa. 1991. Black glaze, red kid-skin and red base. Achieved using resin, the "leg heel" was hand carved.

134. Shoe created by Massaro, 1991

135. Massaro. White mule painted entirely by hand with the Parisian coat of arms. 1997. Creation for the Signé Paris committee.

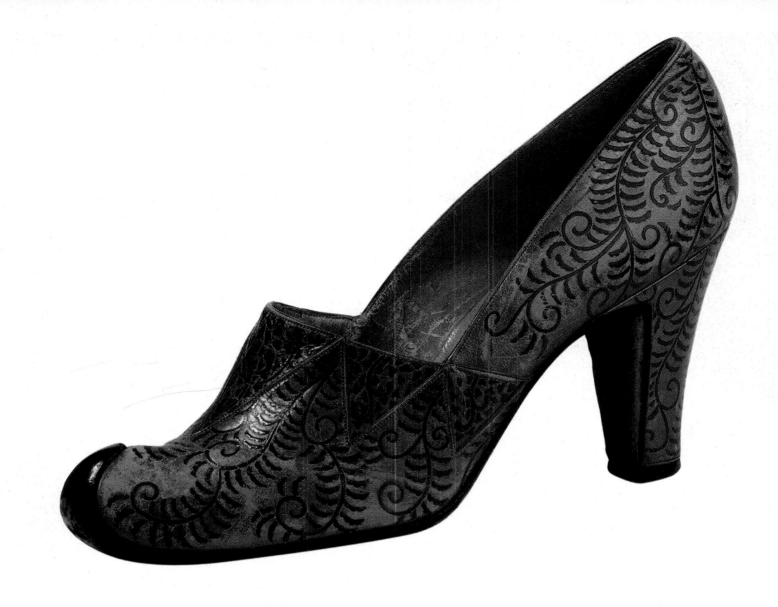

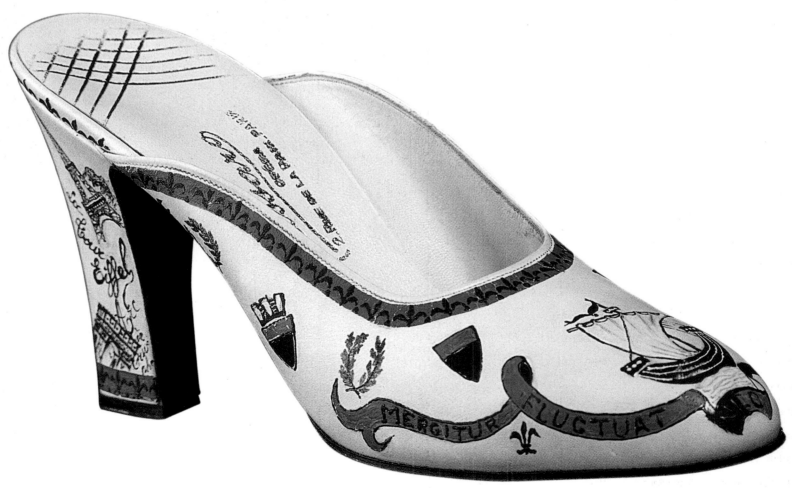

MERGITUR·FLUCTUAT

103

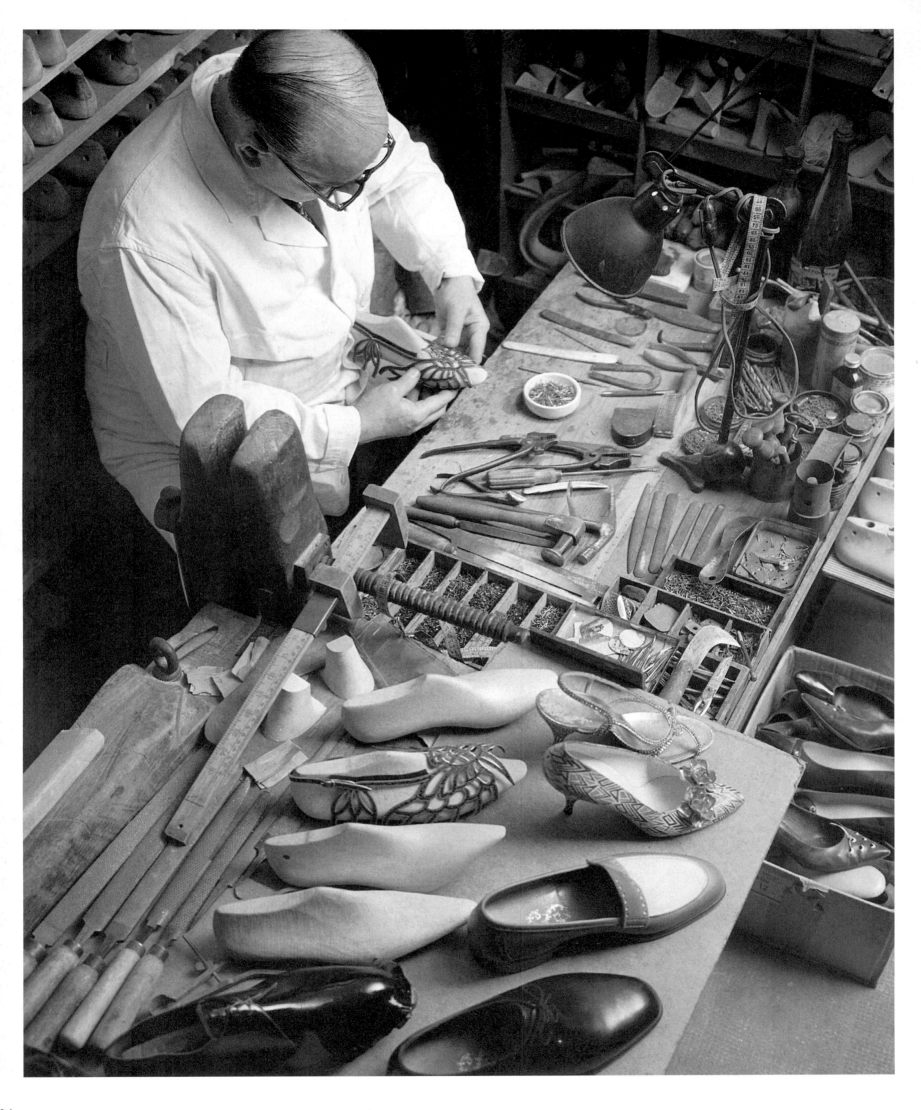

Sarkis Der Balian

The Immortal Shoemaker

Sarkis Der Balian was an Armenian born in the early 20th century in Aïtab Cilicia, Little Armenia. He showed an early interest in shoes. Orphaned at age seven, he was taken in by a regional shoemaker, who gradually taught the craft to Balian while the child went to school. He soon detected within his young apprentice a gifted student and a hard worker who had unusual manual dexterity, so he encouraged the boy to continue.

Full of love for his craft, the child embraced an Armenian saying that "knowing a traditional craft is like having a gold bracelet on your wrist." He arrived in France on March 7, 1929, to practice his craft in the various workshops of Parisian custom shoemakers. Around 1934, he went to work for Enzel, a shoemaker on the rue Saint-Honoré, where he managed a team of forty workers. The famous Charles Ritz managed the firm and he admired Balian's work. During this period he made shoes for Marie Curie, the aviator Hélène Boucher, and Mistinguett, among others.

Balian complemented these productive years designing for Enzel with independent work as a model maker, which allowed him to assert himself more individually. Among the clients he created models for were Max Bally, the factories of Unic-Fenestrier in Romans, the Fougères factories, and the firm Besson, a small Parisian maker of women's shoes. He also technically perfected certain models made for the large couturiers.

In 1935, he toured Italy, taking away from that country an image of perfected beauty that would constantly guide and illuminate his work designing pumps, sandals, booties, and shoes. The events of 1936 lead to Enzel being closed down. His journey then led him to the corner of the rue Rivoli and the rue Renard to "Cecile," a firm specializing in footwear for men, women, and children where he obtained the job of Technical Manager. He turned down an invitation from Delman who offered him the opportunity to make shoes in the United States in 1939. Attached to his adopted country of France, he set up shop on the rue de la Sourdière in Paris from 1943 to 1945. The rococo interiors of his first store, which he designed himself and made with his own hands, remains in place today. Success led him to move into a much larger store at 221 rue Saint-Honoré in 1947. Once again, he left his stamp on the architectural interior and decoration and designed a setting to welcome and seduce a demanding clientele, interested in elegance and comfort. The comfort of his shoes merited the label "Der Balian comfort fit" for this consummate craftsman, shoemaker, boot maker, model maker, and designer, as he described himself.

His need to constantly achieve new heights led him to produce masterpieces such as the history of Cinderella. A true miniature painting, it is made of over five hundred thousand tiny bits of leather. The same technique is found on a shoe depicting the city of Zurich viewed from the windows of the Town Hall. At the time, the city of Zurich persistently tried to purchase the shoe, but Balian refused. The piece represented over a year's work for this craftsman of art objects who never looked at his watch, and who was ready to undo and redo as often as necessary, the result being the only thing that mattered to him.

Throughout his long career Balian made shoes for a wide range of celebrities, including the painters Salvador Dali and Dunoyer de Segonzac; sculptor Paul Belmondo; actors Claude Dauphin, Gaby Morlet, Greta Garbo, and Laurent Terzieff; boxer Georges Carpentier; the artists Henri Salvador and Yehudi Menhin; the writers Jean Anouilh, Aragon, and Elsa Triolet; and the aviator Jean Mermoz.

Internationally known since 1930 he received many prizes and the highest awards in all the national and international exhibitions. In 1955, he won footwear's world cup in Bologna for his masterpiece called "floralie," an extraordinary shoe with a hollow silver heel that was inlaid. The jury was so impressed with this shoe that they named Balian the "Michelangelo of the shoe." For this honour, the city of Paris presented him with the médaille de vermeil. Best worker in France in 1958, his appointment as technical advisor for technical training was renewed five times by the French Ministry of National Education.

Balian's generosity led him to spontaneously transmit his knowledge to the younger generation. He moreover knew how to recognize and admire quality work with total impartiality; doing so was his greatest pleasure. Assisted by his wife and daughter, Astrid, he kept his business going until 1995 and died on March 29, 1996.

This virtuoso of shoemaking, about which he was absolutely passionate, still speaks to us if we stop to contemplate his work preserved and displayed at the International Shoe Museum, Romans.

136. Sarkis Der Balian at his workbench.

Following pages:

137. Zurich, creation of Sarkis Der Balian. Paris, 1950. The upper is of parchment inlayed with naturally coloured leather, with not a stroke of paint.
This view of Zurich is that which one has from the windows of the town hall.

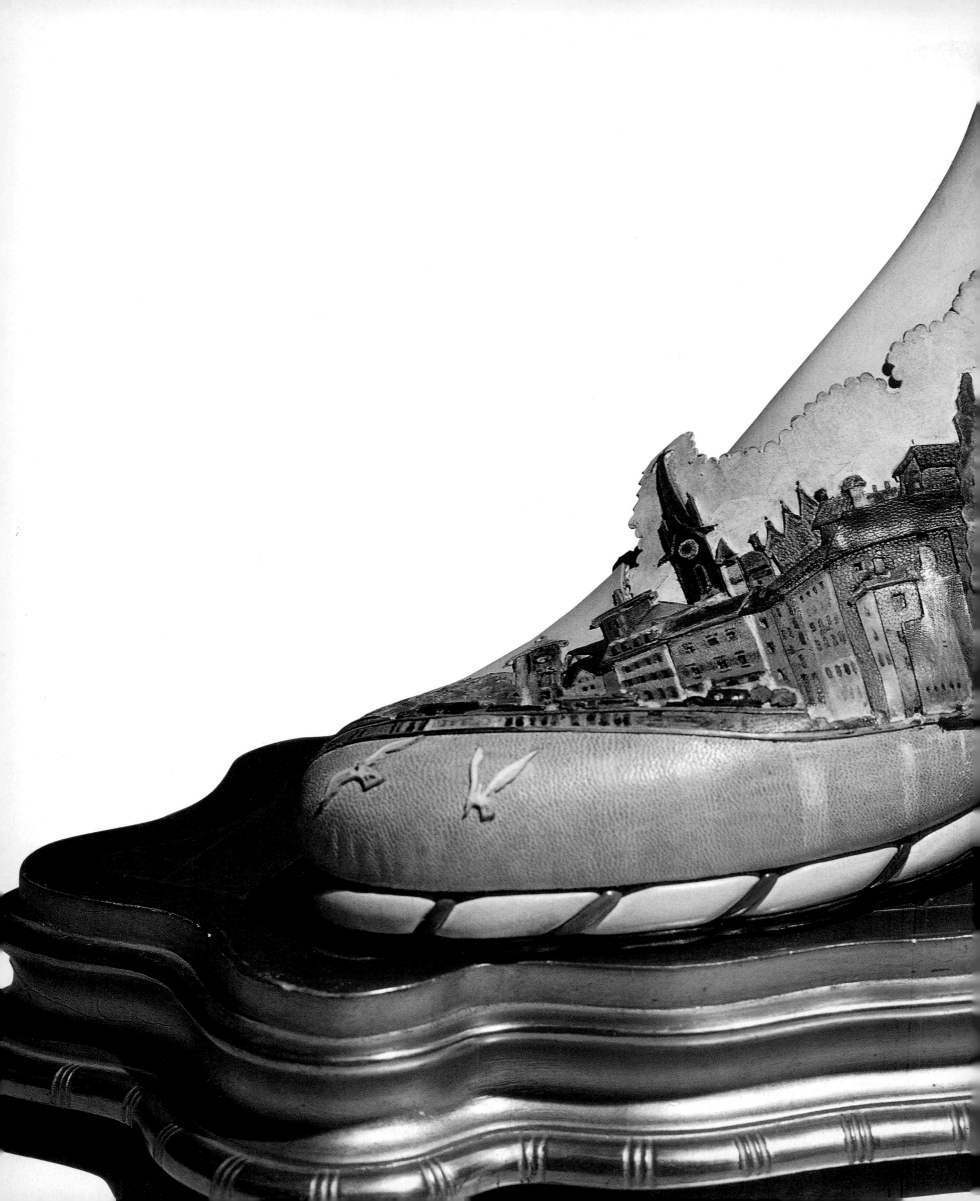

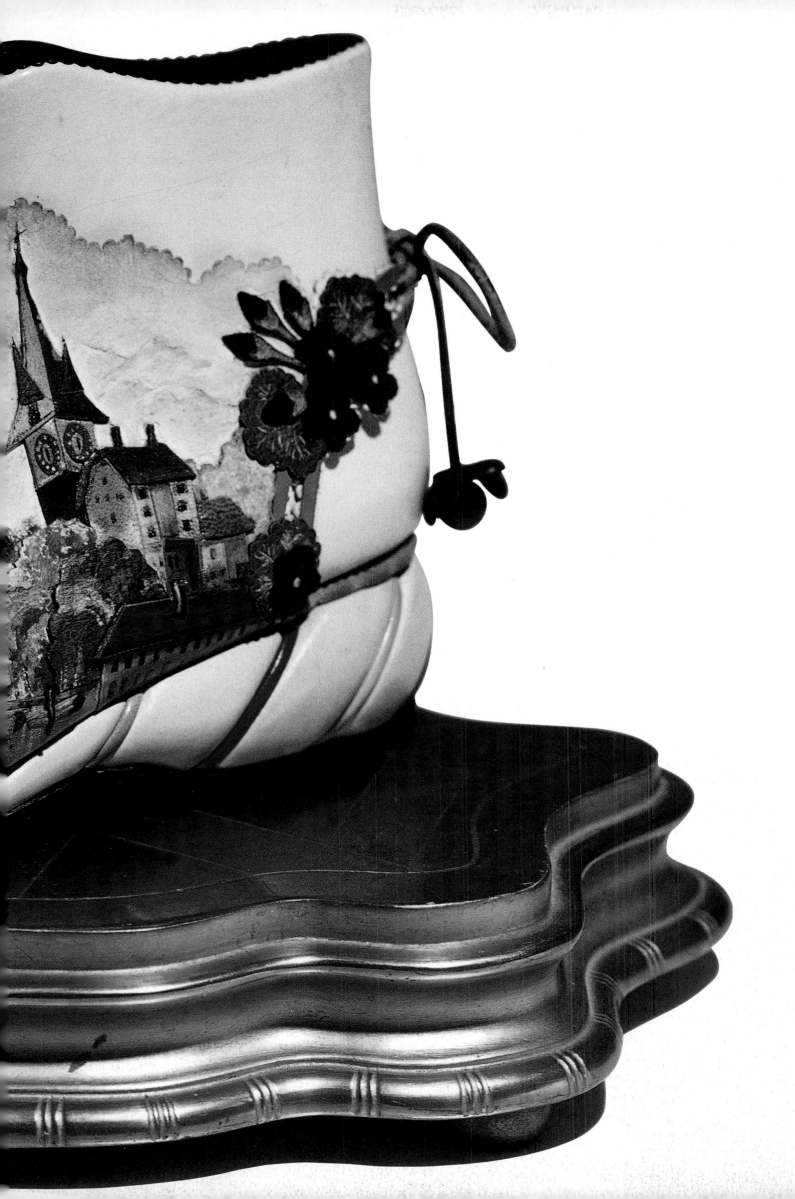

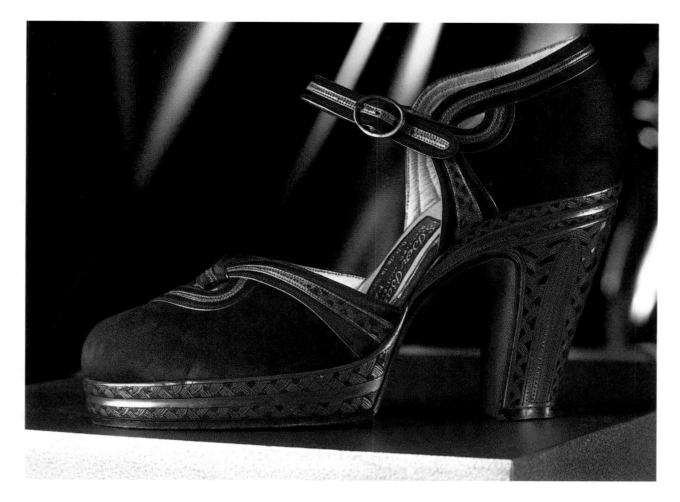

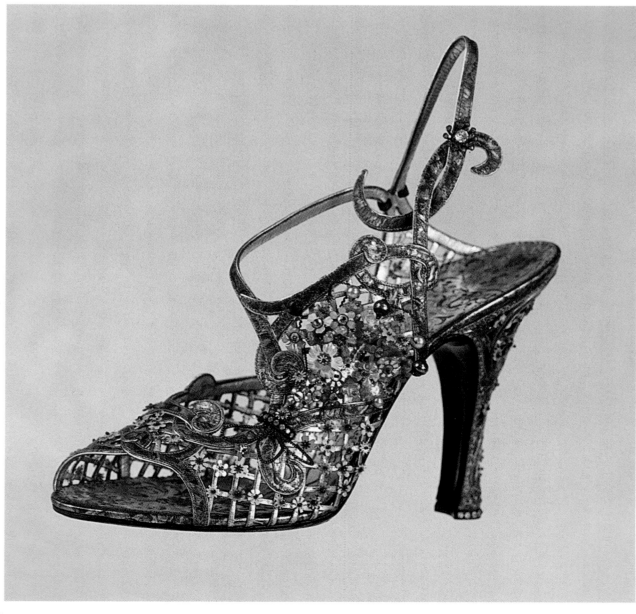

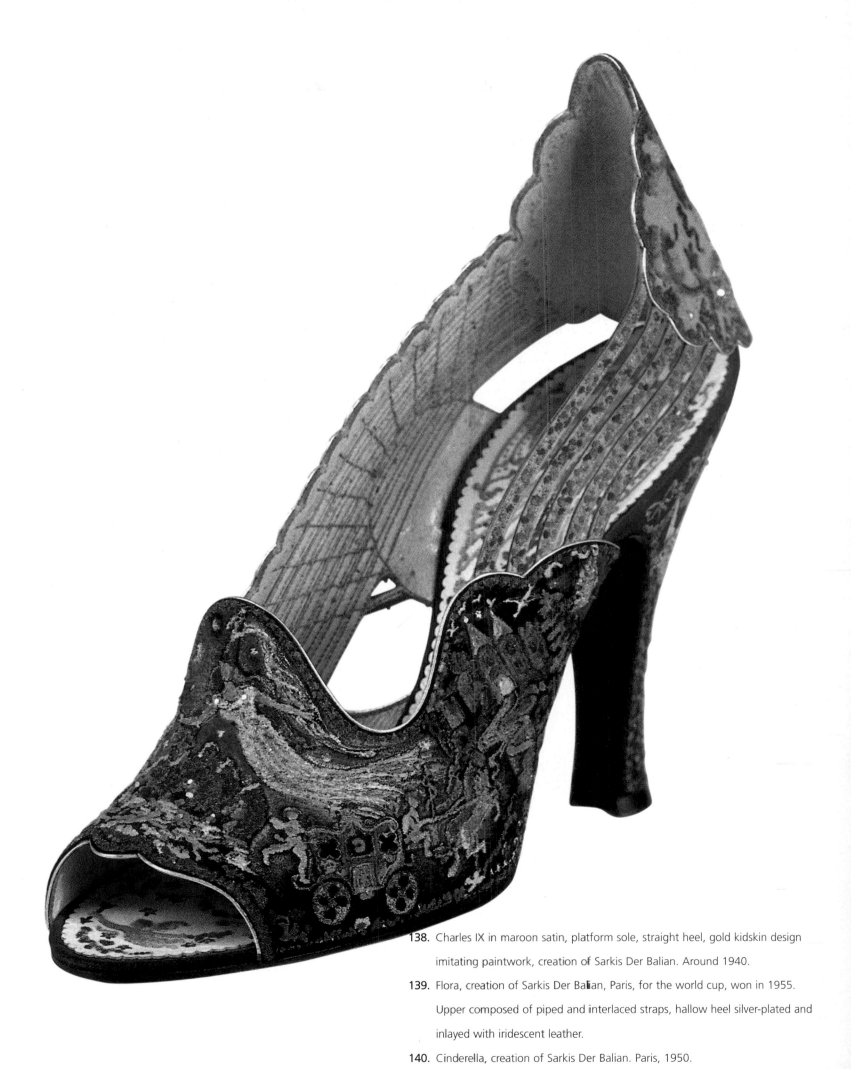

138. Charles IX in maroon satin, platform sole, straight heel, gold kidskin design imitating paintwork, creation of Sarkis Der Balian. Around 1940.

139. Flora, creation of Sarkis Der Balian, Paris, for the world cup, won in 1955. Upper composed of piped and interlaced straps, hallow heel silver-plated and inlayed with iridescent leather.

140. Cinderella, creation of Sarkis Der Balian. Paris, 1950. Fairytale realized on a velvet upper inlayed with tiny, multicoloured sequin.

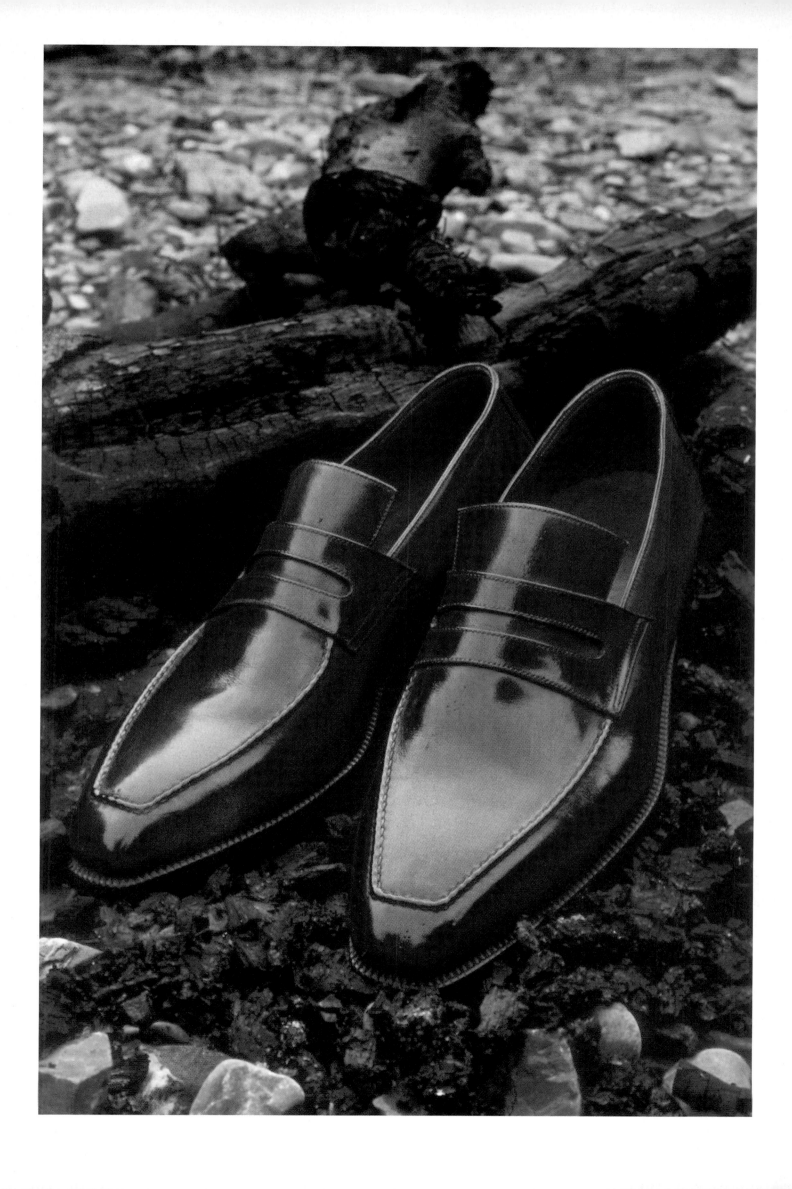

Berluti
Three Generations of Artists

A native of Senigallia, Italy; Alexandre Berluti began his apprenticeship in woodworking as an adolescent. This initial craft cultivated his love of finely worked wood that he would later rediscover in the art of form making for shoes. Possessing great manual dexterity, he acquired knowledge of leather craft that his descendants would inherit. The gripping tales of Ilebrando, an old shoemaker who emigrated to Marseille, reached Berluti's village and put the notion of travel in his head. So, around 1887, carrying Ilebrando's shiny tools as his luggage, he departed for new horizons. Once on the road, he encountered a troupe of saltimbanques that he accompanied for several years, making the shoes for the players in the company.

Arriving to Paris in 1895, he practiced the craft of shoemakers, creating exclusively custom shoes, a tradition maintained today by the Berluti firm. The 1900 World Fair offered him a chance to make himself known to a larger public. Upon his return to his native country, he ran a workshop until his death and transmitted the secrets of his art to his son Torello.

Torello apprenticed in his father's workshop where he showed a predilection for hard work and a desire to get ahead. With a sculptor's skill, his hand measured, cut, polished, and assembled shoes. During the Roaring Twenties, he settled in Paris, opening a boutique in 1928 on the rue du Mont Thabor under the trade name Berluti, exclusive custom-made shoes.

The house style was established by three emblematic types: lace-up pumps (or pope's shoe, a pure form made from a single piece without seams), the flat or moccasin of a single piece called the "Renaissance princess shoe" and finally the Napoleon III, a tall style with elastic on the side, which would one day elicit the following comment from the Duke of Windsor: "Something simultaneously modest and mischievous."

From this time forward, Berluti had a reputation, and attracted a lot of attention from the international clients of the surrounding luxury hotels, resulting in the store's relocation to 26 rue Marbeuf. This elite location became a temple to the shoe and of masculine elegance, decorated in wood and leather, in homage to the family's dual crafts.

In the early 1950s, a variety of celebrities were to be seen at Berluti's: James de Rothschild, Alain de Gunzburg, Sacha Distel, Eddy Constantine, Bernard Blier, Gaston and Claude Gallimard, Charles Vanel, Fernand Gravey, Marcel l'Herbier, Pierre Mondy, Yul Bryner, Marcel Achard, Jules Roy, and André Hunnebelle. These names demonstrate how well Berluti's fame attracted the Jet Set in 1958.

In the early 1960s, the firm was successfully established and Torello's son Talbino took the reigns. Talbino had been introduced to the shoemaker's craft at age fourteen, but he subsequently pursued architectural studies. The roles were immediately shared between the father and son. Talbino, whose talent was rather intellectual and imaginative, had the vision and made the designs, whereas Torello fabricated the stuff of his son's dreams. From this close collaboration was born the laced moccasin in the early 1940s. But in 1959, Talbino disrupted the firm's tradition by inviting exclusive ready-to-wear into the world where the custom-made reigned with its production delays. This new direction satisfied demanding and impatient clients. Immediately available, these "exclusive ready to wear" shoes permitted lower prices, an expanded client base, and the growth of the firm.

But how did one get a perfect fit if measurements were not taken? Talbino and his cousin Olga solved the problem by playfully perfecting five morphological foot types: the pretentious, the intellectual, the fragile, the masochist, and the unpleasant. These portraits corresponded to a "visual chart" that allowed one to visualize the most suitable model once the client's shoes were off.

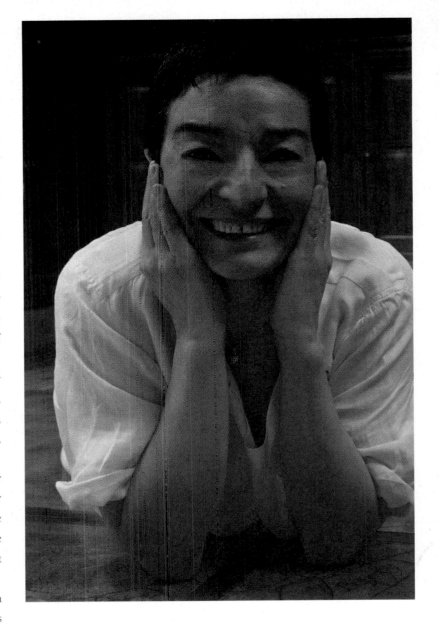

141. Men's shoes executed by Berluti.

142. Photograph of Olga Berluti.

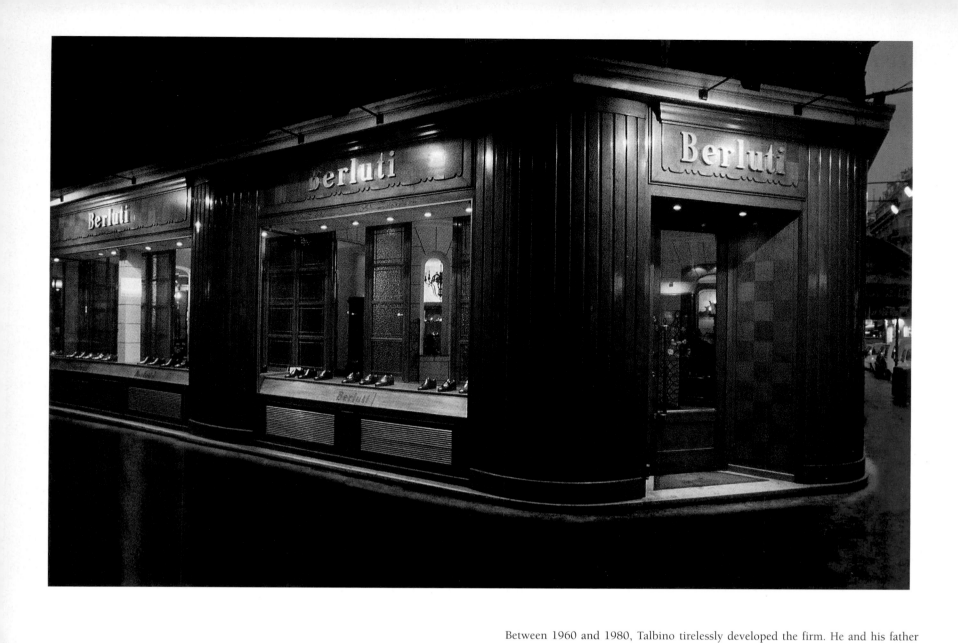

Between 1960 and 1980, Talbino tirelessly developed the firm. He and his father gave clients a warm welcome into a world of refinement.

As for Olga Berluti, Italian by birth, she spent her childhood in Parma and Venice, but became Parisian at heart and in culture. During university she leaned toward philosophy before devoting herself to the art of custom shoemaking. Her arrival to rue Marbeuf in 1959 marked the beginning of ten years of intense and productive apprenticeship in addition to study with surgeons who were clients of the firm. Together, they examined how shoes are used as well as posture and the form of the foot, enabling them to diagnose foot and back problems some people suffered from. This truly "clinical research" led to the physiological line called "Comfort." New ideas were in the air. Olga responded by offering to clients used to wearing classic shoes new designs that had the forms and colours they were dreaming about. Unusual shades of green, gray, and yellow appeared attracting such customers as François Truffaut, Andy Warhol, Roman Polanski, and Jacques Lacan. The boutique became a salon, with hurried people stopping in their tracks to exchange pleasantries with Olga. The shoemaker had become artist and poet. Even the moon's magic, though its whitening effect on shoe leather exposed to moonbeams, cooperated with Olga, who achieved deep tones and a previously unknown shine. As the ambassador of this prestigious brand, the exceptional, exciting, and passionate Olga was in charge of promotion and decoration of Berluti boutiques, which opened throughout the world. The firm's current designs reflect the fashion phenomenon of urban sports shoes, as can be seen in the styles offered in the recently opened boutique on the boulevard Saint-Germain. But our-century's changes are unlikely to alter the time-honoured methods of hand-fashioned shoes, for three generations the symbol of the Berluti.

143. Berluti boutique in Paris, 26 rue Marbeuf.

144. Men's shoes executed by Berluti.

Following pages:

145. Men's shoes executed by Berluti.

146. Men's shoes executed by Berluti.

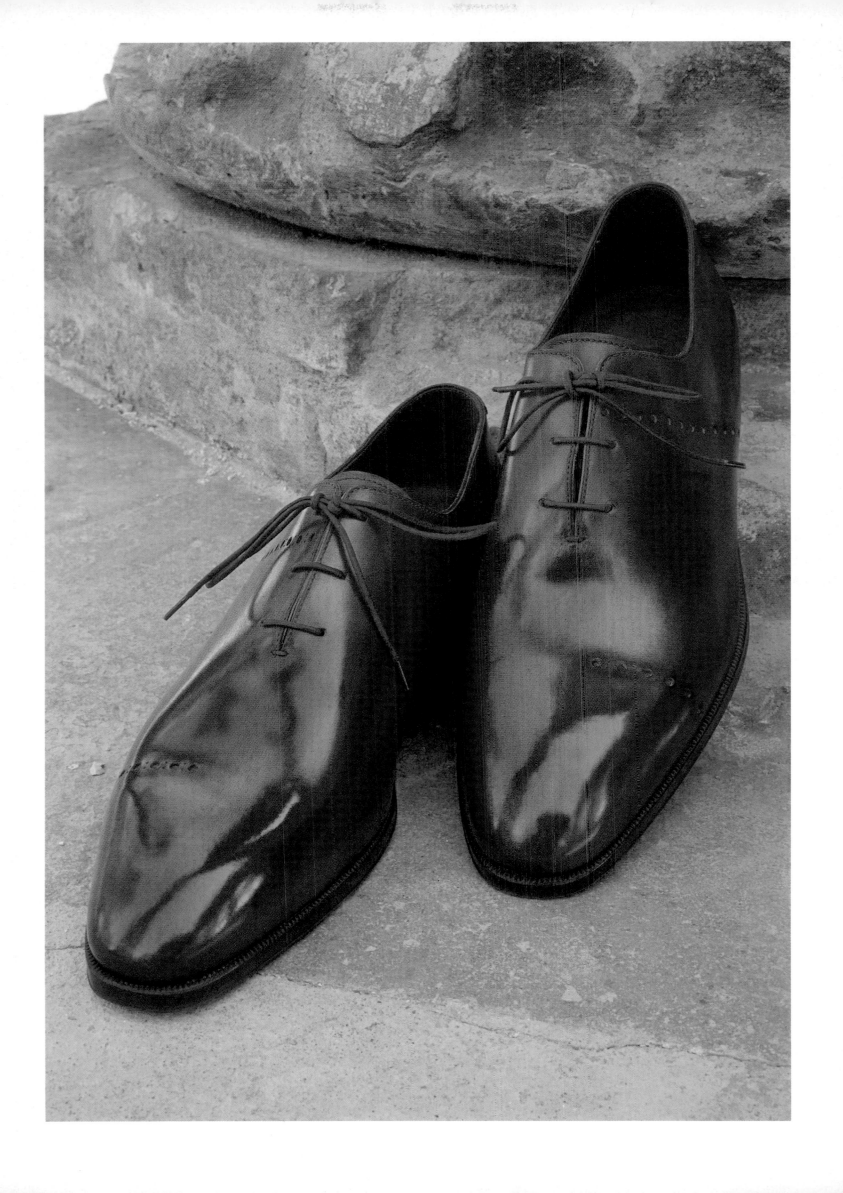

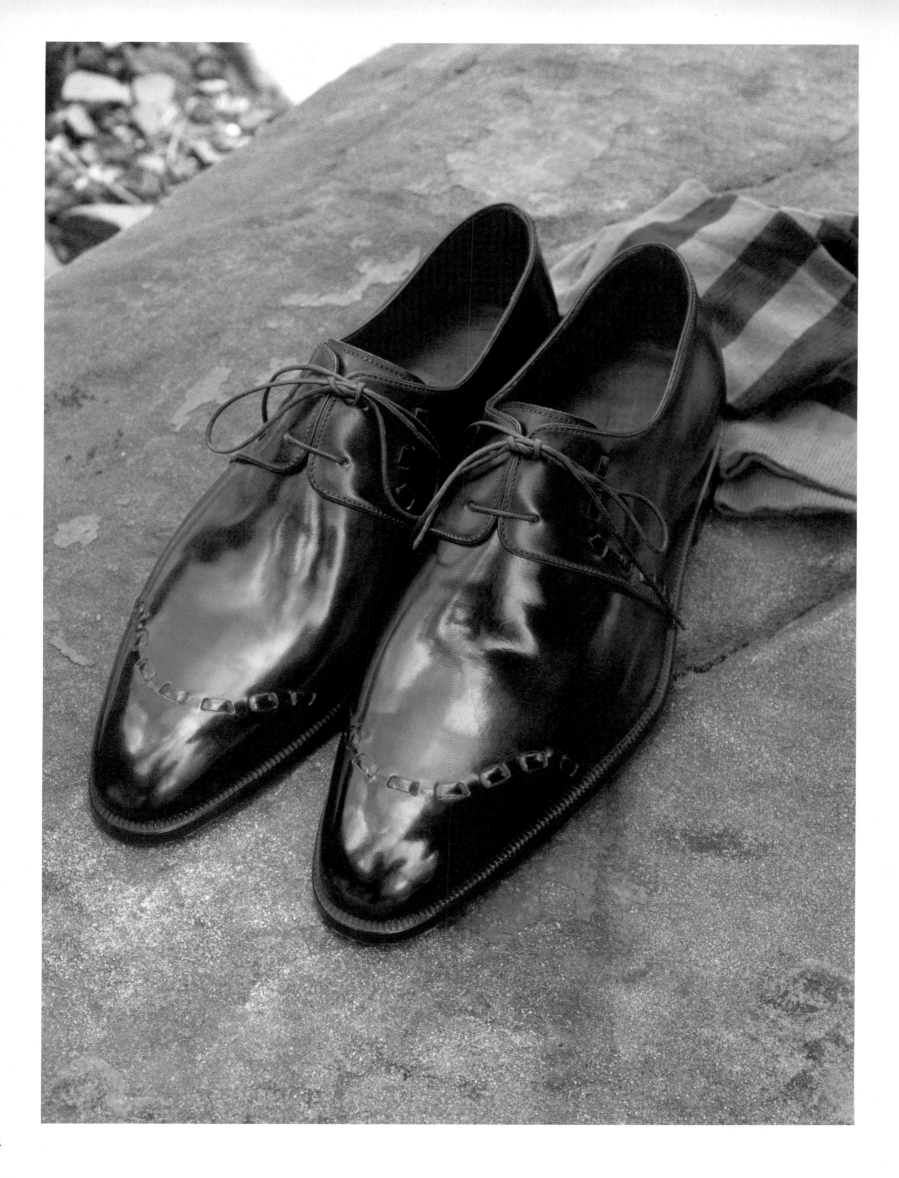

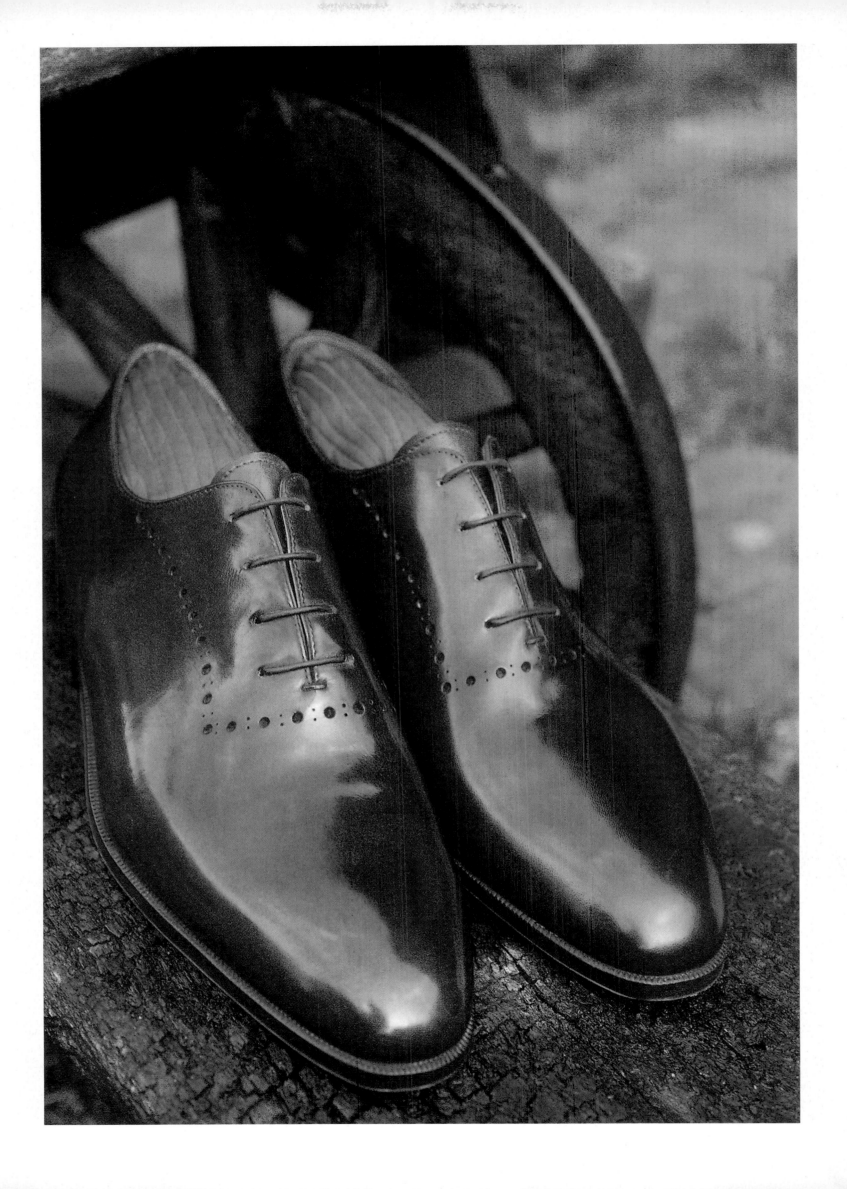

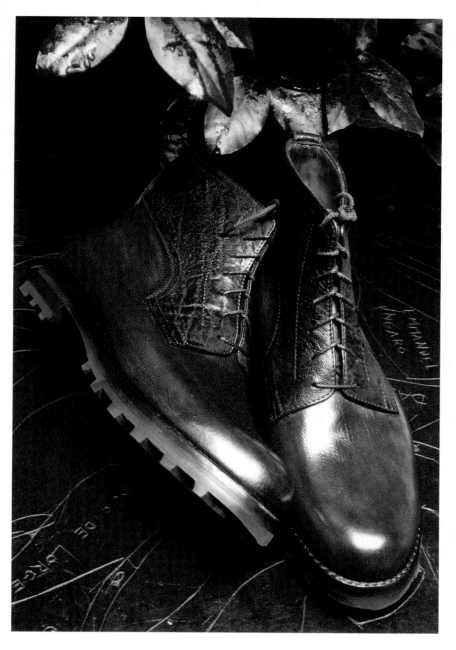

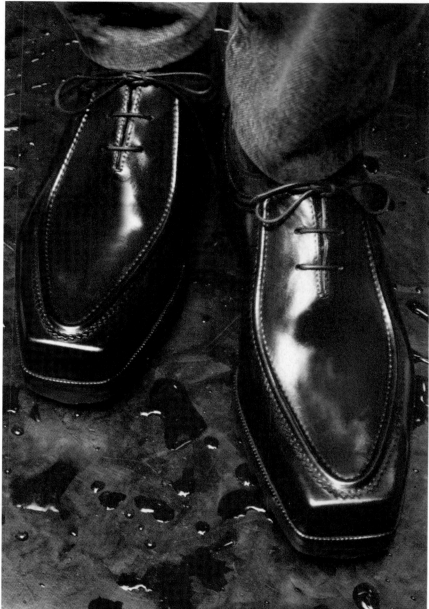

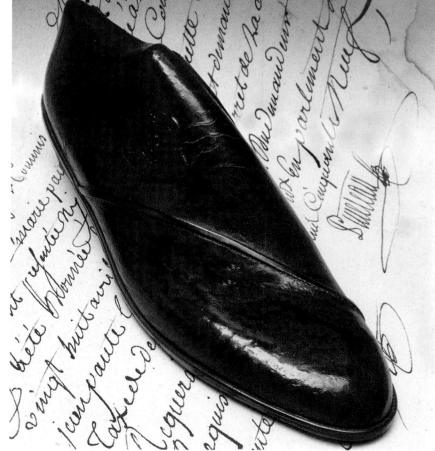

147. Men's shoes executed by Berluti.

148. Shape of shoes created for Gaston Gallimard.

149. Shoe created for Gallimard by Berluti.

150. Men's shoes. Tatoues Collection, House of Berluti.

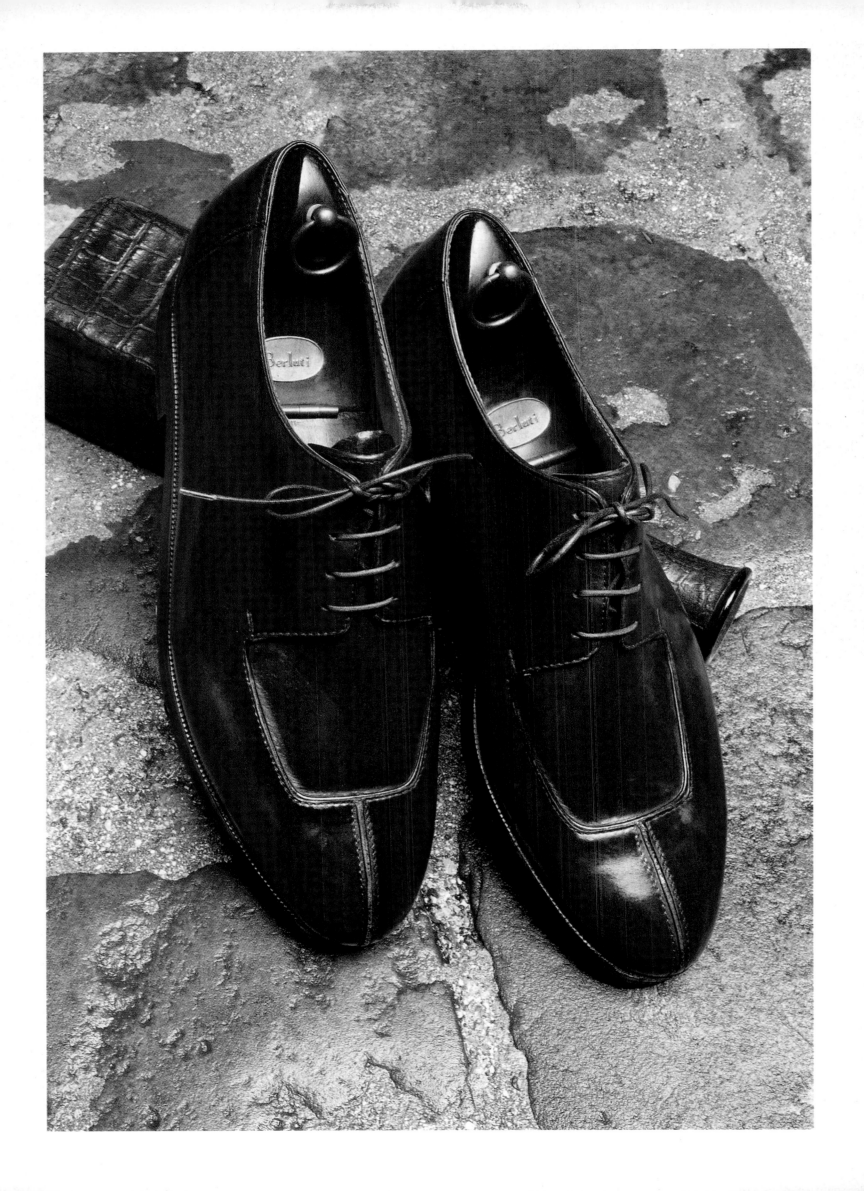

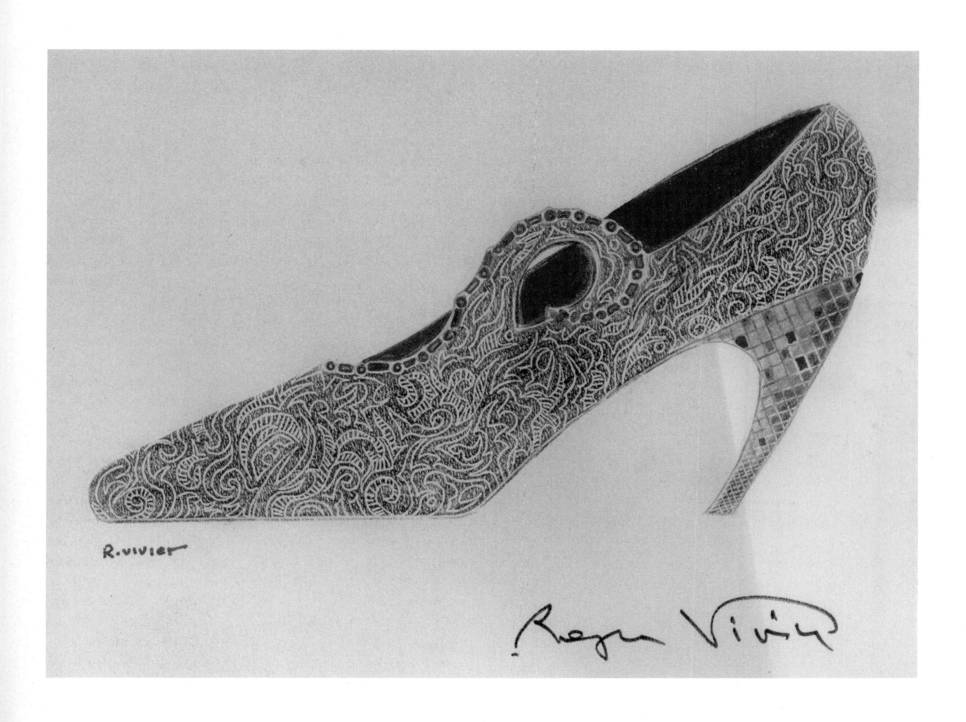

R.vivier

Roger Vivier

Roger Vivier
Couturier of the Shoe

Roger Vivier was born in Paris in 1907. At age thirteen he went to work in a shoe factory owned by family friends where he learned technical basics and the different stages of fabrication.

His artistic abilities naturally led Vivier to the Ecole des Beaux-Arts in Paris where he studied sculpture. Between 1926 and 1927, at age twenty, he decided to devote himself to shoe design. His meeting with theater decorator Paul Seltenhammeur was decisive; with Seltenhammeur, Vivier visited Venice and Berlin, turning his attention to a world closely linked to the artistic and literary avant-garde of his time. Mistinguett ordered Vivier shoes, as did Josephine Baker and Marianne Oswald, who sang Cocteau. Vivier navigated all the avant-garde trends with eclectic taste, immersing himself in the great artistic movements of the time: the decorative arts in France, the Bauhaus in Germany, the Wiener Werkstätten in Austria. His assimilation to this culture was expressed in the decoration of the successive apartments he lived in.

Hired in 1936 as an exclusive designer and maker of shoe patterns for Laborémus, the French division of a major German tannery located under the eaves of 16 place Vendôme, Roger Vivier was responsible for producing a highly Parisian shoe line that would win over buyers and facilitate the quantity sale of leather skins.

In 1937, Roger Vivier opened his first store on rue Royale where his styles, made by his own workshop, were sold to a large French and American clientele. He also designed shoes for the largest manufacturers in the world such as Delman who guaranteed the exclusivity of his designs in America. Vivier also attracted the attention of the fashion world, especially Elsa Schiaparelli.

The war necessitated the closing of his studio on the rue Royale when he joined the army. Discharged in 1940, he was invited by Delman to continue his work in the United States. In 1941, he left for New York on the transatlantic ship L'Exeter. On board he met Suzanne Rémy, the top milliner at Agnès, who was emigrating with her mother. When the United States entered the war, the use of leather was drastically restricted to be able to meet the priority demands of the army. Short on raw materials, Roger Vivier turned to a complementary activity and becoming the assistant to photographer Georges Hoyningen-Huene, who was working for Harper's Bazaar. There he came in contact with the fashion world and met Carmel Snow, Harper's Bazaar's editor at the time. He also formed a close friendship with Fernand Léger and associated with other European artists in exile such as Max Ernst, Calder and Chagall. At the same time, he was working for Bergdorf Goodman and making hats in the evening with Suzanne Rémy. The celebrated milliner from Agnès taught him the art of hat making. A hat store under the name of "Suzanne et Roger" opened in 1942 at the corner of Madison Avenue and 64th Street. Within a year, the store had become the most Parisian destination in New York. In 1947, he went back to Paris where he made the acquaintance of Michel Brodsky, his future collaborator, and Christian Dior. He created all the custom-made shoes for Dior's collections after 1953. That same year he made shoes for the Coronation of Queen Elizabeth II of England.

Two years later, Christian Dior and Roger Vivier had the ingenious idea of establishing a department for "prêt-à-porter" shoes. It was the first time a Parisian couturier associated his label with that of a shoemaker for the purpose of promoting a mass-market line. In 1954, a shoe with a slender heel of seven to eight centimeters deposed the draped shoe and reigned until the appearance and victory of the stiletto heel in 1956, also one of Vivier's inventions. Shoes were adorned with sumptuous 18th-century style embroidery by Rébé. Vivier's collaboration with Yves Saint-Laurent always showed the most innovative forms.

For example, the 1959 choc heel, so named because at first glance it was shocking, was nevertheless a brilliant success. In 1960, the Punchinello heel and the stem heel drew attention. The success of the square toe was confirmed in 1961 when the following women adopted it: Queen Elizabeth II, the Impress of Iran, the Duchess of Windsor, Jacqueline Kennedy, Olivia de Havilland, Marlene Dietrich, Elizabeth Taylor, and Sophia Loren.

In 1963, Roger Vivier opened his own boutique with Michel Brodsky at 24 rue François 1er. The comma-shaped heel was his personal signature on sumptuous shoes. In 1965, he created a shoe with a stacked heel for Yves Saint-Laurent; square, decorated with a buckle of gold metal, this design sold tens of thousands of pairs. The use of synthetic materials, such as transparent vinyl, also aroused great interest.

In 1970, the hippie style inspired Vivier to make thigh-high boots, which were appreciated by Brigitte Bardot and mini-skirt wearers. Vivier made shoes for many celebrities: the Empress of Japan, Princess Grace of Monaco, Claude Pompidou and Romy Schneider, among others. The list of royal highnesses, princesses and actresses is impressive. His international reputation as a virtuoso of shoemakers put him at the feet of clients from all four corners of the globe. One of them even ordered shoes for her toy poodle, Bonbon. Although somewhat surprised by this most unexpected order, Vivier accepted. On the day of the fitting, the shoemaker brought out two models that were fit to the animal's paws; the woman's little "toutou" began to run around the store while his mistress's eyes filled with wonder at the models. However, her look then changed to consternation and she turned to her shoemaker and said, "But my dog has four paws." Roger Vivier hastily amended this oversight to the great pleasure of his faithful client.

Vivier gave his shoes the volume of a sculpture and the contours of a drawing. They can sport daring heels, like the stem heel, or malicious heels, like the Cancan, Guignol, and Punchinella; sometimes they rest on the ground like a scintillating paste sphere, a favorite style of Marlene Dietrich. The variety of materials used created surprise: shoes were adorned with pheasant feathers of gold edged in black, guinea fowl feathers, kingfisher feathers and were even wrapped in panther.

Some of his shoes were covered in pearls, brightly coloured paste, sequins, and sumptuous embroidery from the dazzling collaboration between Roger Vivier and the embroiderer François Lesage. His collaboration with Paris couture ended in 1972, but foreign contracts gave him the opportunity to create relentlessly until the end of his life. His son, Gérard Benoît-Vivier assisted him. The elder Vivier died on October 1, 1998. He was at home in his townhouse in Toulouse, still at his worktable. The most important collections of his shoes (Vivier preferred the French word soulier over chaussure to signify the general category of all shoes) affirming his talent, virtuosity, and tireless work are preserved in the following museums: Fashion and Textile Museum (Paris), Galliera Museum (Paris), the International Shoe Museum (Romans), Victoria and Albert Museum (London) and the Metropolitan Museum of Art (New York). Vivier's timeless shoes were and continue to be the subject of many international exhibitions that pay tribute to the shoe's great couturier.

151. Shock heel by Roger Vivier. 1955.

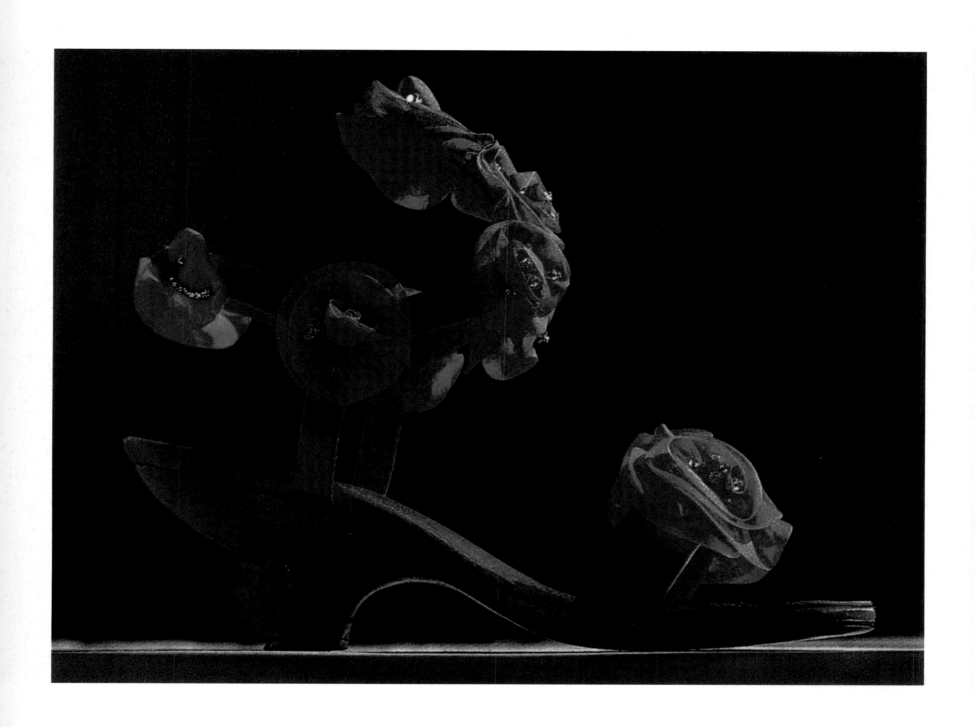

152. Evening sandal. Organza and strass. Created by Roger Vivier. Paris, 1985.

International Shoe Museum, Romans. Photo by Joël Garnier.

153. Poulaine style shoe. Velvet, pendants and beads. "Clown" heel.

Created by Roger Vivier. Paris, 1987. International Shoe Museum, Romans.

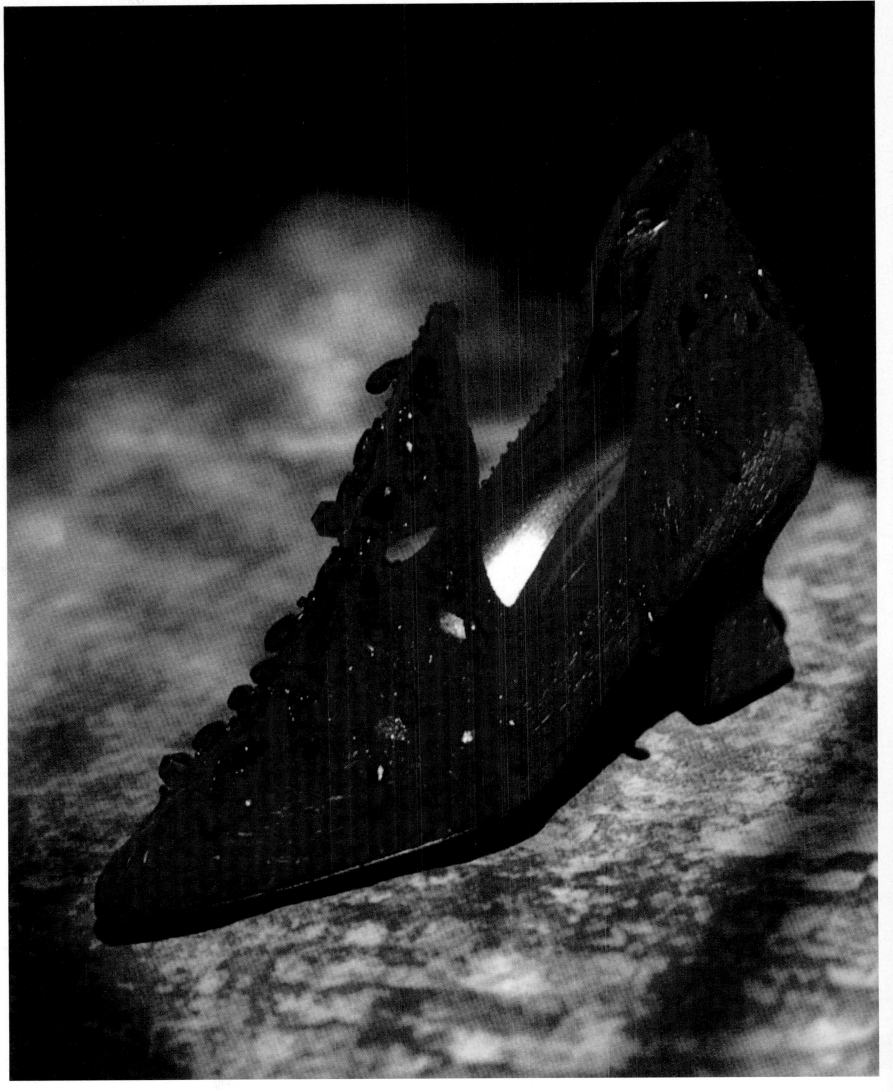

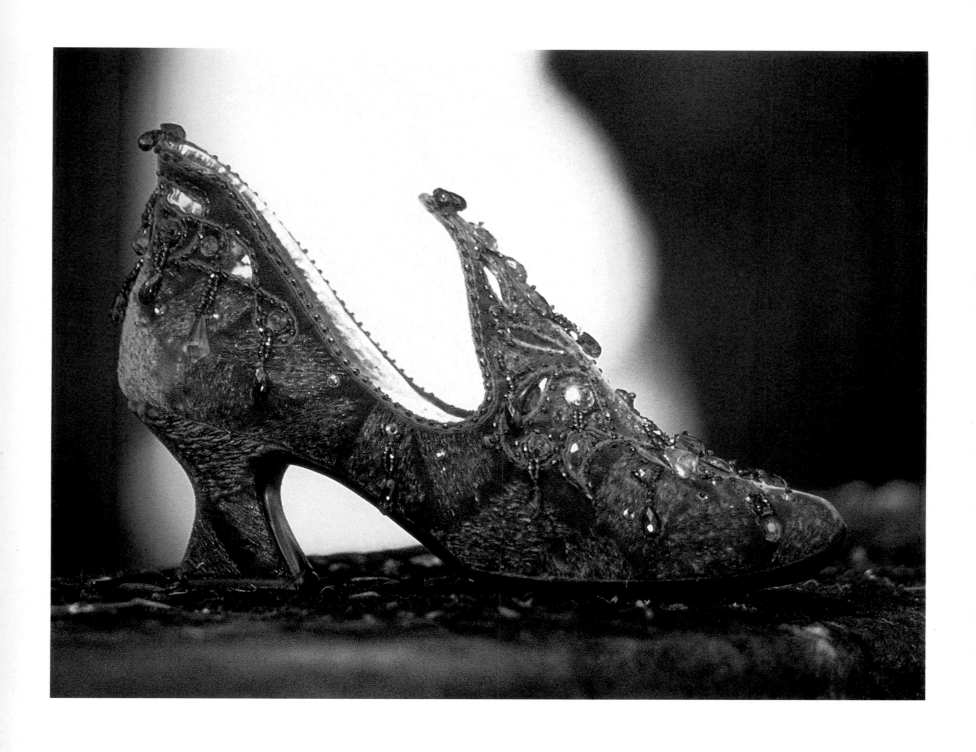

154. Poulaine style shoe. Velvets, pendants and beads. "Clown" heel.

Created by Roger Vivier. Paris, 1987. International Shoe Museum, Romans.

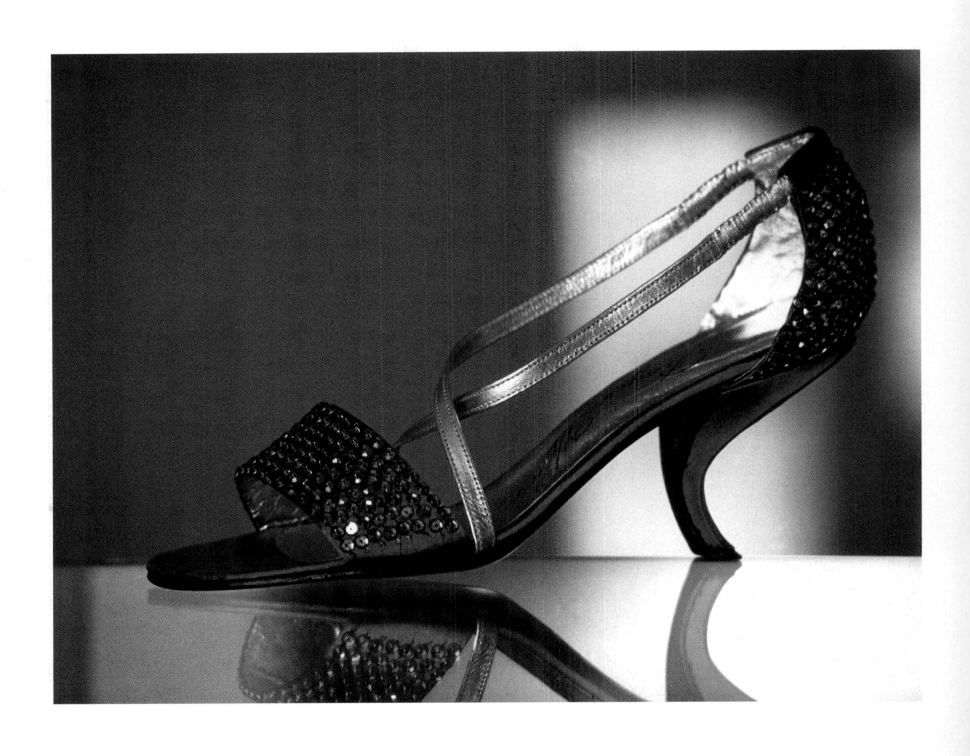

155. Evening sandal. Blue satin, sequin embroidery. "Comma" heel.

Created by Roger Vivier. Paris, 1963. International Shoe Museum, Romans.

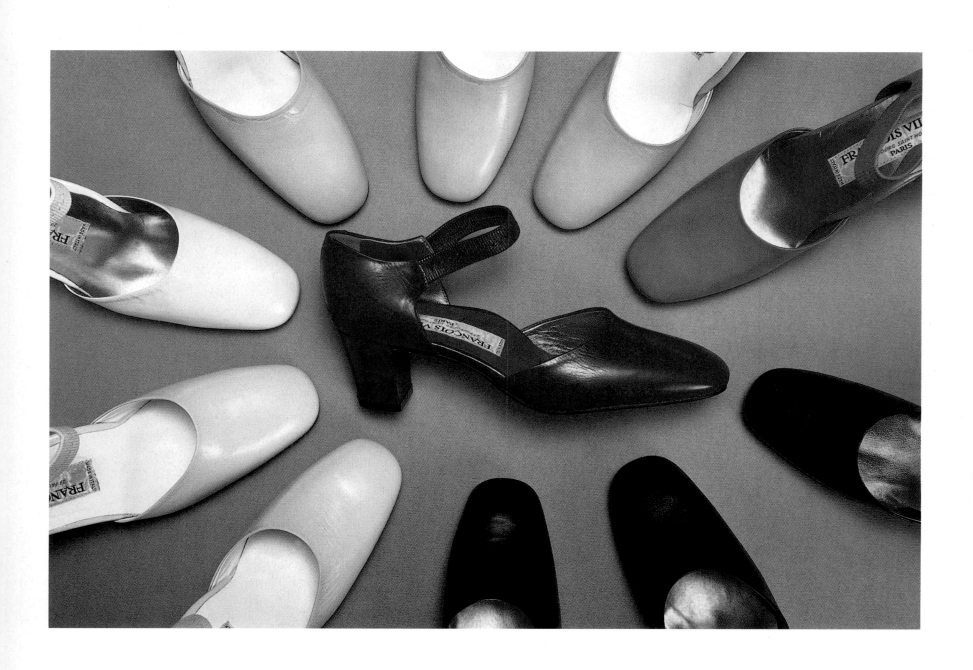

156. Kidskin shoes shown in eleven shades, straight heel. Around 1980.

Creations of François Villon. International Shoe Museum, Romans.

François Villon (1911-1997)

His real name was Benveniste. François Villon was a pseudonym the shoemaker borrowed because he admired the great French poet of the Middle Ages.

After a close collaboration with the firm Perugia, of which he was the chief executive, François Villon created his own design house in 1960. He set up shop at 27 rue du Faubourg Saint-Honoré and worked on the custom-made shoe concept he had already experimented with at Perugia, but adapting it to a larger scale of production. The François Villon label was highly successful around 1965, attracting a refined and famous clientele.

The styles of François Villon did not always keep up with the vagaries of fashion and were sometimes out of step with the times. He made various versions of boots, such as leather thigh-high boots (a red leather version was worn by Sheila for her televised series in 1968), cowboy boots for city dwellers, and riding boots. He also introduced the cut boot in 1970, which coordinated with the dresses of Louis Féraud.

Beginning in 1969, his ballerinas were shown in the same couturier's fashion shows. He created shoes for sport, for town, and for evening with equal enthusiasm. His research led him to create a spiral heel constructed with great complexity.

François Villon quickly opened a number of boutiques abroad in Milan, New York, Singapore, and Hong Kong.

Among the couture firms that chose his shoes for their fashion shoes were Hermès, Chanel, Ted Lapidus, Jean Patou, Nina Ricci, Jean-Louis Scherrer, Louis Féraud, and Lanvin.

François Villon pursued his career tirelessly until his death in 1997.

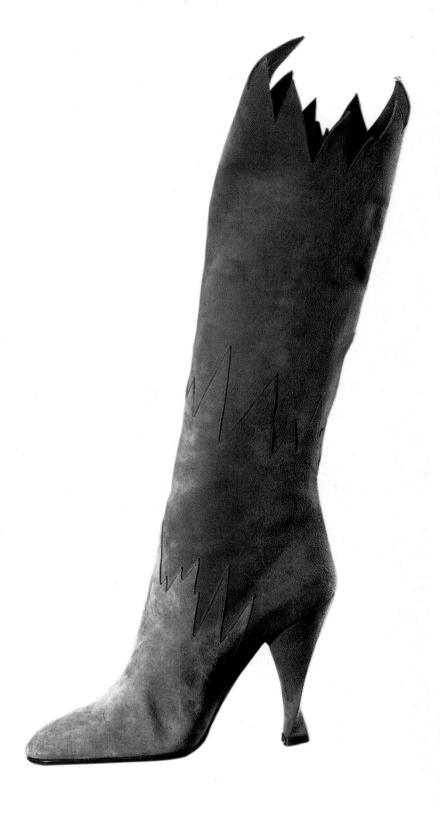

157. Suede boot with tendril heel. Creation of François Villon. Paris, 1980-1981.

International Shoe Museum, Romans.

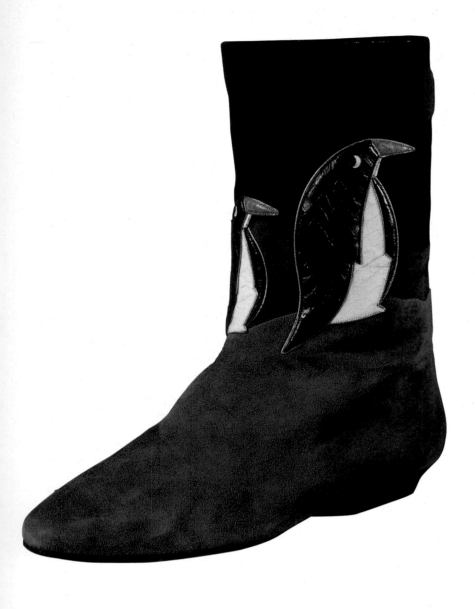

Andrea Pfister
Happy Feet

Born in 1942 in Pesaro, Italy, in the region of the Marches, Andrea Pfister was age eighteen when he entered the University of Florence to study art history. A graduate at age twenty from the Ars Sutoria of Milan, he won first prize in the 1963 international competition for best shoe designer held in Amsterdam, thus beginning a surefooted career marked by the following key dates:

1964: Pfister settles in Paris where he designs shoe collections for the couture firms Jean Patou and Lanvin.

1965: Pfister launches his first collection under his own name.

1967: Pfister meets Jean-Pierre Dupré, who becomes his partner. Together they open the first Andrea Pfister boutique on the rue Cambon in Paris.

1974: Pfister buys his own factory, which produces two hundred pairs of shoes a day and introduces a new development with the creation of bags, belts, and scarves.

1987: Pfister inaugurates a second boutique with a highly symbolic address: via San Andrea in Milan.

1988: Once again Pfister is consecrated best shoe designer, winning the Grand Fashion Medal of Honor from the Fashion Footwear Association of New York and the Fashion Media Association.

1991: Pfister begins collaboration with Anaconda tanneries (specialists in reptile skins) and Stefania (specialists in kid leather and suede) to create a chromatic line of his design. The styles he envisions combine reptile and kid leather with suede in perfect harmony.

1993: The International Shoe Museum, Romans, gives him a retrospective. The exhibit traveled to the Bata Shoe Museum in Toronto in 1996 and the FIDM in Los Angeles and San Francisco in 1998.

Always interested in the alliance of aesthetics and comfort and known for his research on shoe shapes and heels, Pfister improvises on diverse themes with great panache: fruits, flowers, animals, the starry night, the ocean, music, the circus, Las Vegas, et cetera.

Classic and baroque, opulent and unusual, daring and visionary, decorated with multi-coloured glass pearls, paste, sequins and even embroidery, Pfister's shoes seduce his clients. Among his clientele one can find such stars as Ursula Andress, Candice Bergen, Jacqueline Bisset, Claudia Cardinale, Cher, Catherine Deneuve, Bo Derek, Linda Evans, Madonna, Lisa Minelli, Diana Ross, Barbara Streisand, Elizabeth Taylor, and Sylvie Vartan.

As Jean-Claude Carrière has so aptly written: "Feet in Andrea's shoes have style. To walk in Pfister, is to wear always-smiling shoes; it's to invent a look everyday. It's to walk lightheartedly even under gray skies. It's near bliss."

158. "The North Pole" farandole of penguins in snake skin on suede ankle boot. Andrea Pfister. Winter 1984-1985. International Shoe Museum, Romans.

159. "Tomato" mule by Andrea Pfister. Spring-Summer 2002. International Shoe Museum, Romans.

160. "Carrot" sandal by Andrea Pfister. Spring-Summer 2002. International Shoe Museum, Romans.

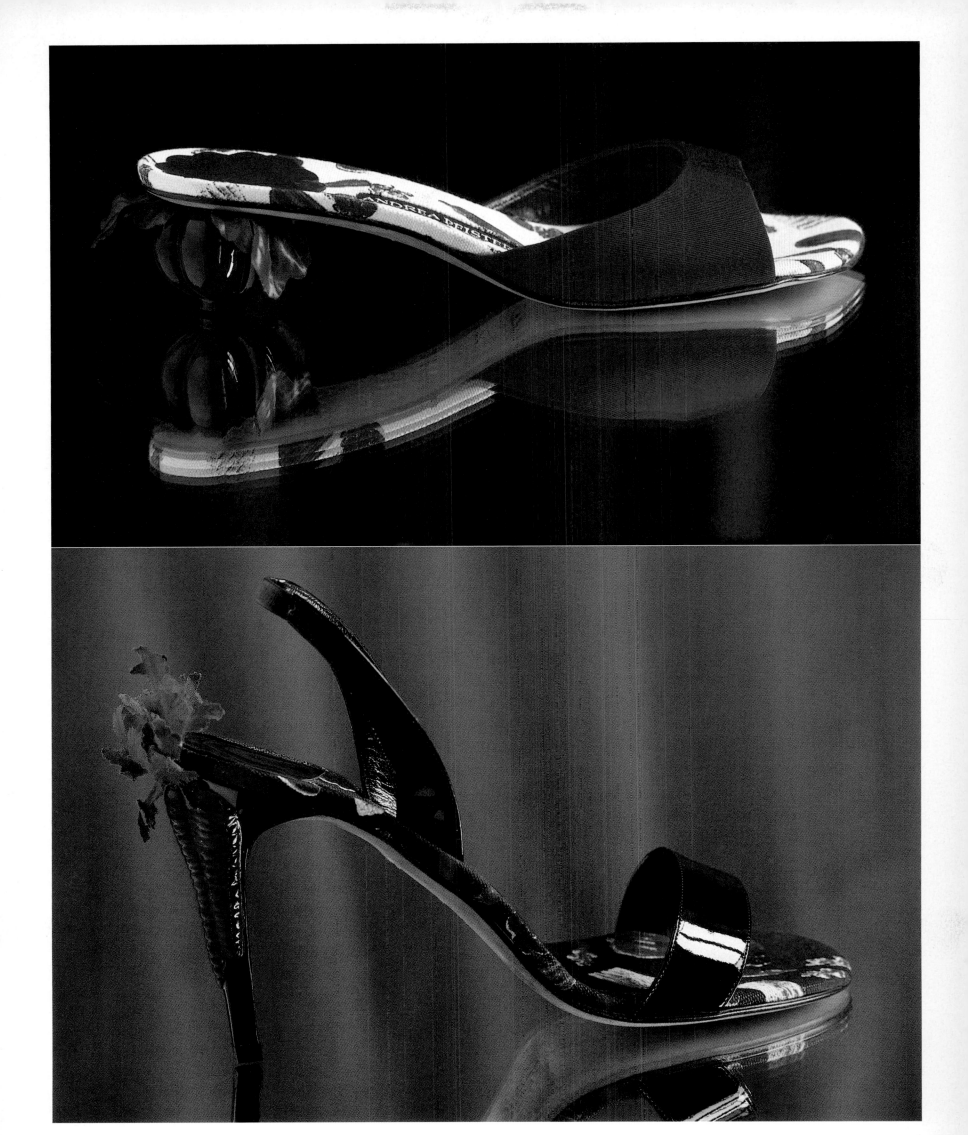

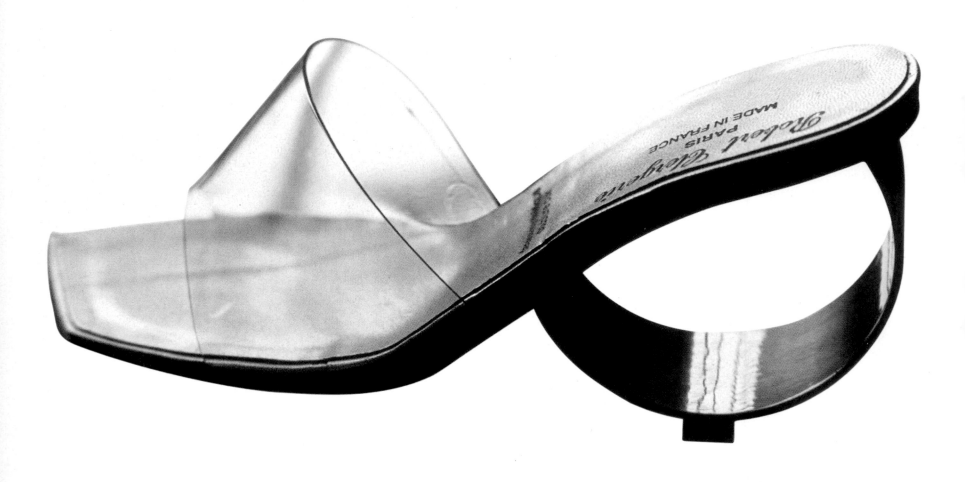

The rise of the Shoe Industry
Romans is the city of fine shoes

The two great names of the 20th century:
Joseph Fenestrier
Robert Clergerie

In the Middle Ages, the tanners of Romans were highly prosperous. Around 1850, François Barthélemy Guillaume got the idea of using the city's tanneries that were already in place to create the first factory for shoes mounted on wood.

Beginning in the 19th-century, Romans shoes acquired a certain fame. The train station, open since 1864, permitted long-distance shipping. At the same time, industries related to shoes were being established and expanded, especially factories for shoe forms. The great industrial revolution, beginning in 1890, gathered momentum with the use of electrical-powered engines and propelled breathtaking expansion of mechanization, completely changing the face of the industry.

But Romans had a significant reservoir of highly qualified labourers who knew how to perform each stage of production by hand. These workers did not welcome the arrival of technical modernization. They feared this change would eliminate work for a certain number of workers in the profession.

Early in the century, large shoemaking centers like Limoges and Fougères adopted machines that increased production more cheaply and with fewer workers. Romans suffered from this extra-muros factor, but continued to stand for quality production.

After putting a lot of effort into development, around 1900 all the factories of Romans (thirty-five factories and three thousand workers) were equipped with finishing machines and produced one hundred thousand pairs of shoes a month. Out of the three thousand workers, one-third worked in the factory, while the others performed their jobs at home. During this period there were three kinds of workers:

– Preparation men and women included the workers who cut the uppers and soles, those who stitched the uppers, buttonhole makers and eyelet and button fitters;
– The workers involved in making the shoe itself were divided into assemblers and finishers;
– The workers who trimmed the shoes, prepared shoes for boxes and were responsible for steaming and shipping.

The average salary for workers in these categories came to about three francs per day for men and two francs for women. However, highly skilled seamers working on pieces in the fabrication process earned twenty francs a week; other less skilled workers, even though more hardworking, could not earn more than ten francs a week.

Those working at home were also involved with their household. Their workday was therefore not as productive as a factory worker's.

The First World War disrupted the city's economy and production had to be increased to met the needs of the military. Men called to the front were replaced by female laborers who demonstrated their adaptation to manual dexterity. Many a small business came into being at the impulse of a skilled and adventurous labourer, sometimes assisted by a traveling sales representative, with one managing the workshop and the other managing sales.

In 1920, many firms were like families and were still structured like traditional craft organizations rather than industrial companies. But the workers of Romans defended and always produced quality articles. Firms such as Sirius, Bady, Will's, and Barnasson had considerable reputations and knew how to create a true brand image for their shoes. But the most typical Romans-style factory was the work of a pork butcher called to a higher destiny and fame.

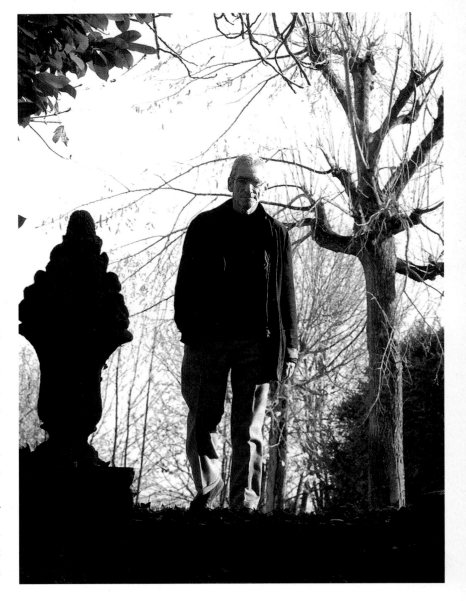

In 1895, Joseph Fenestrier, age twenty-one, bought a small rubber boot factory near the train station. A novice to the industry, he partnered with M. Pervillat. The business had a very craft-based structure, and despite an unfavorable business climate, it produced eighty pairs of shoes a day. From 1890-1901, the industrial sector slowed down and during this period many factories closed their doors. But from 1901, lack of space on the premises justified the construction of a new factory on the boulevard Gambetta, with immense possibility of future expansion. Joseph Fenestrier launched the then innovative idea of specialization and made expensive men's shoes, an idea that would remain the foundation of his future concepts. To this end, he introduced a new assembly technique: Goodyear Stitch construction. To do this, he set up the most modern machine available, which he leased from the United Shoes Machinery Company, an American trust. Well aware that abundant skilled labour was located in situ, Joseph Fenestrier proceeded to risk mechanizing. In 1904, he launched the first advertising campaign in the history of the shoe throughout France under the following brand names:

161. Mules by Robert Clergerie. Spring-Summer 1998.

International Shoe Museum, Romans.

162. Photograph of Robert Clergerie.

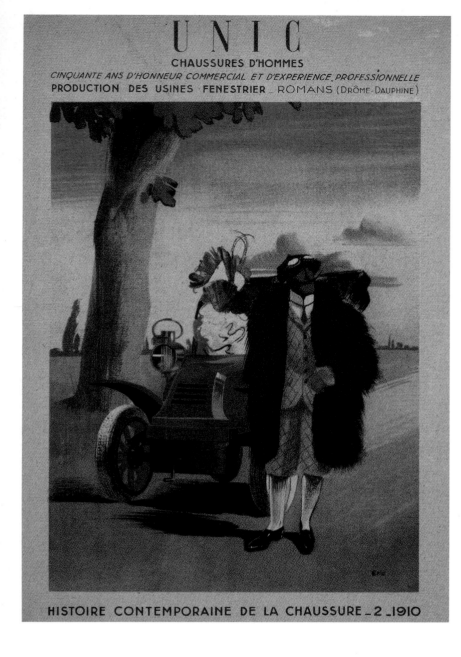

UNIC
CHAUSSURES D'HOMMES
CINQUANTE ANS D'HONNEUR COMMERCIAL ET D'EXPERIENCE PROFESSIONNELLE
PRODUCTION DES USINES FENESTRIER _ ROMANS (DRÔME-DAUPHINE)

HISTOIRE CONTEMPORAINE DE LA CHAUSSURE _ 2 _1910

163. Advertisement UNIC. 1910. International Shoe Museum, Romans.

– Excelsior chaussures moderne
– Good Taste American Fashion
– Chaussures supérieures Fenestrier

The Unic brand established in 1907 crowned his career. Posters six meters square displaying six legs dressed in Unic carried this prestigious brand to the height of its glory. Then, in 1910, Unic was awarded a true victory with the grand prize from the World Fair in Brussels. Joseph Fenestrier nevertheless expressed the following motto: "In ten years, ten times better, ten times bigger."

Shortly after the Brussels World Fair, production exceeded five hundred pairs a day. New extensions were made to the factory. Fenestrier constantly fanned the flames of Unic's loyal following among an elegant clientele with intelligent advertising, the creation in Paris of an independent sales division, and by the inauguration in 1912 of a sales system based on imposed prices. Throughout this period, the firm shone most brightly in all the international sales exhibitions. Between 1910 and 1914, Unic won the highest awards at the World Fairs. The prizes came one after another: 1911 (Turin), 1912 (London), 1913 (Ghent), and 1914 (Lyon). Unic became a member of the exhibition's jury (outside of the competition) in the 1915 San Francisco World Fair. The brand expanded throughout continental Europe, Russia, Egypt and the Middle East.

Just like French cities, major cities in Germany, Belgium, Italy, and Switzerland had an elite Unic retail store. After the premature death of its founder in 1916, at age forty-two, his widow took over managing the firm. In 1917, a fire destroyed the factory. A second factory established in Saint-Marcellin the year before enabled production to continue while the factory in Romans was rebuilt.

In 1922, the couple's son, Joseph Emile-Jean Fenestrier, took over. In 1926, eight hundred workers working in two factories produced one thousand two hundred pairs of shoes per day.

Exports grew in the countries still free of protectionism: Australia, the Netherlands, India, and the Far East. Alongside increased sales, the company developed internal social programs: a mutual aid society, allocations to families with more than two children, playgrounds and fields for sports. The factory had its own autonomous division of fully equipped fire engines, which sometimes reinforced the town's numbers. The firm also had its own maintenance division, which included shops for spare parts and wood working, among others.

An office of design and testing came up with the new styles. The first collection of women's sports shoes came out in 1930. Joseph Fenestrier briefly considered making Louis XV shoes, but abandoned the idea for technical reasons.

From 1935, Sarkis Der Balian, talented Parisian custom shoemaker established at 221, rue Saint-Honoré, lent his experienced hand to the design of certain styles and often traveled to Romans. Unic called on the best artists and artisans for advertising, including Cappiello, Cassandre, Laure Albin-Guillot, and Van Moppès. The company's motto summed up the guarantee it gave to its clientele: Unic uniquement (exclusively unique). In 1938, a new-patented design called the "new crêpel" appeared for men and women. Its immense success lasted thirty years.

During the Second World War, designers and technicians used their ingenuity to make "portables," shoes out of wood, felt and raffia. In 1945, Joseph-Emile-Jean Fenestrier was appointed president of the Fédération Nationale de l'Industrie de la Chaussure de France, a French shoe industry group. He died in 1961. The company remained in existence and merged with Maison Sirius in 1967.

In 1969, the André group bought Unic, which became Société Romanaise de la Chaussure. Robert Clergerie took over the company in 1977, giving it new life.

Robert Clergerie graduated from the École Supérieure de Commerce of Paris and came to shoes from the government sector. He took over the management of Xavier Danaud (a Charles Jourdan subsidiary) in 1971 and his work there with Roland

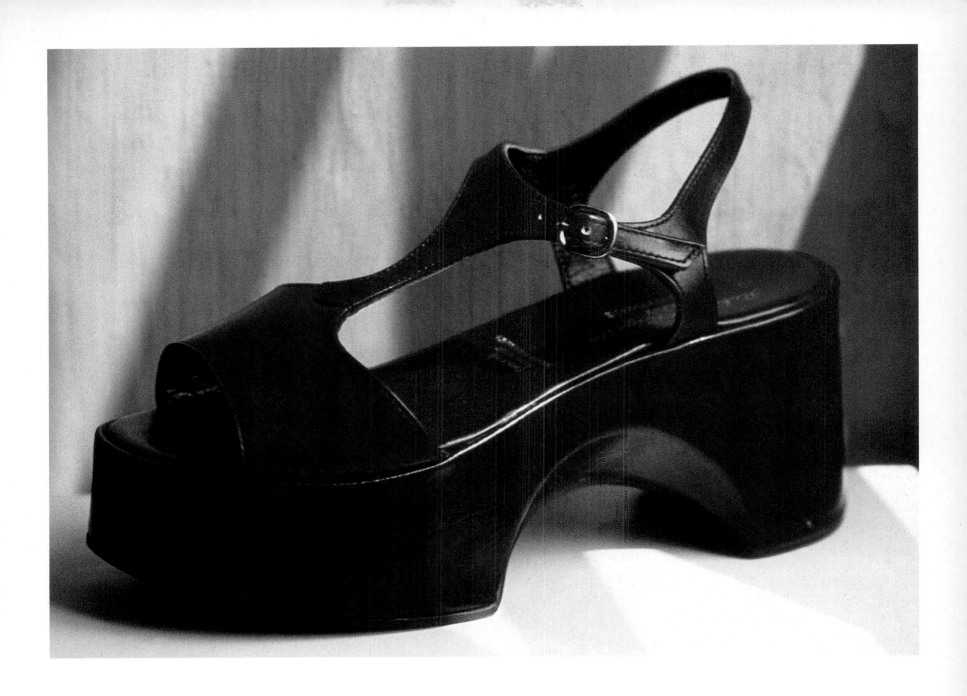

Jourdan gave him solid experience. While continuing to make men's shoes in the tradition of the Goodyear Stitch construction and distributing under the name of Joseph Fenestrier, Clergerie launched his own line of ankle boots and boots. At the same time, he made even more sophisticated styles by studying volume and heels. His shoes took on the look of sculpture, true accessories to feminine elegance. But in this approach, Clergerie always remembered the words of André Perugia, who told him one day: "Young man, never forget that although someone may wear an article of clothing, a shoe wears you: therein lies the whole problem."

Clever public relations with a network of press attachés contribute to the international reputation of Clergerie's designer label. He collaborates with couturiers and creates styles for Thierry Mugler, Anne-Marie Beretta, Chantal Thomas, and Yohji Yamamoto. The leader's talent has three times earned him the Award for best designer from F.F.A.N.Y. in the United States. Many boutiques under the sign of Robert Clergerie were opened in France and around the world between 1981 and 2002. He established his first boutique in 1981 in Paris at 5 rue du Cherche Midi, followed in 1982 by a shop at la place des Victoires (a symbolic location for a successful product). Additional boutiques opened in Tokyo, New York, Madrid, London, Brussels, Los Angeles, and most recently Chicago in 2001.

164. Sandal by Robert Clergerie. Spring-Summer 1998.

International Shoe Museum, Romans.

165. Pump in lilac satin with metal heel by Robert Clergerie.

Spring-Summer 1995. International Shoe Museum, Romans.

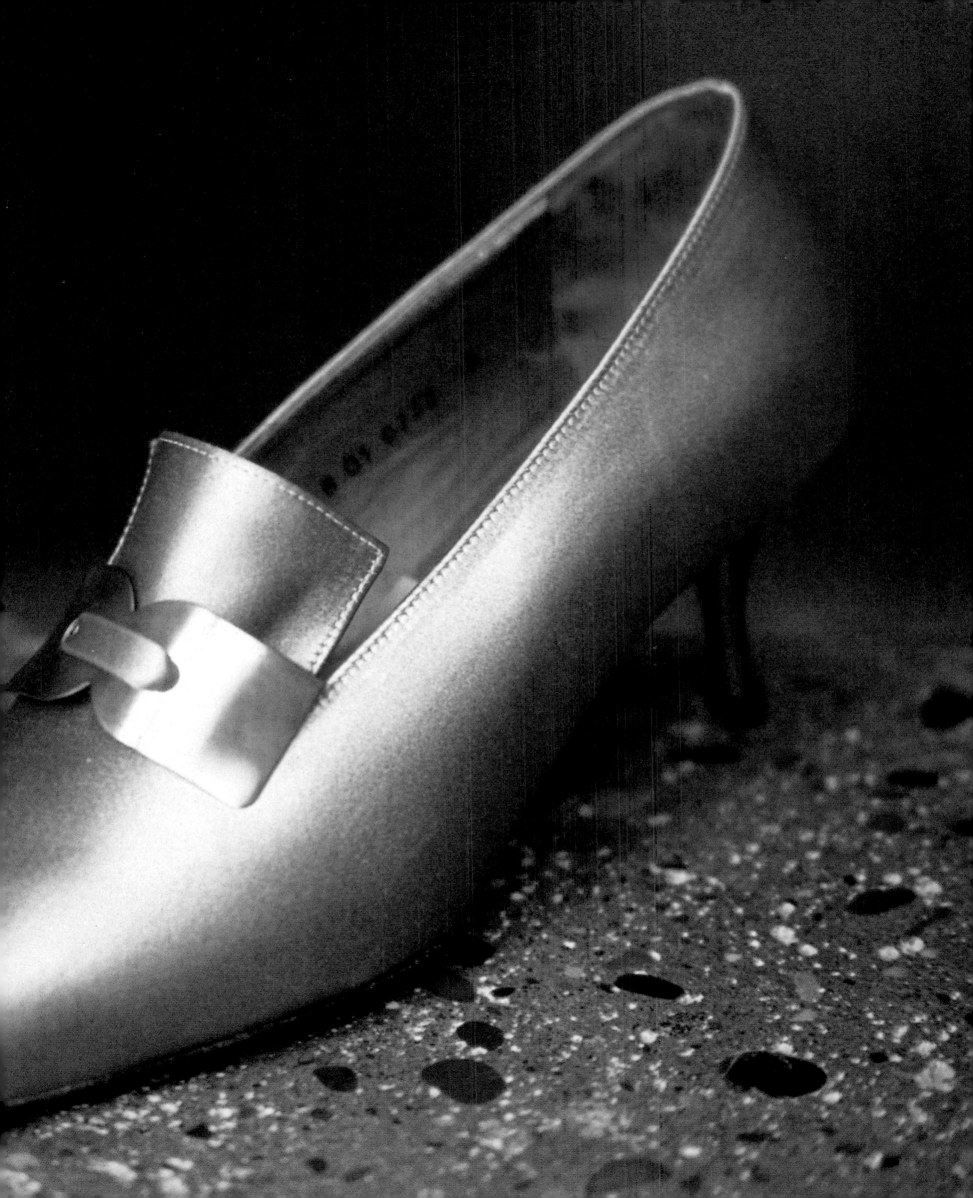

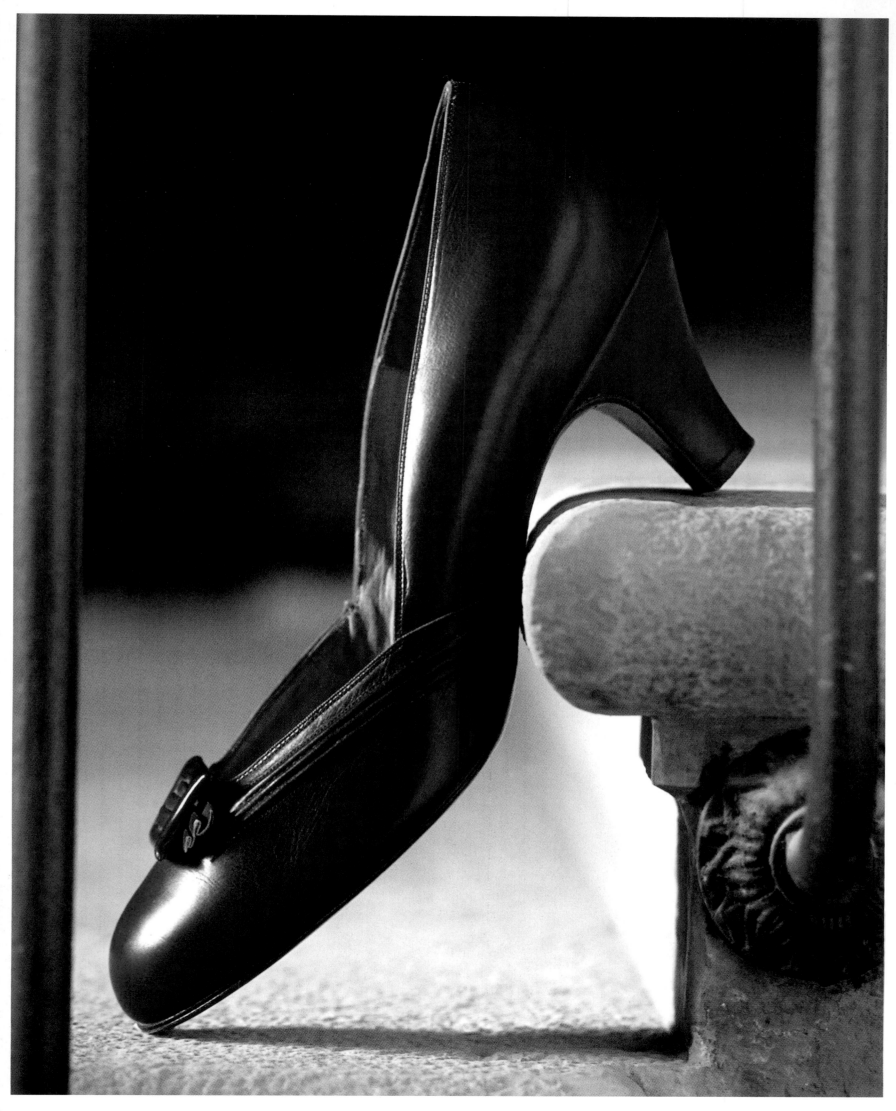

Charles Jourdan
From a workshop on Côte Macel (Butchers' Hill) in Romans to the Empire State Building in New York

Charles Jourdan undoubtedly ranks among the most accomplished individuals in the world of shoes. His stellar rise began in 1917 at the age of thirty-four. Cutting-room foreman at Etablissements Grenier, he lacked the necessary capital to set up his own business. His workday done, Jourdan would withdraw into his tiny workshop on côte Macel where he made women's shoes. His wife Augusta and two colleagues lent him a hand until late into the night. The results of these nocturnal creations were already worthy of the Jourdan quality label.

When the war ended in 1919, Jourdan's customers became numerous enough to enable him to leave his employer and go into business for himself in a larger studio with 10 workers. His diligence as a craftsman paid off, resulting in a large volume of orders. In 1921, he relocated his workshop to the boulevard Voltaire and hired thirty workers.

By 1928, the business had outgrown the small factory and new buildings were constructed. During the 1930s, Jourdan expanded his product's distribution throughout France by deploying "official sales reps." He also launched his new label Séducta, which was promoted by a national advertising campaign that appeared in *L'Illustration* magazine.

The name Séducta sprang from Jourdan's imagination and derives from the French word for seduction. The emblem is a type of doe, a hybrid animal with the coat of a deer and the antlers of a stag. This leaping animal, reproduced under the soles and on the boxes of the shoes, symbolizes the beauty of the elegantly shod foot, with the accent on the doe's light-footed nature.

The metaphor is found in the Bible in the Second Book of Samuel where David addresses the Lord in a Psalm of Thanksgiving: "God is my strength and power, and He makes my way perfect. He makes my feet like the feet of deer, and sets me on my high places." This image of the female foot is also found in the 7th-century Buddhist legend of Padmavati. The daughter of a Brahmin and a doe, she was born with doe hoofs hidden inside silk wrappings. How interesting to note that from Antiquity to the 1st-century of our era, beauty and lightness of foot were compared to that of a doe. In our case, the biblical and Buddhist connection evokes Jourdan's refinement in the art of dressing the foot in charming heeled pumps, emblematic accessories of feminine seduction.

The stock market crash in New York cast a shadow over the 1930s. Parisian haut couture was hit hard by the world economic crisis and Jourdan was affected as well. Nevertheless, he responded by creating two sub-brands, Feminaflor and Qualité garantie. Three hundred workers produced four hundred pairs of shoes.

When World War II broke out, Jourdan, like other manufacturers, had to make use of alternative materials such as felt, raffia, rubber, wood, and cardboard due to the leather shortage. After 1945, Jourdan, assisted by his three sons René, Charles, and Roland, expanded the firm, which thenceforth had one thousand two hundred workers. Nine hundred pairs of shoes were leaving the factory daily in 1948.

In 1950, Roland set out to capture the American market and opened a sales office in the Empire State Building in New York. In 1957, the first Charles Jourdan boutique opened in Paris on the boulevard de la Madeleine. An instant hit, sales clerks had to give out numbered admission tickets to customers in the long waiting line. This extraordinary success was the starting point for the creation of an international chain of Charles Jourdan boutiques.

Recognition was at a zenith when Charles Jourdan signed a licensing agreement with Christian Dior. During the 1960s the brand went international as boutiques were

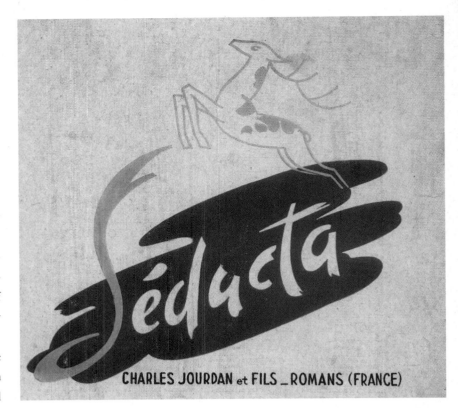

opened in London, Munich, New York, Los Angeles, Miami, and Tokyo. Charles Jourdan directed a series of advertising campaigns with photographs by Guy Bourdin that changed the art of advertising. No longer was the shoe the main subject, but portrayed in a strange, even surrealist situation.

In 1971, Roland Jourdan was appointed Chairman of the group, while his brothers sold their shares. Karl Lagerfeld entrusted Roland with the production of his shoes in 1980. That same year, the Séducta label was revived. When Roland Jourdan stepped down in 1981, the Swiss group Frantz Wasmer assumed the honor. The 1990s saw the launch of the Charles Jourdan Bis line for men and women and collaboration with the designers Michel Perry and Claude Montana.

With Emile Mercier at the helm and Hervé Racine as the current CEO, Charles Jourdan's star continues to shine in Paris and throughout the world. Its global prestige is based on the following: a production system invested with exceptional know-how and engineered to respond effectively to the needs of the marketplace, marketing communications in sync with trends set by the stylists, a network of seventy boutiques under the Charles Jourdan trade name, and over a thousand loyal retailers. But above all, the firm continues to offer its customers products continually renewed in the spirit of its founder, Charles Jourdan.

166. Seducta pump. 1954. International Shoe Museum, Romans.

167. Seducta logo, taken from a 1949 advertisement.

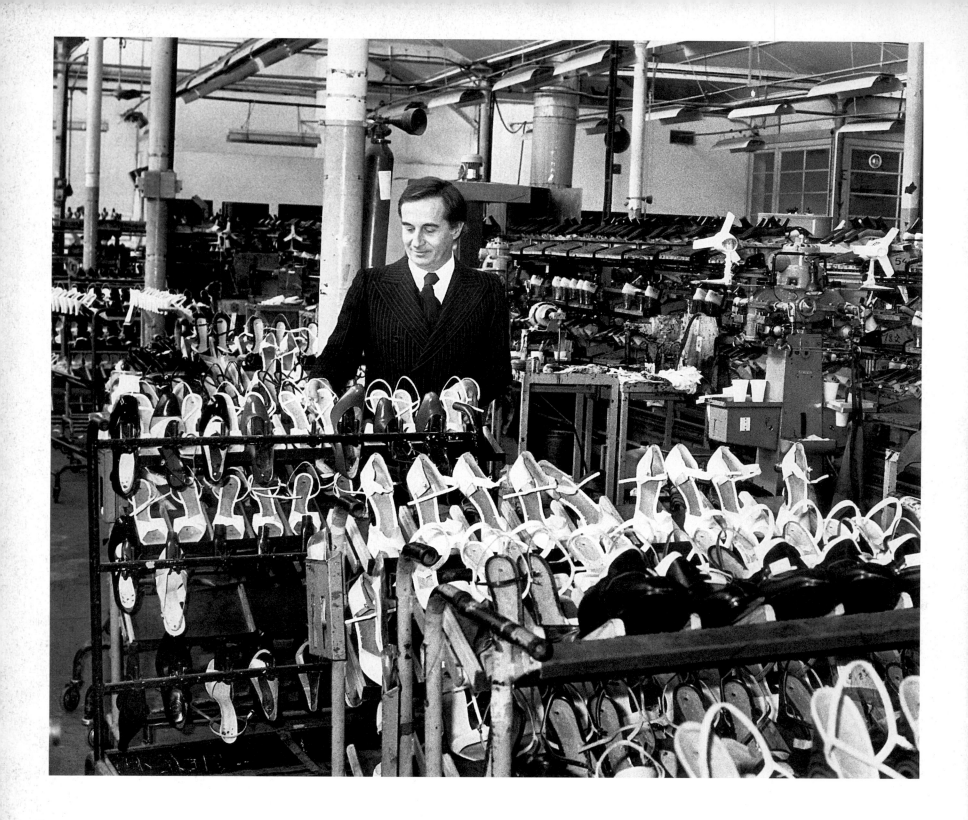

168. Charles Joudan in his factory.

169. Evening shoes created by Patrick Cox in honor of the Golden Jubilee of Queen

of England Elizabeth II in 2002. Creation limited to fifty copies.

Gift of Patrick Cox, International Shoe Museum, Romans.

Following pages:

170. Hand woven boot, Winter 1994. Hand woven shoe, Winter 1998.

Hand woven sandal. Stéphane Kélian. International Shoe Museum, Romans.

171. Sandal by Stéphane Kélian. Summer 2001. International Shoe Museum, Romans.

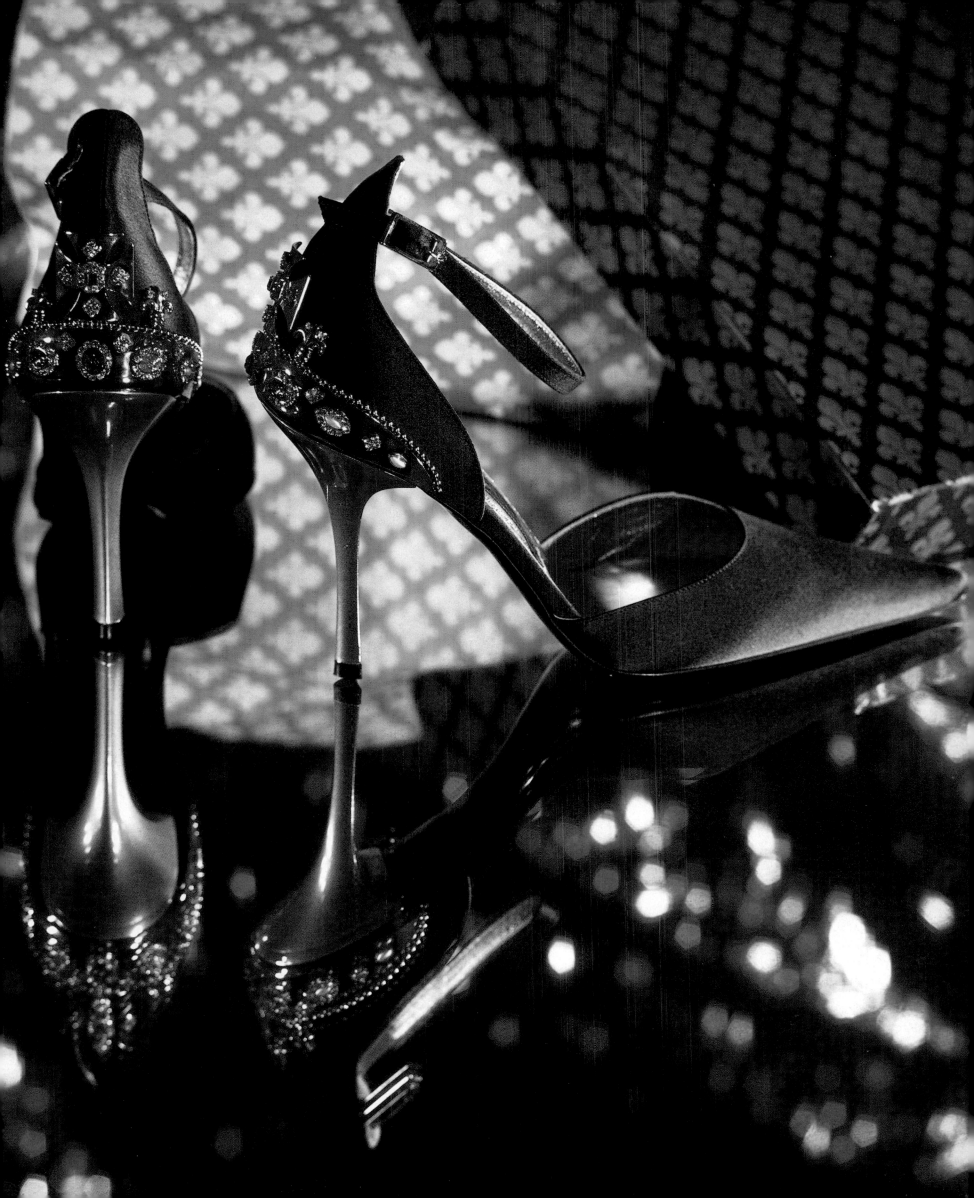

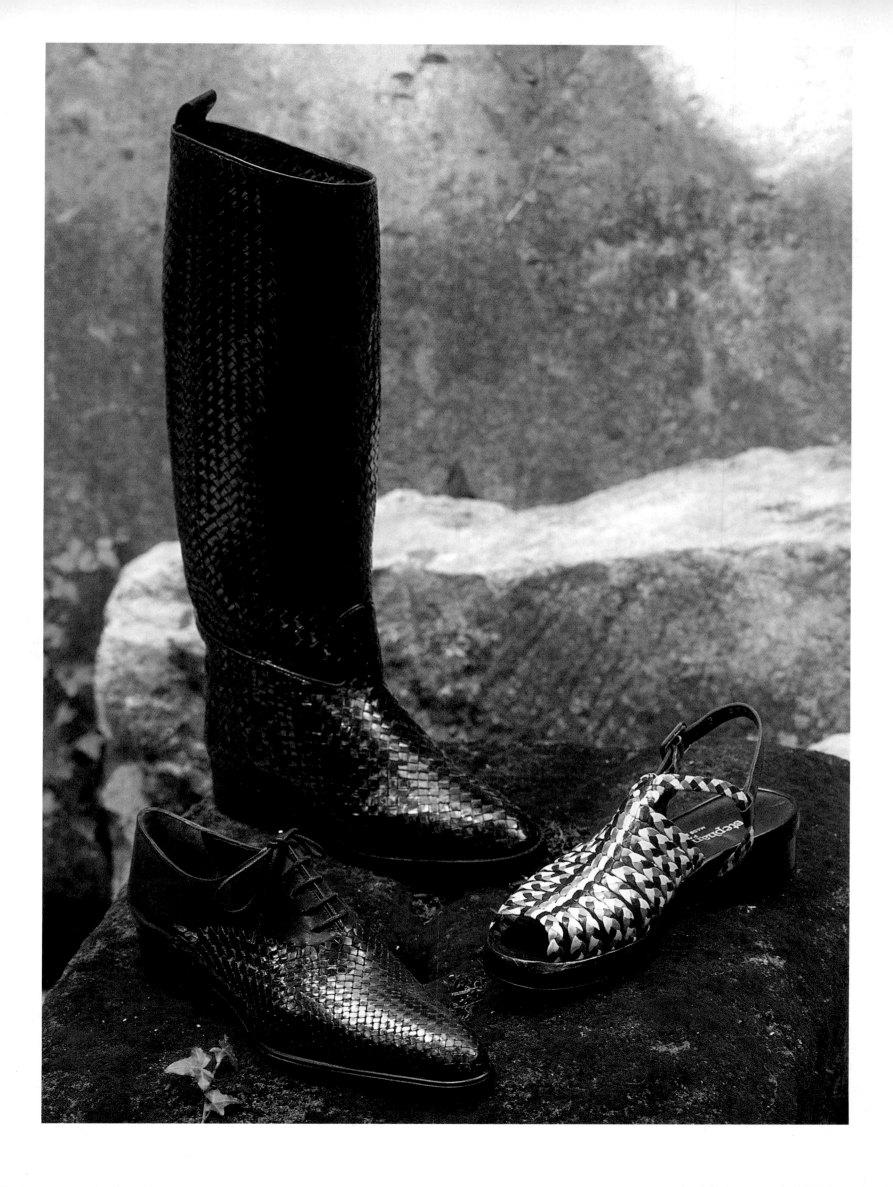

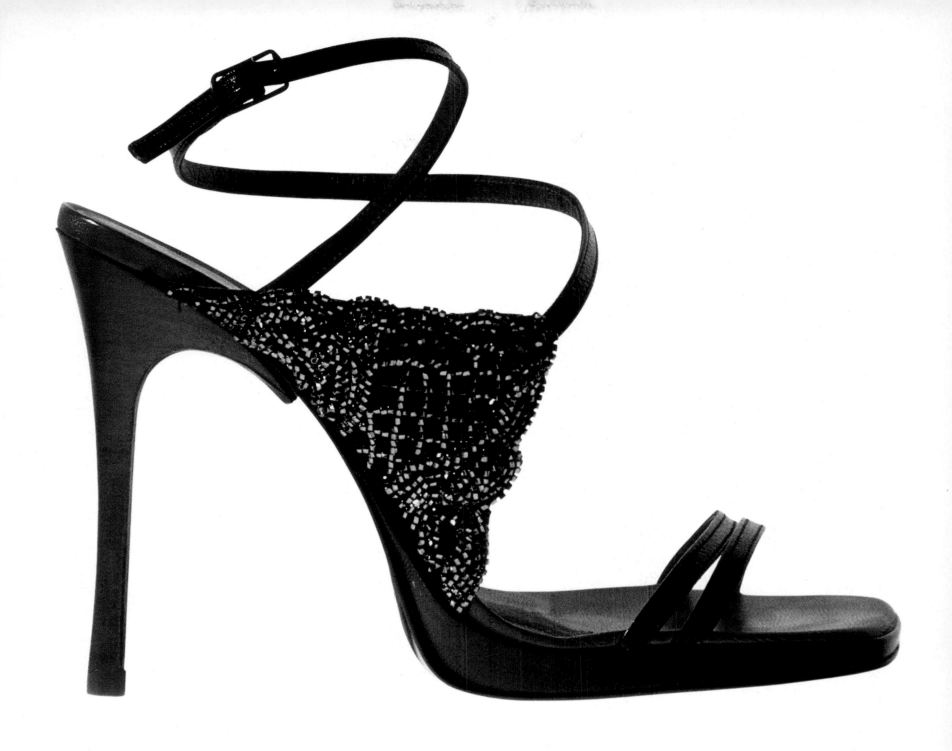

Stéphane Kélian
Specialist in Elegant Hand Braiding

In 1920, there were one hundred and twenty factories in Romans. Many companies that flourished between the wars gradually disappeared over the years. Others sprang up, such as the firm Kélian, founded in 1960 by Georges and Gérard Kéloglanian, men's footwear specialists. Stéphane, the brother of the two founders, launched in 1978 the first women's collection under the label Stéphane Kélian. Talented specialists in elegantly braided styles, their superb quality shoes quickly acquired an international reputation. Listed on the stock exchange since 1985, the company has two factories (Romans and Bourg-de-Péage) and employs four hundred.

Jean Tchilinguirian
Tradition and Know-How

Léon Tchilinguirian, an Armenian immigrant, worked in Romans' shoe factories before opening his own workshop in 1945. In 1955, his son Jean joined the family business, which included his two brothers and sister. This compact manufacturing unit combines tradition and know-how.

Additionally, several large ready-to-wear designers, including Agnès B, have eagerly entrusted the manufacture of part of their collection to this small company with big league status. Today, Jean Tchilinguirian produces designs under his own label "Tchilin" and markets them in his own boutique in Romans.

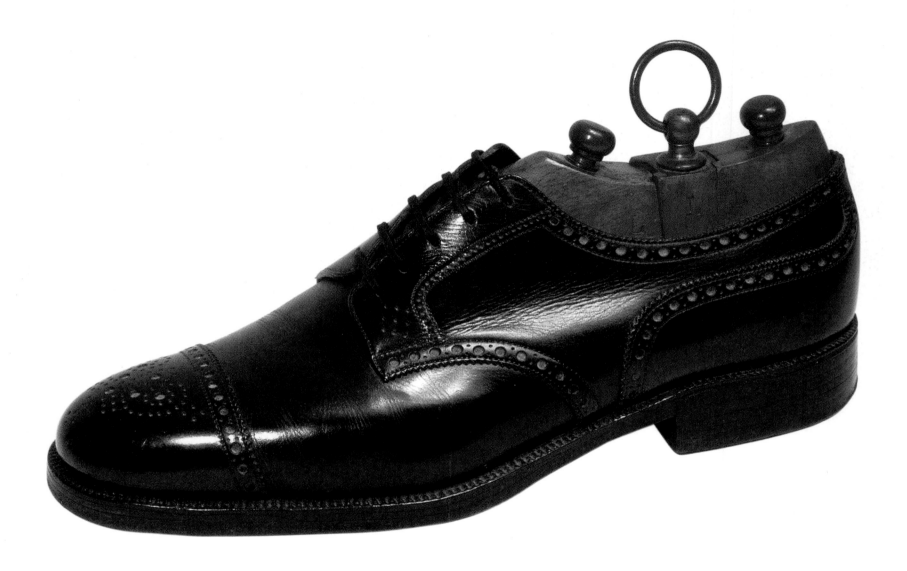

172. Shoe by John Lobb. Ledermuseum, Offenbach.

173. Shop of shoemaker John Lobb, 24 rue du Faubourg Saint-Honoré, Paris.

174. Shop of shoemaker John Lobb, 9 Saint James Street, London.

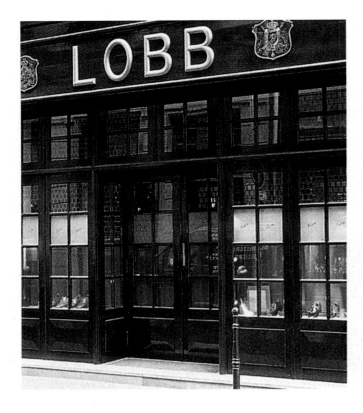
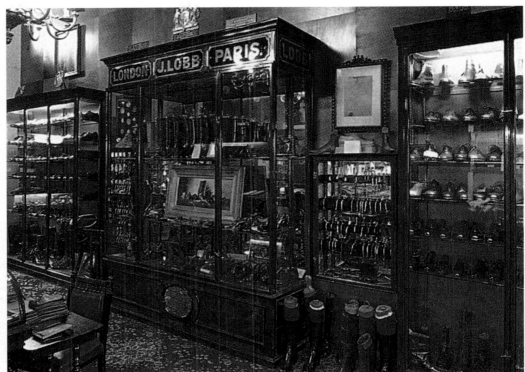

John Lobb

This firm, founded by John Lobb in 1849, is based in London on Saint James Street. During the Victorian era, the custom shoemaker won the highest honors in international exhibitions.

In 1901, John Lobb formed a Paris division. The firm remains a family business. It can take up to six months to achieve the exceptional quality of these made-to-order shoes, which are hand sewn.

Lobb primarily appeals to a wealthy and famous masculine clientele, for whom he makes golf shoes (brogues), Oxfords (Richelieu), and moccasins (loafer).

Official supplier to Her Majesty Queen Elizabeth II, His Royal Highness the Prince of Edinburgh, and His Royal Highness the Prince of Wales, this family firm upholds tradition and quality.

Weston

In the early 20th century, the Blanchard company was making expensive men's shoes in Limoges. Eugène Blanchard traveled to the United States in 1904 to learn the "Goodyear Stitch" construction process and other American manufacturing methods. His idea was to adapt his newly acquired methods to the business in Limoges, but the project did not materialize until after the war of 1914-1918. The year 1926, however, marked a significant step: the Weston brand was launched based on the techniques and philosophy of custom shoemaking. Many of the mechanical tasks went back to being done manually and styles were offered to customers in five widths.

The change in fabrication method thenceforth limited production, which went from six hundred to sixty pairs a day. This is how the brand acquired the characteristics that make it famous even today.

The first Weston store opened in Paris at 98 boulevard de Courcelles. Because of its English identity, the brand was an immediate success. A second store opened in 1932 at 114 avenue Champs Elysées.

In the 1960s, Weston shoes were mainly aimed towards an older clientele. But eventually young people came to appreciate the exceptional quality of the shoes and were willing to pay for it. The shoes stood out from machine-made varieties through the attention given to the following: proper fit and shape, a range of full-grain leathers, a leather inner lining, welt construction, cork filling and leather tanning of hand-crafted soles. Clients were also offered personalization of their orders and repair service. In 1994, Weston had seven stores in France and stores in the following three cities: Geneva, New York, and Tokyo.

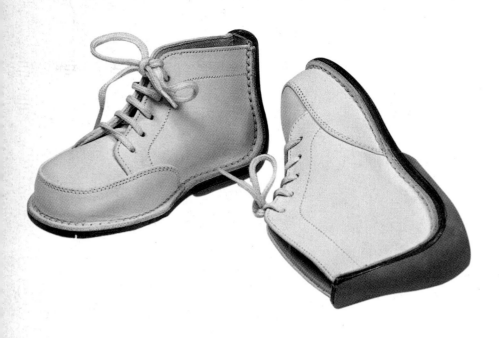

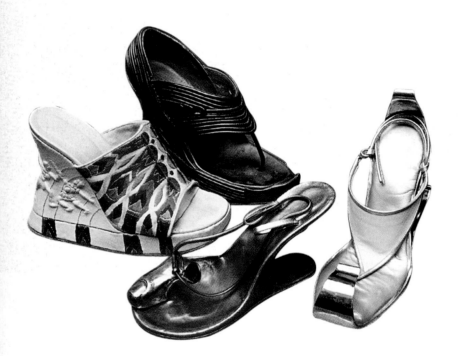

Babybotte Baby Booties

In 1949, the Bidegain company located in Paris launched a revolutionary model called the Babybotte bootie becoming the baby shoe specialist. The company made the shoes for Princess Caroline of Monaco, as well as for Margotte, the heroine of the French animated children's film *The Magic Merry-Go-Round*.

The company became known for the advanced technology of its products, which were designed in close collaboration with pediatricians and chiropodists.

Around 1954, the rear guard was invented, giving better support to the baby's ankle.

It also manufactured and marketed "Le loup blanc," the leading brand of children's medical shoes established in 1959.

It has manufactured and developed children's shoes for its "Kenzo Jungle" line since the summer of 2000, when it entered into a licensing agreement with Kenzo.

Pompeï, Shoemaker for the Stage and Screen
The Pompeï workshop was a family affair

Born in 1912 in Fermo, Italy, Ernesto Pompeï received professional training to work in the shoe industry. The central Italian town of Fermo, located in the region of the Marches, was home to skilled leatherworkers. In 1930, he left his native village for the capital where he became shoemaker for the theater of Rome, specializing in stage shoes. After that, Ernesto's career would take a new direction.

In 1932, with his brother Luigi, he founded the firm Société Pompeï on the via Cavour, close to Saint Mary Major Basilica in Rome.

At the outset, the brothers supplied theaters before entering the cinema world with the celebrated film Scipio Africanus (Scipio the African) by Carmine Gallone, produced in Italy in 1937. Pompeï's workshop soon was Cinecitta's regular shoemaker, as evidenced by Pompeï's dazzling history of collaboration with great costume designers like Sanilo Donati (favored by Federico Fellini) Piero Tosi (for Luchino Visconti), Lila de Nobile, Marcel Escafier, and Alberto Verso.

Ernesto's son Carlo was born in Rome in 1938. A graduate of Rome's political science university, nothing had indicated that he would enter the family business. Nevertheless, he was deeply involved in the world of theater as well as becoming an assistant film director from 1963-1970 and working on American films such as Otto Preminger's *The Cardinal*. In 1971, Carlo joined Société Pompeï and collaborated closely with his father until his father's death in 1973.

From 1974 to 1990, the firm grew and established branches in London, Brussels and the United States. In 1988, Société Pompeï's takeover of the Galvin firm (rue Meslay in the third arrondissement in Paris), which had worked for everyone in the world of Paris entertainment, led to a new development: thenceforth known as Société Pompeï-Galvin, the new firm moved to the boulevard Bourdon in the fourth arrondissement in 1993.

For theater, opera and cinema, the house of Pompeï designed styles ranging from the simplest to the most extravagant; from Ancient Rome to the Court of Versailles, passing through the First World War and the barbarian invasions in the process.

All of these designs involved the cooperation of talented and demanding costume designers. As shoemaker to the stage and screen, Carlo Pompeï received an encouragement award for theatrical crafts in 1995 and the gold medal for craftsmen in the arts in Munich. These distinctions awarded Carlo's specialties as a shoemaker: professionalism and preservation of traditional craftsmanship. These qualities are the same as those of a shoemaker for town shoes: both are preoccupied with historical accuracy. It should be noted that extraordinary care was given to making shoes that only had to give the illusion of period fashion. Unfortunately, the morphology of the

175. Baby booties, 1954.

176. Shoes worn by Monica Belluci in *Astérix and Obélix: Mission Cleopatra*. Created in the Pompéi workshop in 2001.

177. Shoes worn by Anita Ekberg in the role of Sylvia in Federico Fellini's *La Dolce Vita*, 1960. Shoes created at the Pompéi workshop. International Shoe Museum, Romans.

Following pages:

178. Shoes for movie extras created by the House of Pompéi.

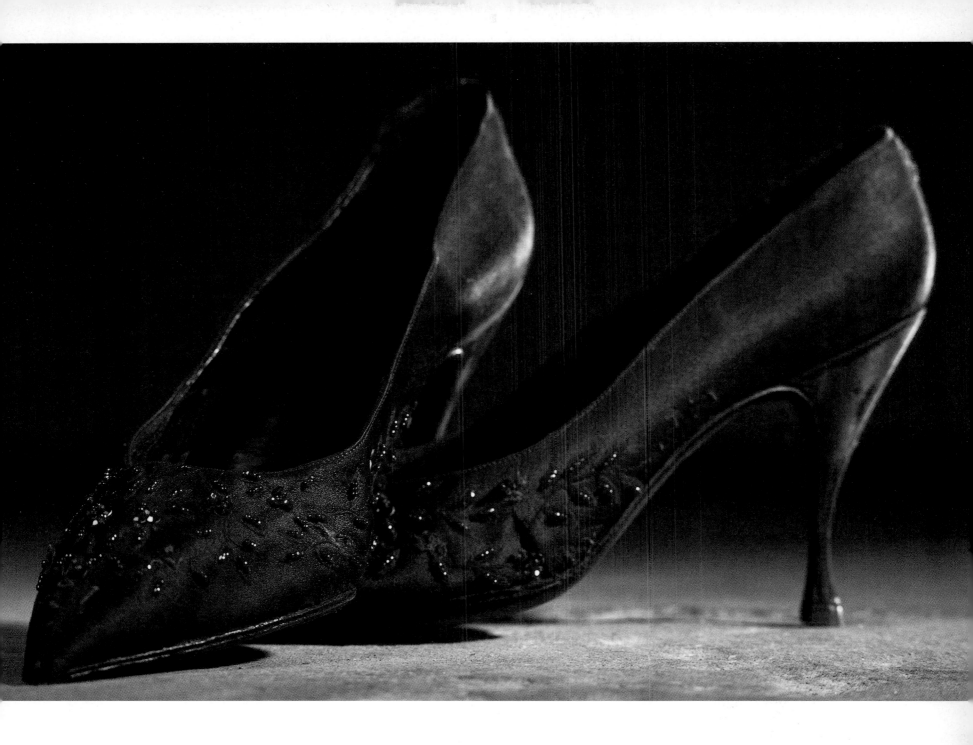

foot had changed. Longer and larger, it could not wear the short shoes from the time of Louis XVI, or the long, pointed ankle boots from the beginning of the century. Still, it is always possible to the lower the heel, to round the upper, to reduce the leg, without necessarily changing the shoe's appearance.

In addition to being concerned about historical accuracy, Carlo Pompeï was also concerned with the comfort of the actor's feet. Some celebrities received special treatment: custom-made styles of which Carlo Pompeï tried to keep a few copies for his collection. Sometimes the shoes needed for a film, a musical or theatrical entertainment were chosen from among existing stock and adapted as needed. After being used, the loaned shoes were returned to the studio where they were checked and arranged according to period and style. There were close to eight hundred thousand. Before being re-used, the shoes were "refreshed," dyed if necessary, and always fit with an inner sole worthy of Pompeï's nickname, "number one in cleanliness." When it is a matter of supplying hundreds of pairs of shoes, the shoes are not actually fitted; selections are made from the sizes provided by the costume maker. It also happened that the production company retained ownership of the shoes and costumes. Who knows why the actors sometimes kept their shoes: personal attachment, a souvenir, or in the spirit of collecting?

Carlo Pompeï's Paris studio was for receiving, conservation, and fabrication. Approached by individual clients, but most often by costume designers or the theater artists themselves, the shoemaker responded to extremely varied requests. Fabrication was often done in a rush. If the Paris studio was overwhelmed, the Rome studio took over for it. There were also Carlo Pompeï workshops in London, Brussels, and Avignon, where Carlo Pompeï supplied the operas of Aix, Orange, and Marseille.

Famous actors put themselves in the hands of this shoemaker. But Carlo Pompeï was also shoemaker for the following companies in the performing arts: the Opéra Garnier (Paris), the Opéra Bastille (Paris), the Comédie Française (Paris), and la Scala (Milan). To these should be added many other theaters and opera companies in Paris and in France (Lyon, Marseille, Toulouse, Nancy, Montpellier, Reims, Metz, Rennes, Limoges, Tours, Angers, and Villeurbanne), as well as in other European countries and the United States.

Finally there is one other specialty among Carlo Pompeï's activities that deserves mentioning: making shoes for fashion shows, including those of Thierry Mugler. For the 100th anniversary of the cinema, the International Shoe Museum, Romans, devoted an exhibition to the Maison Pompeï, which was re-shown and updated by the Bon Marché on the left bank in Paris.

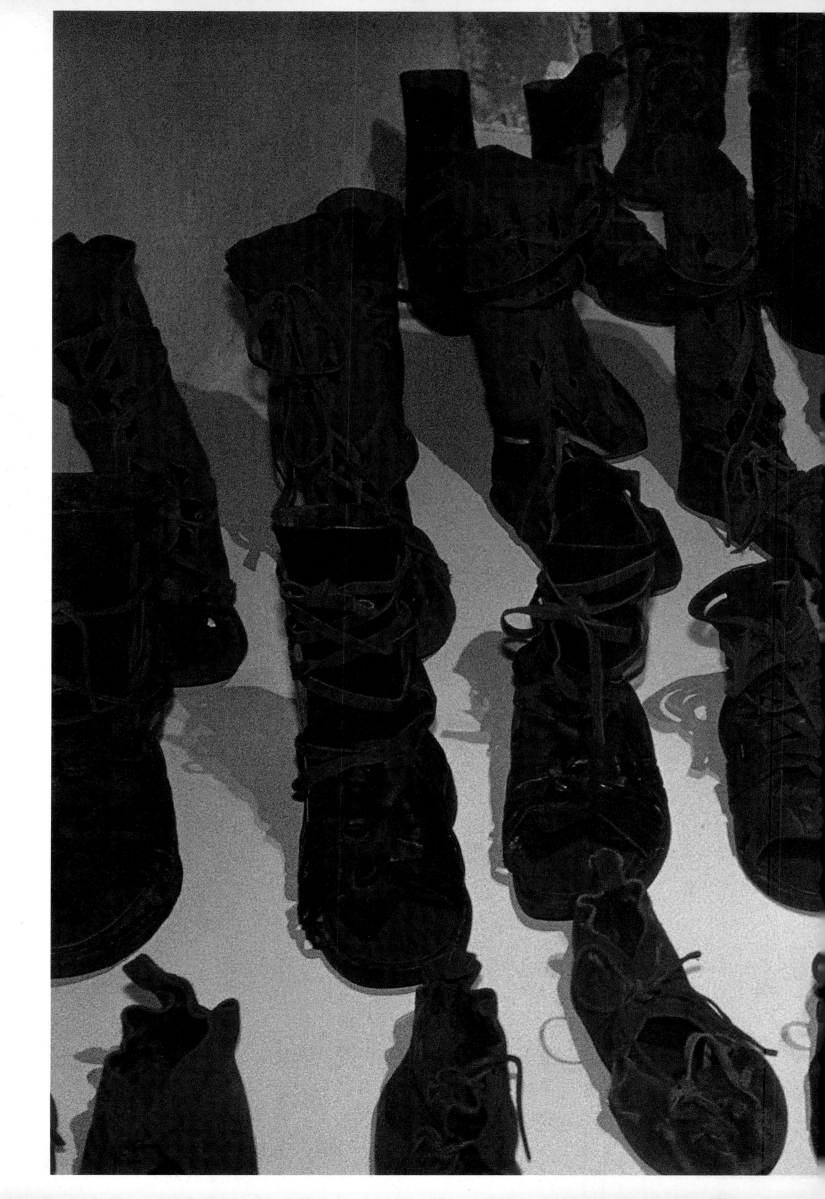

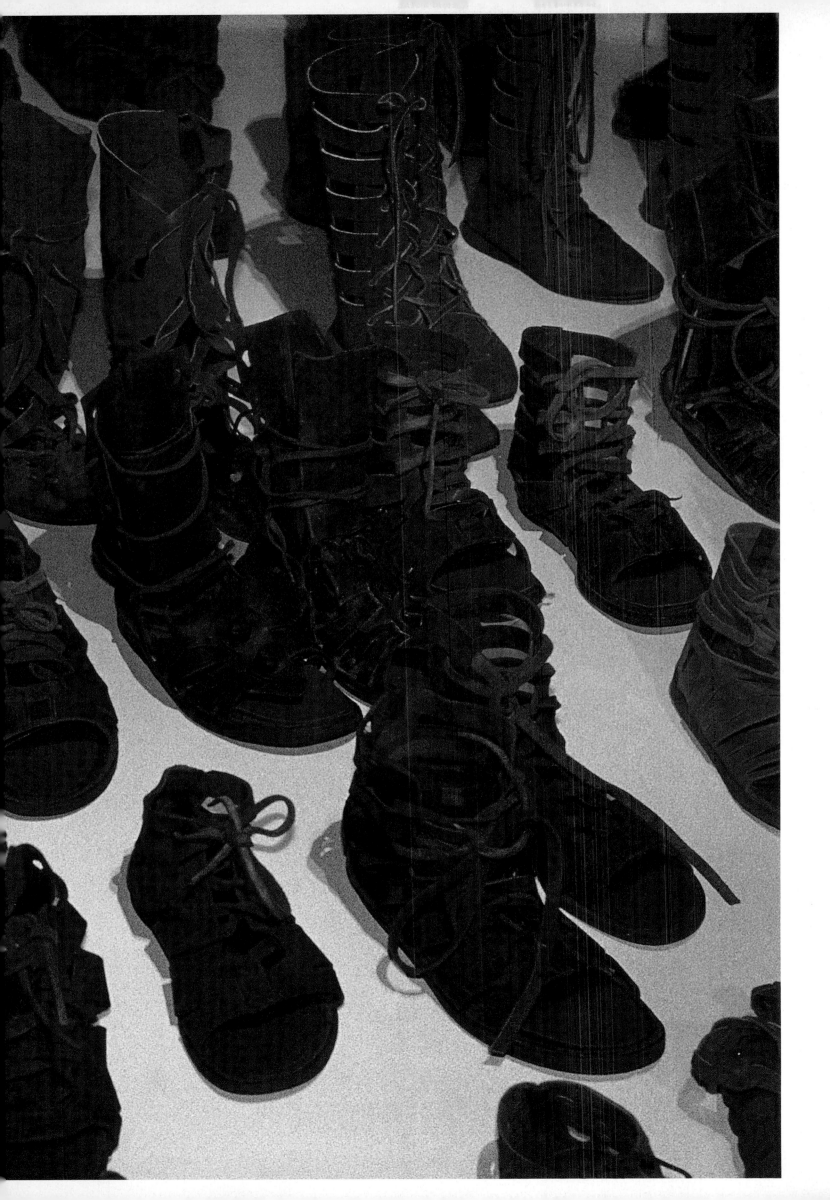

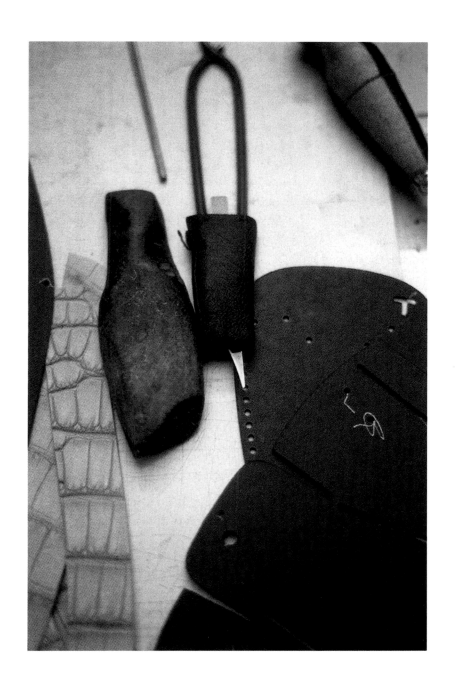

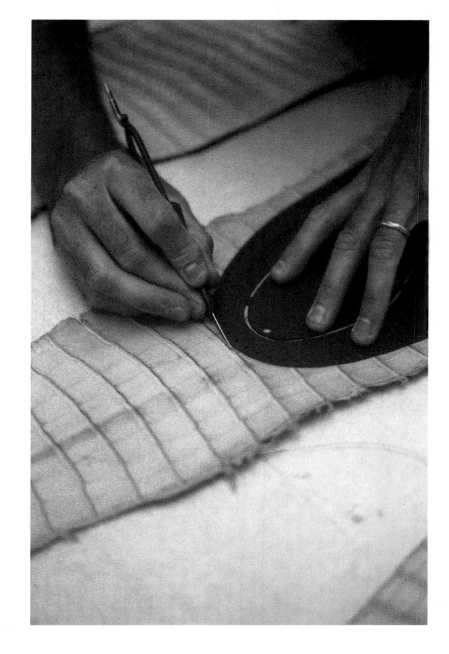

179. Manufacture of Tod's treaded moccasins: the tools.

180. Manufacture of Tod's treaded moccasins: the cutting out.

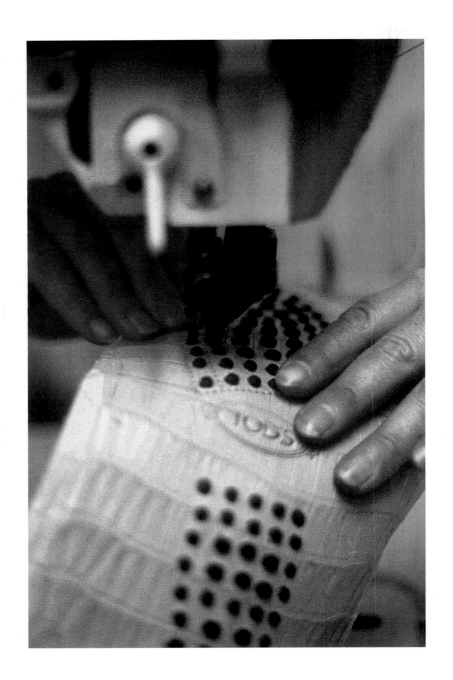 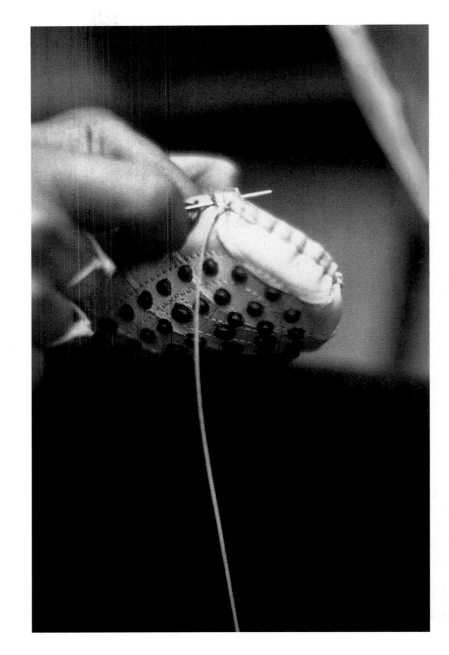

181-182. Manufacture of Tod's treaded moccasins.

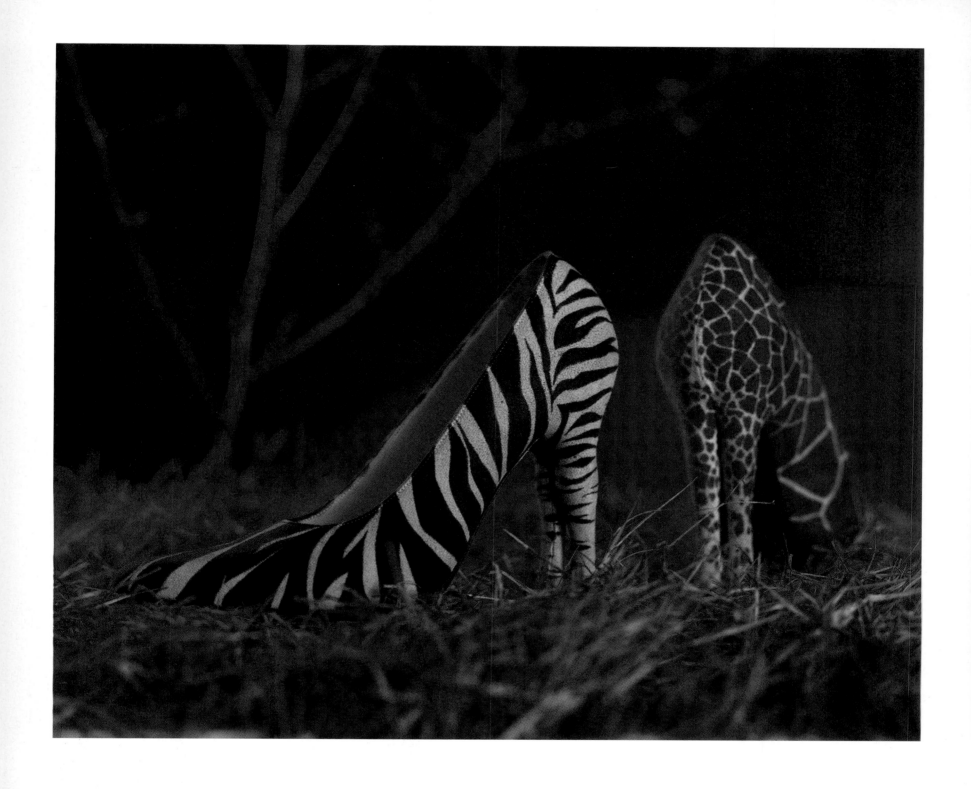

183. Giraffe shoe and zebra shoe in kidskin and velvet painted entirely by hand. Heels of carved wood covered with hide evoking the hind legs of a giraffe and a zebra. Created by Stéphane Couvé Bonnaire, winner of the competition under the category for the stiletto heel organized by the Style Bureau of the National Federation of the Shoe Industry in 1995. International Shoe Museum, Romans.

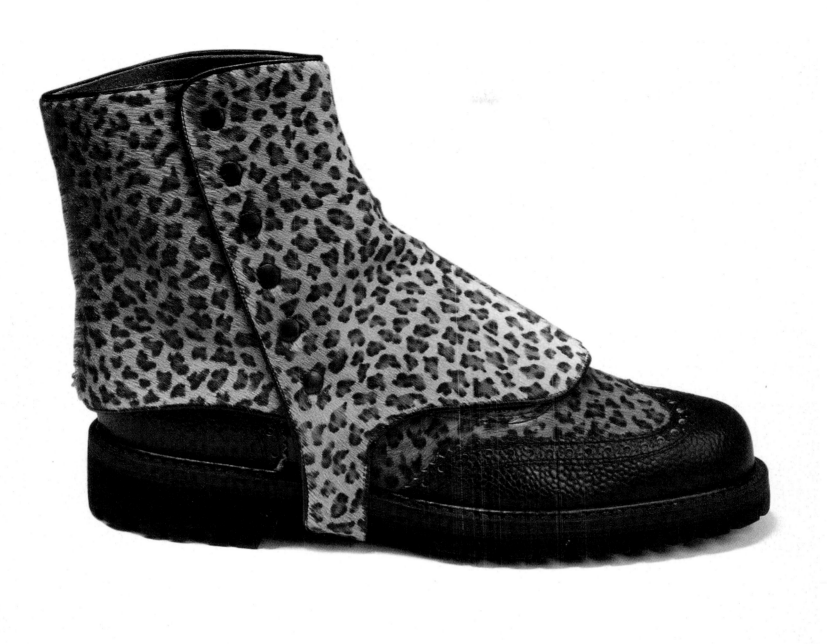

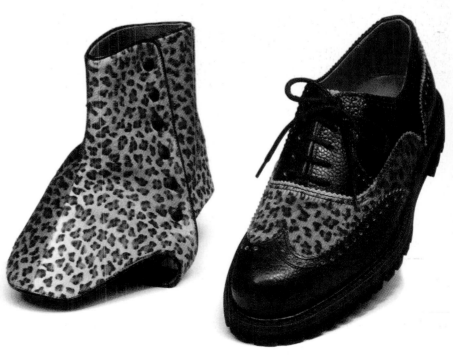

184-185. Leopard shoe and gaiter.

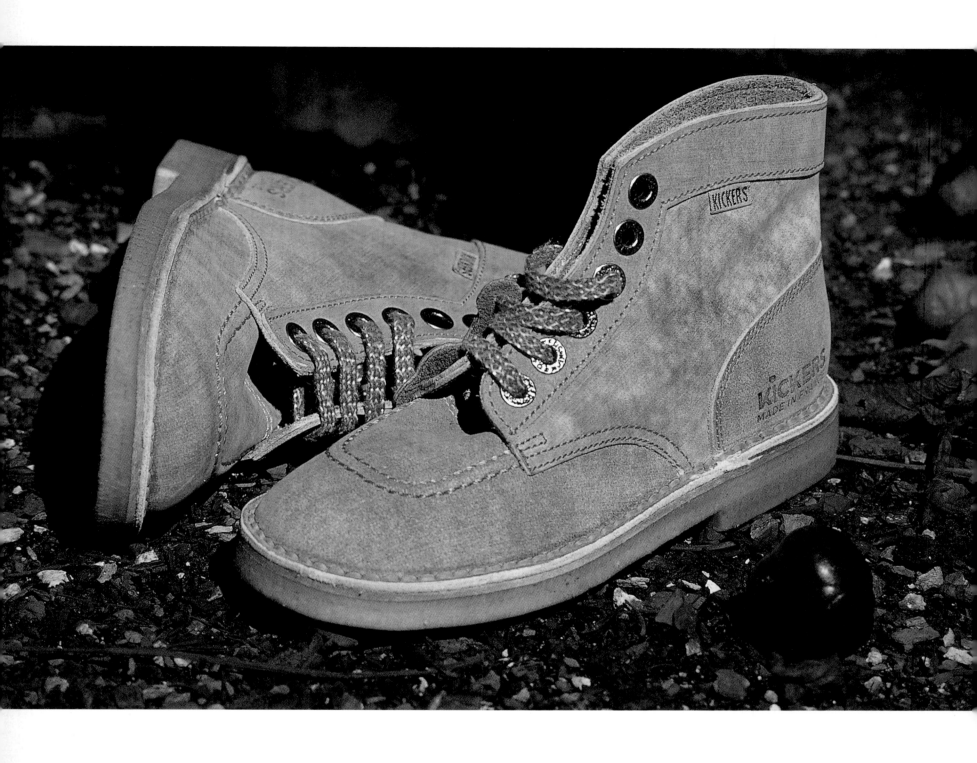

186. Children's boots, Kickers, 1971.

International Shoe Museum, Romans.

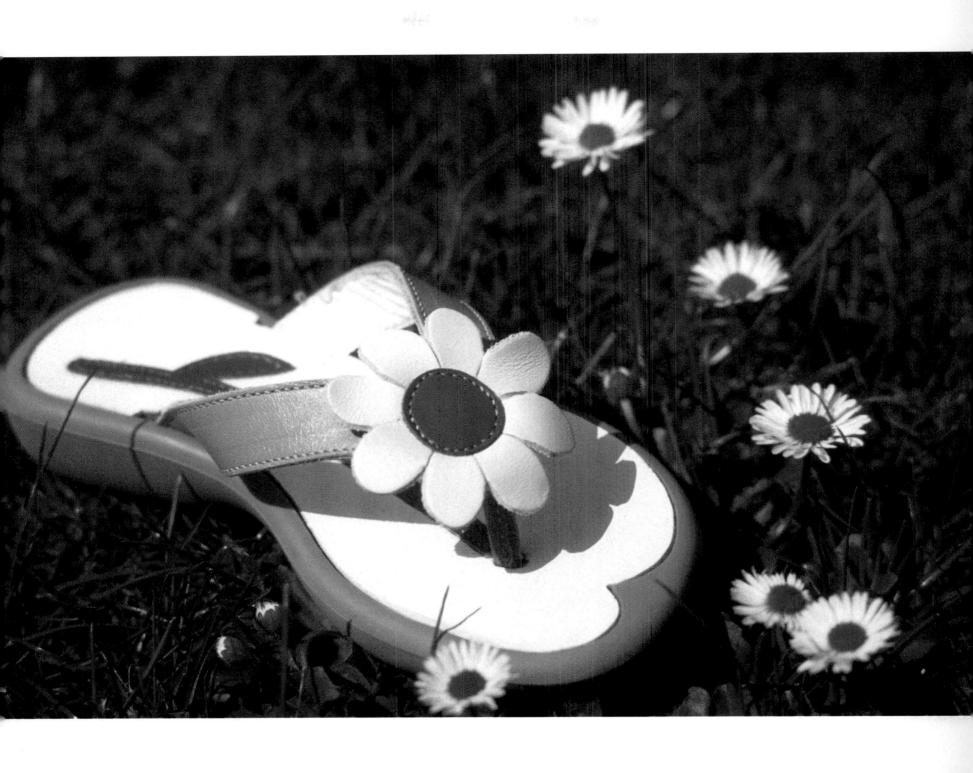

187. Child's mule decorated with a marguerite, synthetic sole.

Summer 2002. International Shoe Museum, Romans.

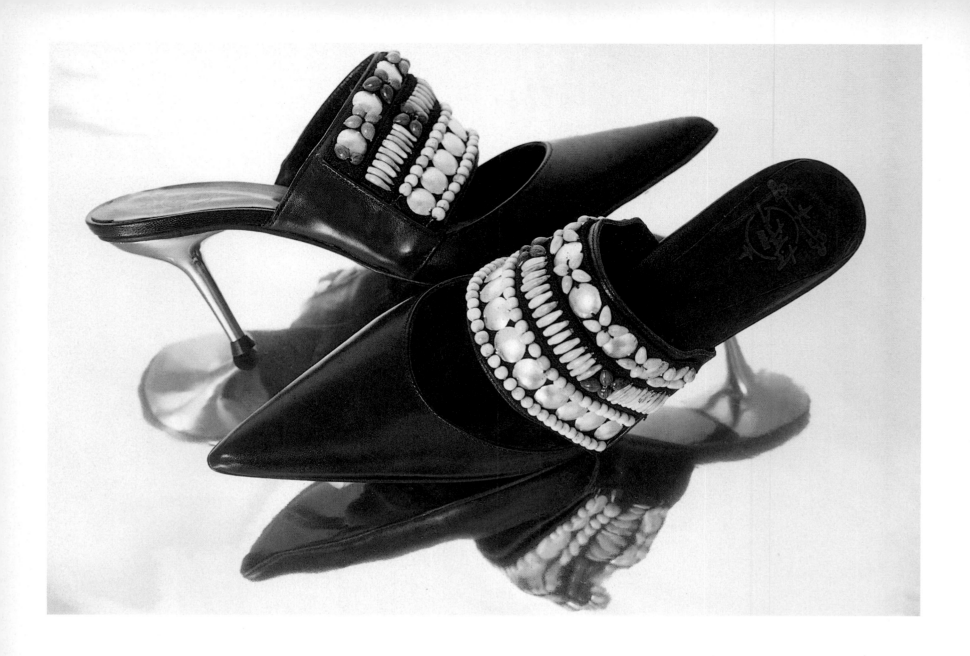

Le Salon Midec
International Footwear Fashions

Salon Midec-Paris, a fashion showing entirely devoted to shoes, is held at the Porte de Versailles in March and September. Established by a French industry group called the Bureau de Style Chaussure, Maroquinerie, Cuir and aimed at promoting design, Midec exhibits the collections of young international designers inside a "Fantasy" space. It also organizes the annual competition "Exercises de Style" which is open to budding fashion designers to nurture new talent and a fresh approach to the future.

L'Escarpin de Cristal (The Crystal Pump)

An initiative of the magazines Hebdo Cuir and Chausser, in partnership with professional sponsors, the escarpin de cristal (the crystal pump) has rewarded creativity and originality since 1999. It looks for footwear innovation in the following areas: image, design, technology, performance, communication, and distribution. This event promotes excellence and unites the profession.

The C.I.D.I.C. Grant

188. "Opium" mules, dress of the Akha tribes of the Golden Triangle (box of recycled coca and jungle seed, 6 cm steel heel, leather). Trikitrixa, Paris.

Creativity in footwear is also honored by the C.I.D.I.C. (The French interprofessional development committee for the leather, leather goods and shoe industries). Each year

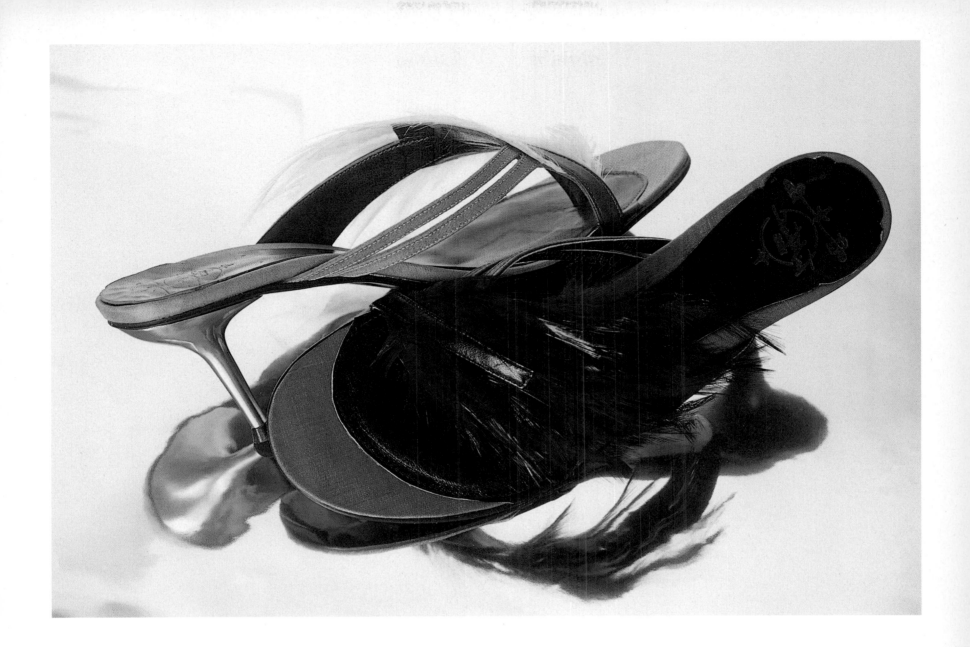

it selects an especially innovative leather accessory designer to receive a grant from ANDAM (National Association for the Fashion Arts). The European Grand Prize in Shoe Design was instituted by the Saint Crispin association. The purpose of the prize is to stimulate creativity. The award also aims to discover and promote young talent entering the professions of shoe and fashion design. The young applicants are asked to design a fashion illustrating a given theme. Twenty finalists selected by a jury make a prototype from their design. The five winners are awarded during the festivities honoring Saint Crispin, patron saint of shoemakers. The work of all the participants is exhibited at the International Shoe Museum, Romans. This competition is under the aegis of the Romans firms Charles Jourdan, Robert Clergerie, and Stéphane Kélian, with the support of the Conseil National du Cuir (French national leather council), the C.I.D.I.C. (Comité interprofessionnel de développement des industries du cuir, de la maroquinerie et de la chaussure, or the French interprofessional development committee for the leather, leather goods and shoe industries), and the C.T.C. (centre technique cuir, chaussure, maroquinerie, or the French technical center for leather, shoes and leather goods). The city of Romans and the International Shoe Museum jointly organize the event. All of these different awards have allowed many, now internationally recognized, talents to emerge in France, mother of the avant-garde. They are steps in the right direction that need to be continued and applauded.

189. "Gall" heeled sandals with rooster feathers and steel heel of 6 cm. Trikitrixa, Paris.

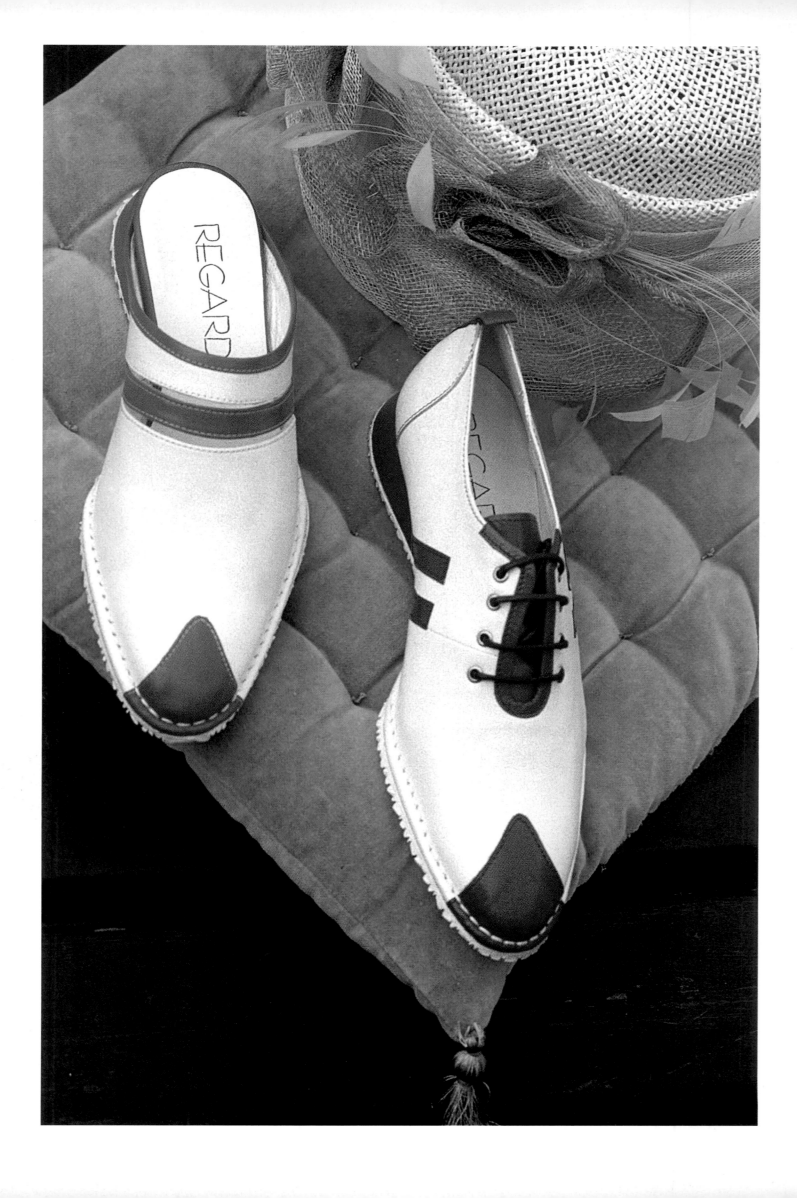

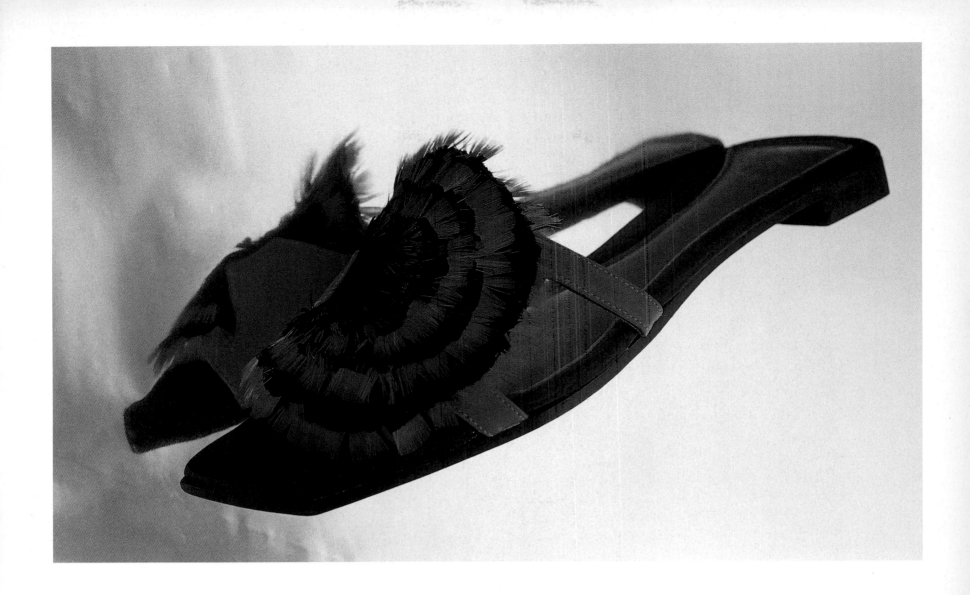

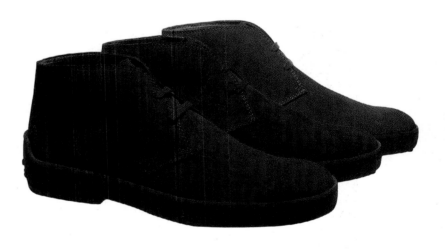

190. Look shoes. Summer 2002.

191. "Rosette" sandals with pheasant feathers. Trikitrixa, Paris.

192. "Double T" shoes, created by Tod's. Spring-Summer 2003.

Following pages:

193. Shoes created by Sara Navarro. Summer 2002.

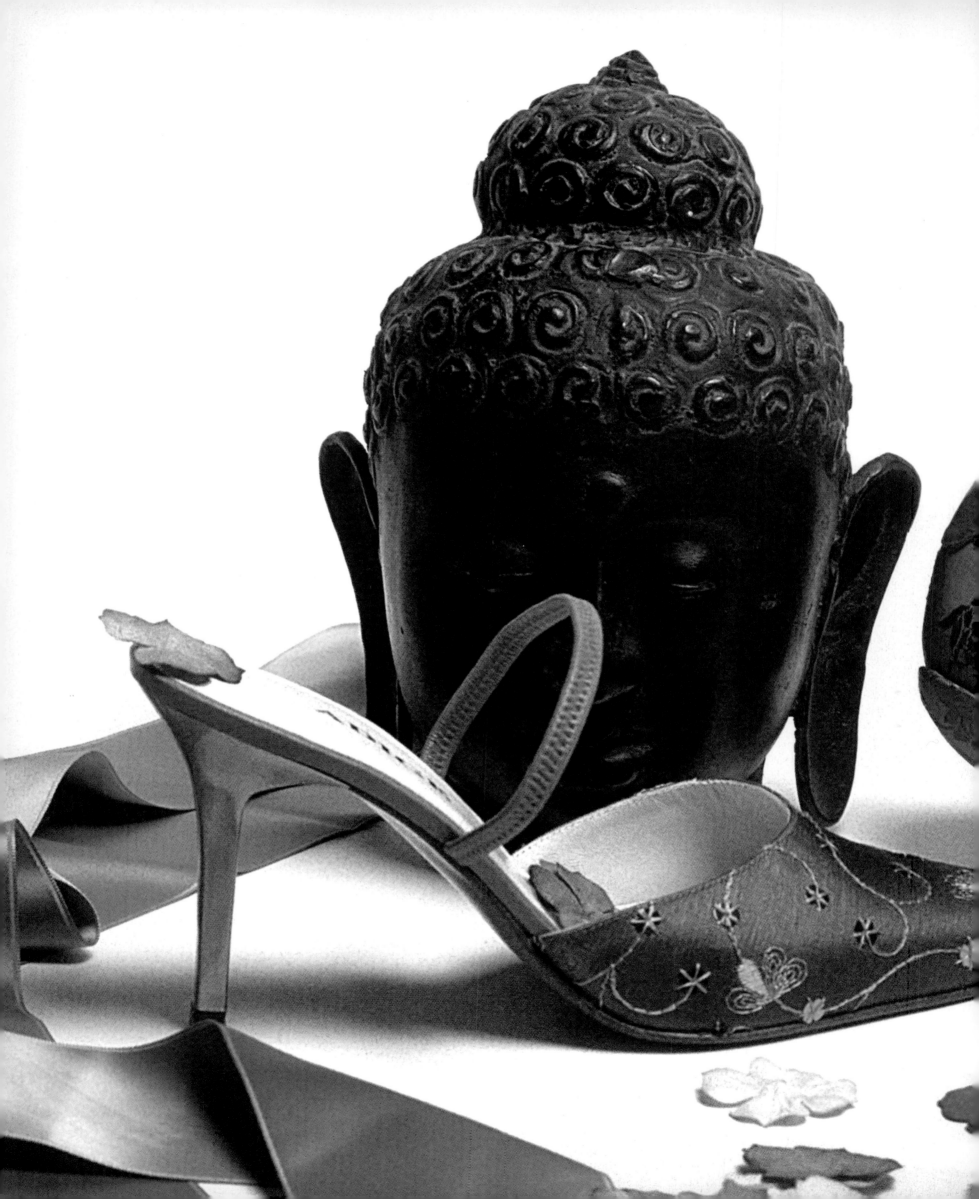

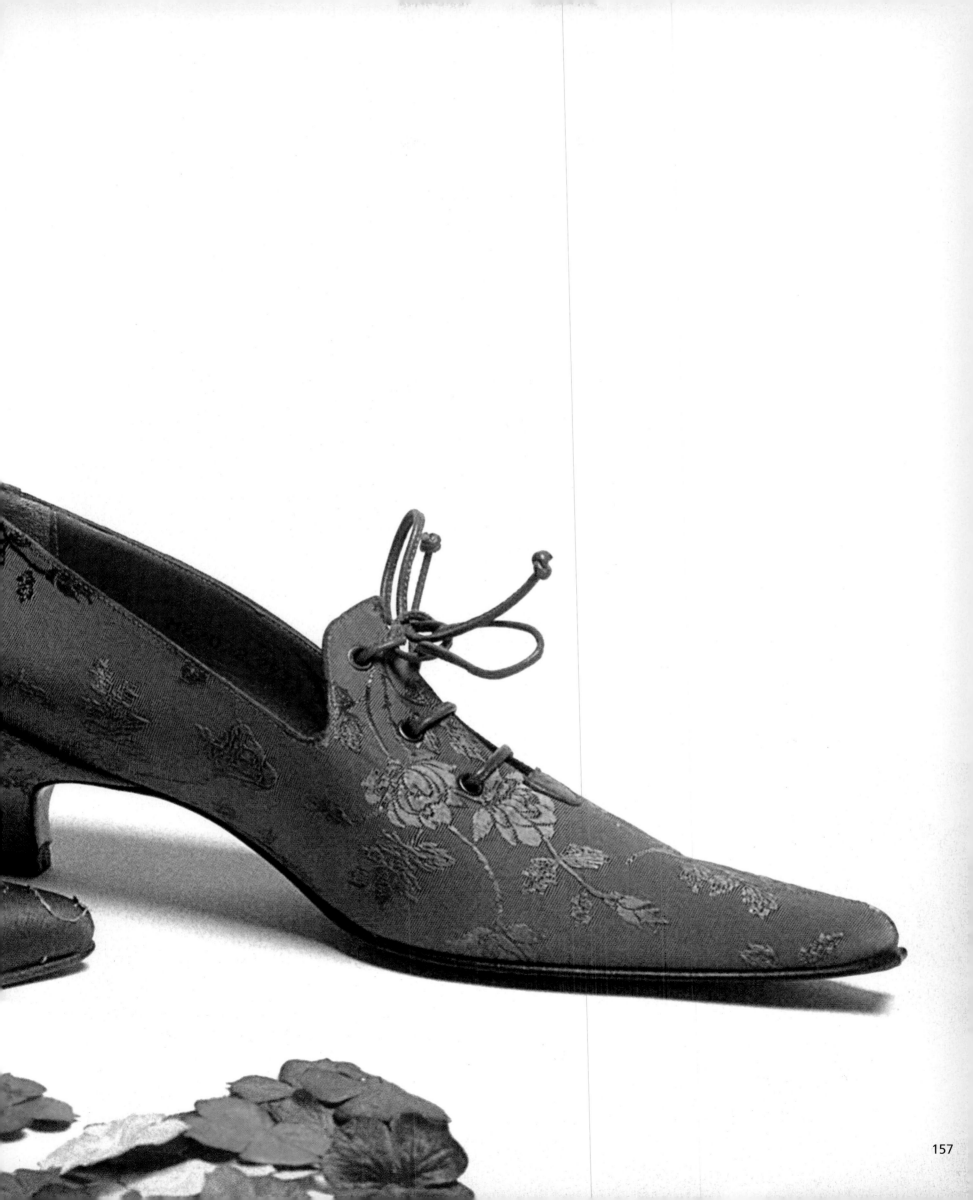

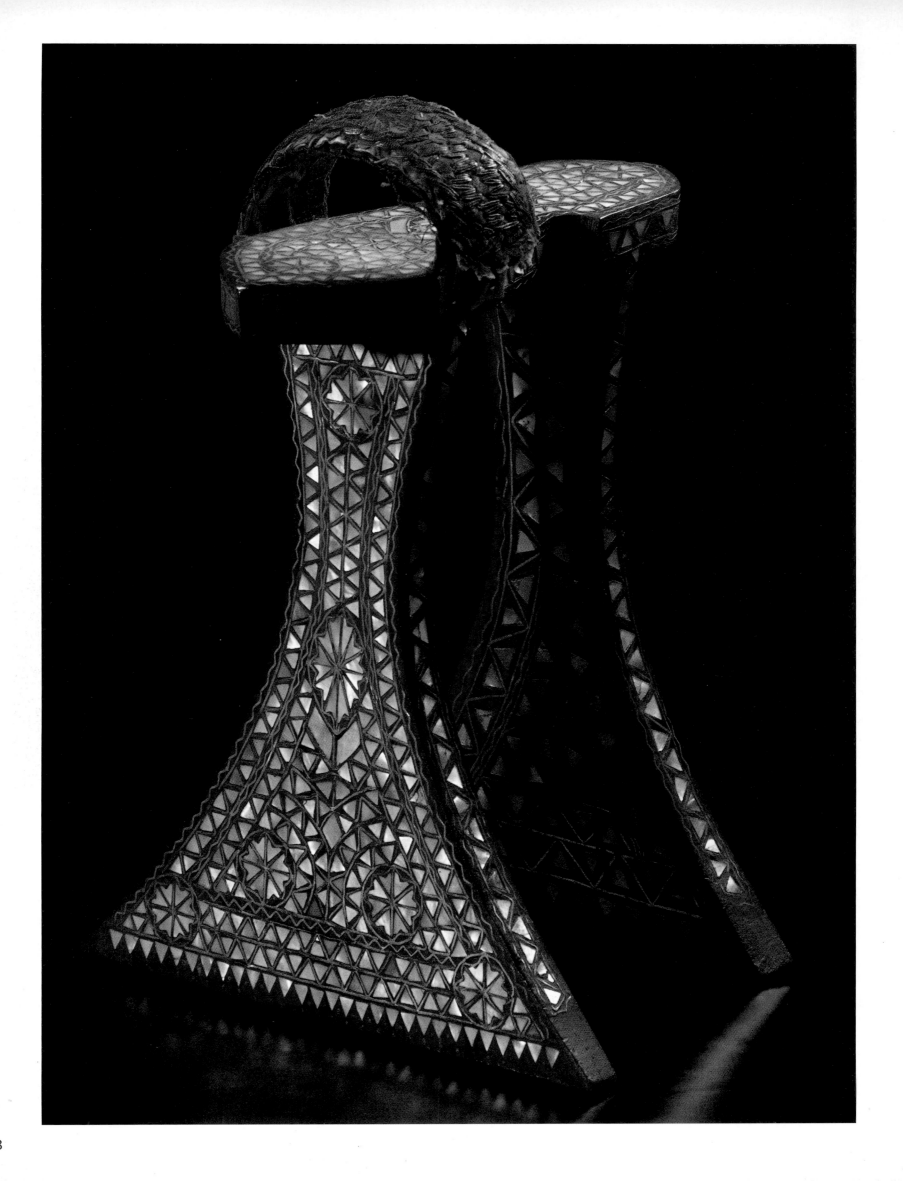

158

Shoes from Around the World

The Ottoman Empire

An avid traveller, Jean-Etienne Liotard set sail for Constantinople in 1738. His carefully observed paintings and drawings of the individuals he encountered earned him a reputation as the Enlightenment's "Turkish painter." In this portrait of almost photographic detail, the woman's pattens are accurately depicted being used to protect her from the damp. Note also that the painting depicts the slave without shoes, in contrast to the mistress: the slave must make do with henna-painted feet.

It was common for women in Turkey and many other oriental countries to wear pattens of variable height inside the bath. Women's pattens were of wood, inlaid with mother-of-pearl or ivory and covered with silver; the strap was richly embroidered with silver and gold thread. Such pattens carried a comprehensive range of the opulent ornamentation found in these countries. As Jean-Paul Roux rightly emphasizes, the inlaid decoration found on these shoes is quite similar to the decoration found on door and window casements, furniture, and Muslim pulpits.

In the early 19th century, the Ottomans formed one of the world's largest empires, encompassing the whole Balkan Peninsula, all of western Asian to Persia, Africa, Egypt, and Tripolitania, and the suzerainties of Algeria and Tunisia. Situated at the crossroads of three continents, between the Mediterranean and the Indian Ocean, the Ottoman Empire occupied a key position. This vast geographical area sometimes produced an interactive synthesis of decorative styles that is perceptible in the ornamentation of shoes from its different countries.

In some oriental countries, women enjoyed an "elevated" status – for a day. To remind them of their superiority to their husbands, brides were hoisted onto excessively high pattens such as these, but the women had to come down from their pedestals the very next day. This way of thinking is confirmed by the Koran: "Men are superior to women, due to the fact that Allah has raised many of them above the others" (Montet translation, Payot, 1954). On the other hand, the woman ruled the home and the presence of a pair of men's babouches at the door forbid any other man from entering.

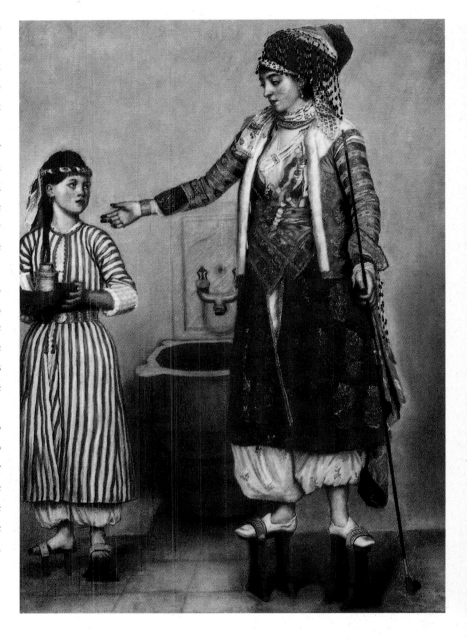

194. Marriage shoes of wood inlayed with windows of mother of pearl, and metal. Middle East, 19th century.
Cruller Collection, International Shoe Museum, Romans.

195. Jean-Etienne Liotard. *Turkish Woman and Her Slave*, 18th century.
Art and History Museum, Geneva.

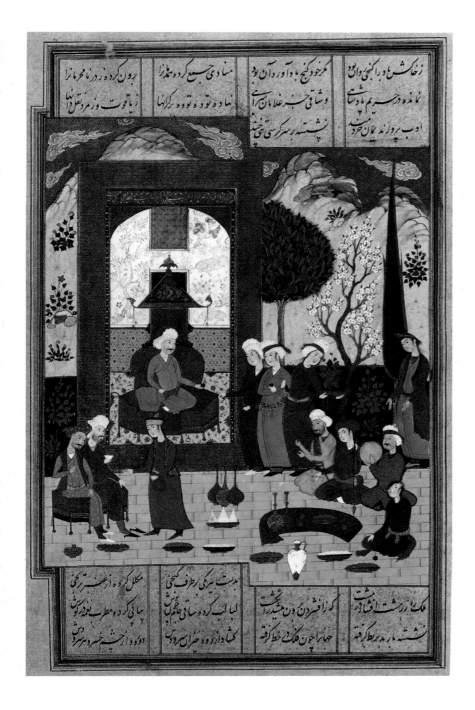

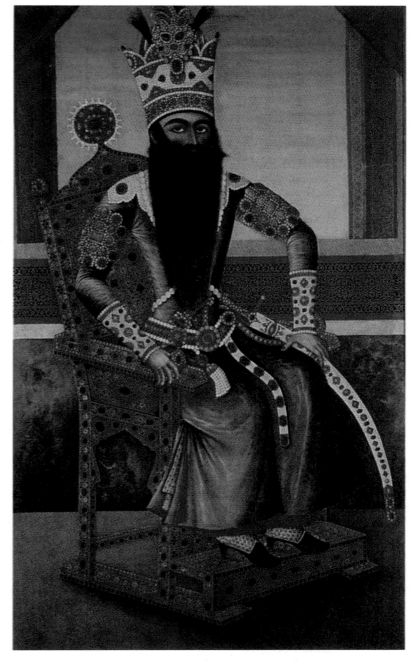

Persia

After the death of Alexander in 323 BC, Iranian culture entered a period of dormancy. The breakdown of the Sassanian and Byzantine empires paved the way for Islam's takeover.

During the golden age of the Safavid dynasty (1501-1736), Persian still dazzled western travellers. The French painter Chardin (1699-1779), who spent ten years in Persia around 1660, was among those impressed. According to Chardin, even the poor were well dressed and wore silver ornaments on their arms, feet and neck.

Unlike shoes in the Hellenized West, the shoes of oriental countries exhibit a continuity of forms whose decorative grammar was transmitted from one century to the next. For example, 17th- and 19th-century ceremonial boots from Persia display on their soles the same stylized floral motifs found on garments worn by Ashurbanipal in the 7th century BC. The motifs are visible on a narrative relief from

Ashurbanipal's palace entitled, "The King killing a lion," now in the British Museum.

Another significant example of continuity is the similarity between the 16th-century heeled shoes with raised tips now in the International Shoe Museum, Romans, and the mules worn by the Persian Emperor Fath' Alī Chāh in his portrait painted around 1805, now in the Louvre Museum. These shoes were worn to best advantage with stockings richly embroidered with gold motifs based on those shown on Ashurbanipals's clothing.

According to Jean-Paul Roux, the babouche, a slipper without a rear quarter or heel worn by men in the orient, probably originated in Iran. The Persian word papoutch comes from the words pa (foot) and pouchiden (to cover). This form of footwear was especially suited to the Islamic custom of removing shoes before entering a mosque or a private home.

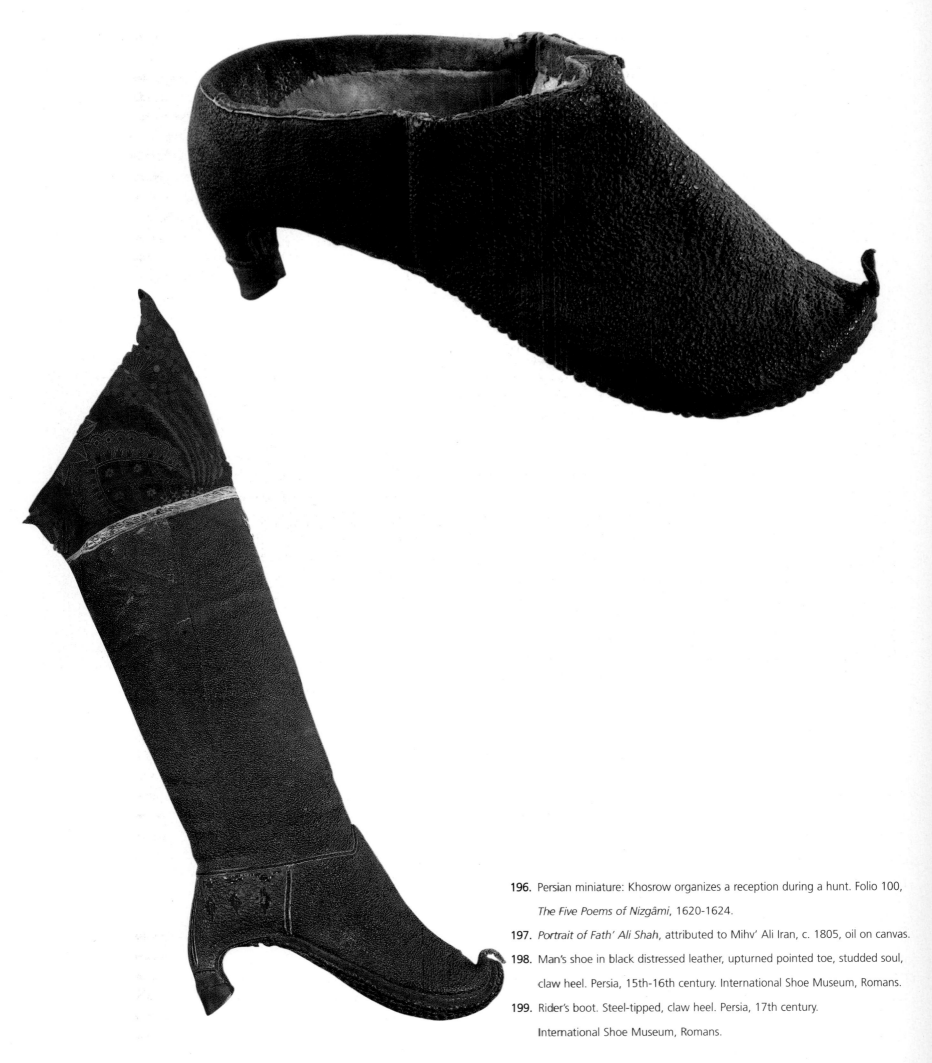

196. Persian miniature: Khosrow organizes a reception during a hunt. Folio 100, *The Five Poems of Nizgâmi*, 1620-1624.

197. *Portrait of Fath' Ali Shah*, attributed to Mihv' Ali Iran, c. 1805, oil on canvas.

198. Man's shoe in black distressed leather, upturned pointed toe, studded soul, claw heel. Persia, 15th-16th century. International Shoe Museum, Romans.

199. Rider's boot. Steel-tipped, claw heel. Persia, 17th century. International Shoe Museum, Romans.

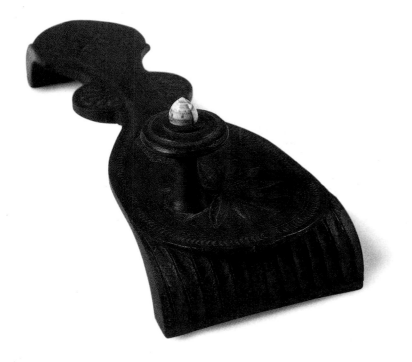

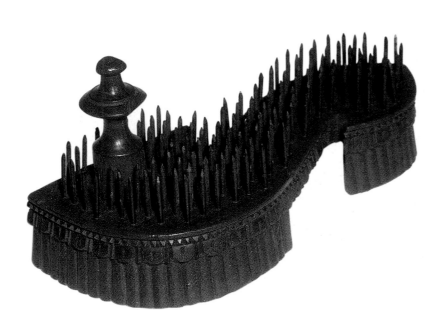

India

A great civilization developed in the Indus valley around 2500-2000 BC. Excavations at Harappa (Punjab) and Mohenjodaro (Sindh) have yielded seals contemporary with the Akkadian period of King Sargon's reign, proof of cultural links between Indian and Sumerian towns well before the Buddhist period. Does this mean the traditional raised tip shoe originated in India? The question remains unanswered. We do know, however, that wearing a raised tip shoe with a pompon became a privilege reserved for the king in both Mesopotamia and India.

Ancient Indian literature makes frequent reference to shoes, but there is little Indian shoe iconography, perhaps because the lower portions of narrative reliefs, standing sculptures and wall paintings are often deteriorated. Additionally, visual images generally illustrate events taking place in locations where wearing shoes is either prohibited or unnecessary. In India, as in many Asian countries, shoes were not worn inside private homes, palaces, or temples.

Valmiki, the legendary author of the Ramayana, tells how King Rama (one of the incarnations of Visnu in Hindu mythology) was exiled to a forest and had his gold-incrusted shoes represent him in his capital. During his three-year absence, the shoes presided in his place. All the decisions delivered by his regent brother were proclaimed before these shoes. A Buddhist variation of the same theme adds an additional detail: when the decisions pronounced before the royal shoes were just, the shoes remained still, but when the decisions broke the law, the shoes rose up in protest.

When the king moved in a procession outside his capital, he was preceded by a servant who carried in her hands the royal sandals, which were the sovereign's emblem. This is affirmed by Buddhist iconography, in particular the Great Stupa (No.1) at Sanchi, which dates from around the Christian era. The material of traditional Indian shoes varies according to historical period and region. Basket makers made sandals out of rush, date palm leaves, and lotus leaves.

In northern India, kings, noble warriors, hunters, and stable boys wore boots and sandals made of leather from the tanned skins of oxen, cow, buffalo, ram, and sheep.

The priestly Brahmin caste considered leather impure and who thus wore wooden sandals instead. Literary descriptions indicate that sandals were made in a variety of colours in shades of blue, yellow, red, brown, black, orange, and sorrel; there were even "multi-coloured" sandals.

Boots, which were sometimes laced, had cotton linings that likewise came in a variety of colours. Boots could be pointed, decorated with ram horns, embellished with scorpion tails, or even have peacock feathers sewn on. To prevent Buddhist monks from giving in to the temptation of these novelty shoes, Buddha was quoted in religious texts as strictly forbidding monks to wear them. Only sandals with simple soles or used shoes received as an offering were approved.

Indians often walked barefoot. The age-old Hindu craft tradition was handed down for generations and stifled innovation.

Men, women, and children continued to wear a type of leather slipper with a raised tip and an exposed heel. Often highly ornate, it displays the Hindu preference for filling. Finally, Islam's influence in India even touched footwear where Turkish-Persian borrowings are evident in certain decorative motifs.

200. Sandal of carved wood. India, 19th century. Collection of the National Museum of the Middle Ages, Thermal Baths of Cluny in Paris, allocated to the International Shoe Museum, Romans.

201. Fakir's sandal. India. International Shoe Museum, Romans.

Page 163:

202. Hooked toe shoes. India. Bally Museum, Schönenwerd, Switzerland.

162

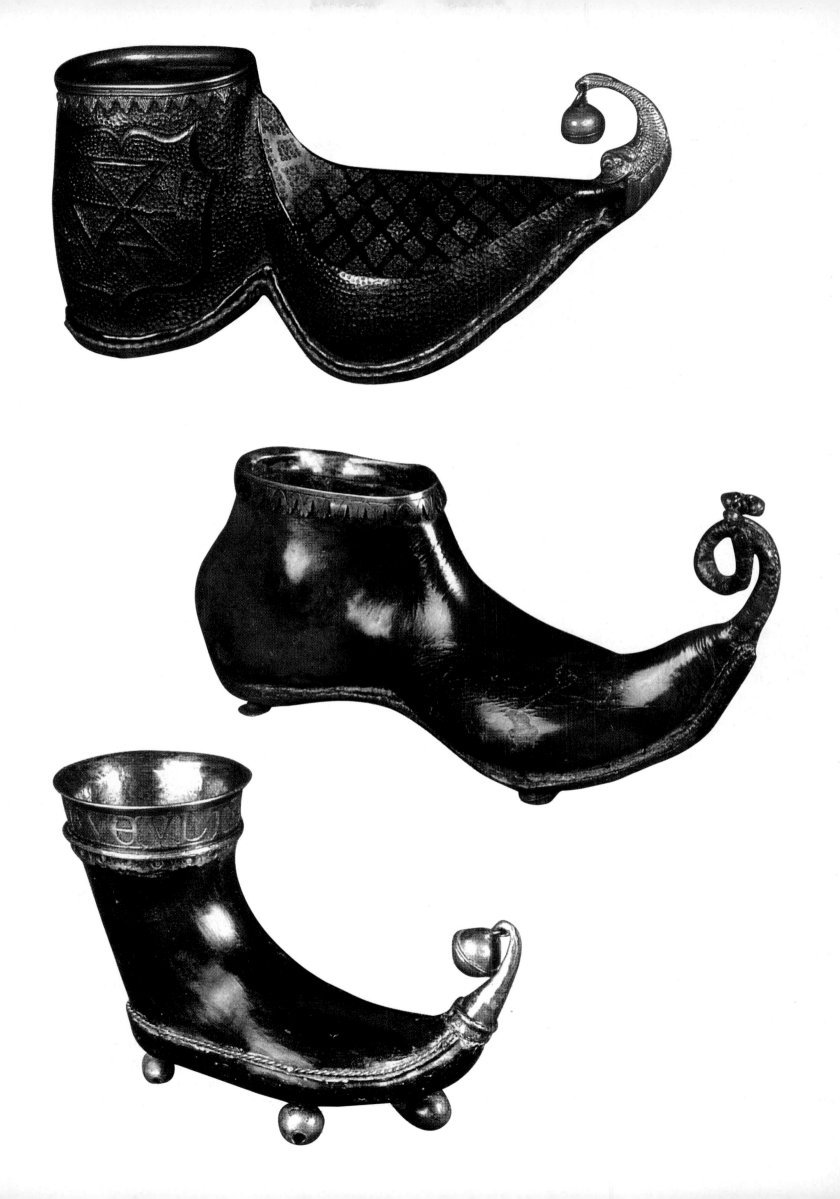

China

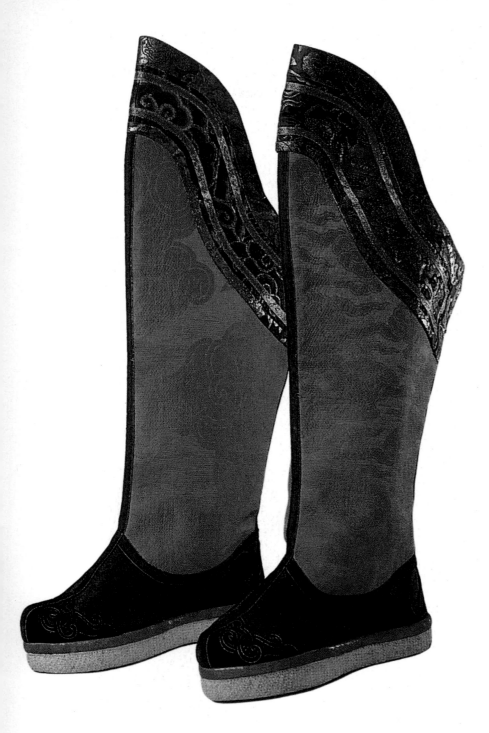

Surely the most unique aspect of Chinese footwear is the tradition of binding women's feet. This ancient Chinese practice deserves specific analysis. Foot deformation was invented in an aristocratic milieu. According to a Chinese historian, in 1100 BC, the Empress Ta Ki had clubfoot. She convinced her husband to order the compulsory compression of all little girls' feet so that they would resemble those of their sovereign, who had become the standard for beauty and elegance.

Five hundred years before Christ, during the era of Confucius (555 BC-479 BC), the beauty of small feet was already being praised as proof of a wellborn status, whereas large feet were synonymous with low birth. Other sources attribute the invention of foot binding to the courtesan Pan Fei, a favorite of Emperor Xiao Bao Kuan (ruled 499-501). Reality was nothing of the sort, although we do owe the expression "golden lotus" to this Emperor.

One day, while Pan Fei was dancing over a floor inlaid with gold lotus flowers for the enjoyment of her imperial lover, the ruler cried out in astonishment: "Look, a golden lotus springs up from her every step!" This metaphor has since come to stand for small Chinese feet.

Another tradition attributes this custom to the 10th century AD in Peking where the Emperor Li Yu (937-978) held his court. Yao Niang, the Emperor's favorite, was famous for her talented dancing. The Emperor gave her a splendid lotus decorated with pearls and then he asked her to wrap her feet in white silk in such a way that their ends came to a point like a crescent moon and dance around the lotus. All the men there watched in rapture as this elegant silhouette twirled on the points of her feet. This lotus dance and the expression "golden lotus" probably originated in a Buddhist legend in which Padmiavati, the daughter of a Brahmin and a doe, made a lotus flower bloom wherever she stepped. In yet another version dating to the 7th century, the story specifies that the young girl had doe hoofs concealed under silk wrappings. The influence of this Indian legend in China was no doubt due to the spread of Buddhism in the early 5th-century. Europeans who began arriving in China in the 13th century showed great discretion concerning the custom of foot binding.

All the same, Marco Polo (1254-1324) noticed the peculiar walk of Chinese women and wrote in his memoirs that:

"Young women always walk so docilely that one foot follows the other by no more than a half-finger length…"

Young girls in very poor families shared the chores of a difficult material existence; having bound feet was a luxury they could ill afford. Scorned, these girls with "big feet," a distinct sign of their modest origin, were called "barefooted" in the Guang Dong. Only girls with banded feet could serve the mistress of the house in her apartments; the others were condemned to the most humble kitchen jobs. In the 13th-century, during the last years of the Song dynasty, it was customary to drink out of a special shoe whose heel contained a small cup.

Later, under the Yuan dynasty, one drank directly from the shoe. This strange custom is attributed to Yang Tieai, a wealthy man of loose morals, who amused himself by planning banquets where guests drank out of the shoes worn by prostitutes attending the party. This practice was called "toasts to the golden lotus," by its author and it had enthusiasts until the end of the 19th century. This is why lotus lovers consider Yang Tieai the patron saint of the brotherhood of drinkers from the little shoe.

203. Silk mandarin boots, from the reign of Kangxi (1662-1722). Gugong Museum, Beijing.

204. G. Castiglione. *Equestrian Portrait of Emperor Qianlong Passing the Troops in Review.* Gugong Museum, Beijing.

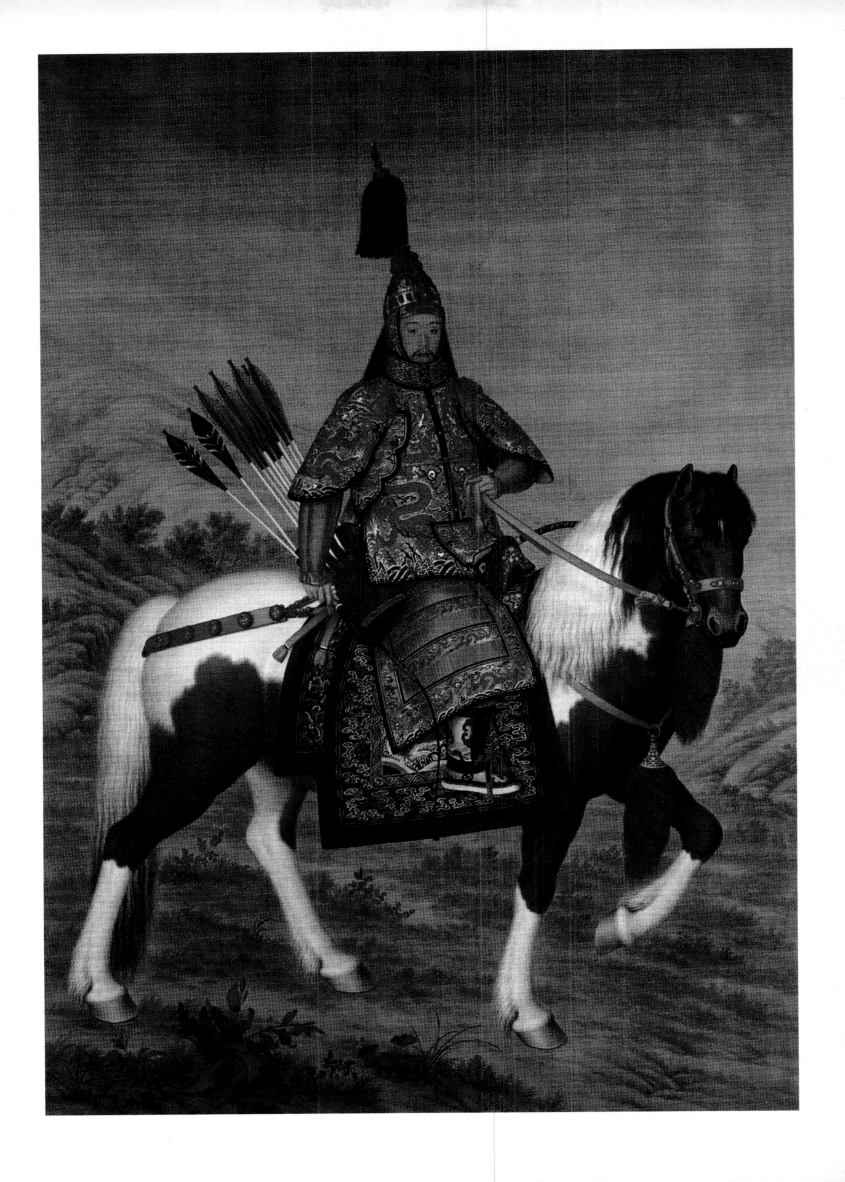

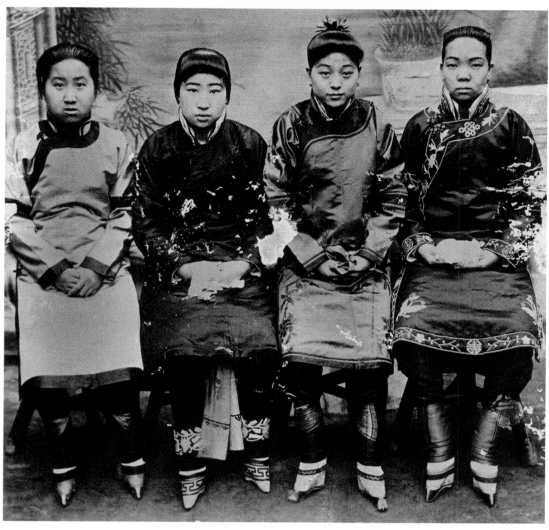

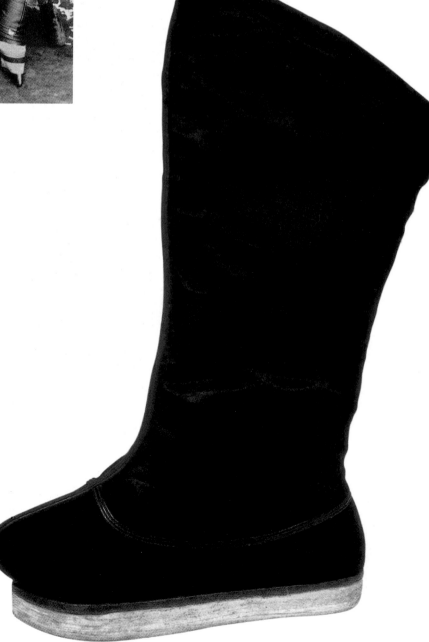

205. Photo of four Chinese prostitutes. Collection of Beverley Jackson.

206. Man's boot in ribbed black satin. Thick sole with sewn leather. Guillen Collection, International Shoe Museum, Romans.

207. Woman's boot in pink satin, embroidery of gold and black thread tracing a dragon. China, 19th century. International Shoe Museum, Romans.

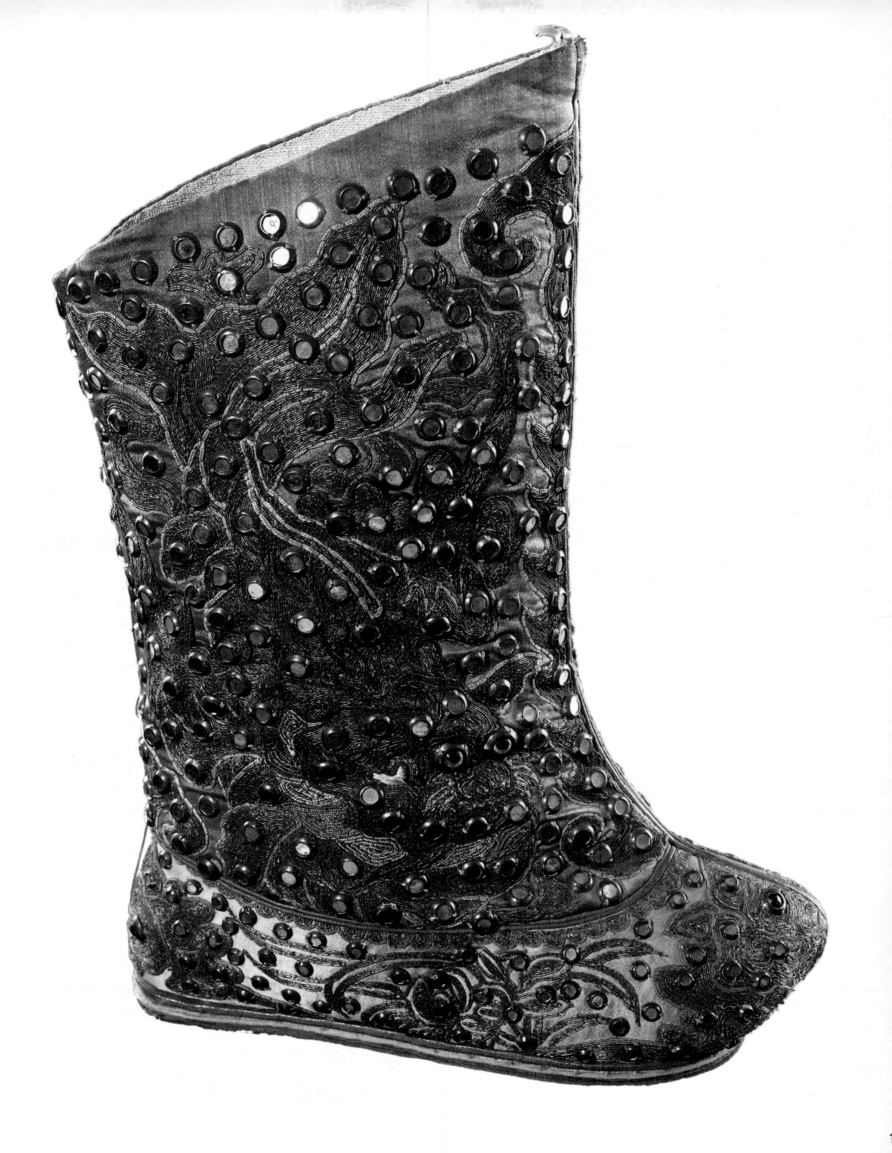

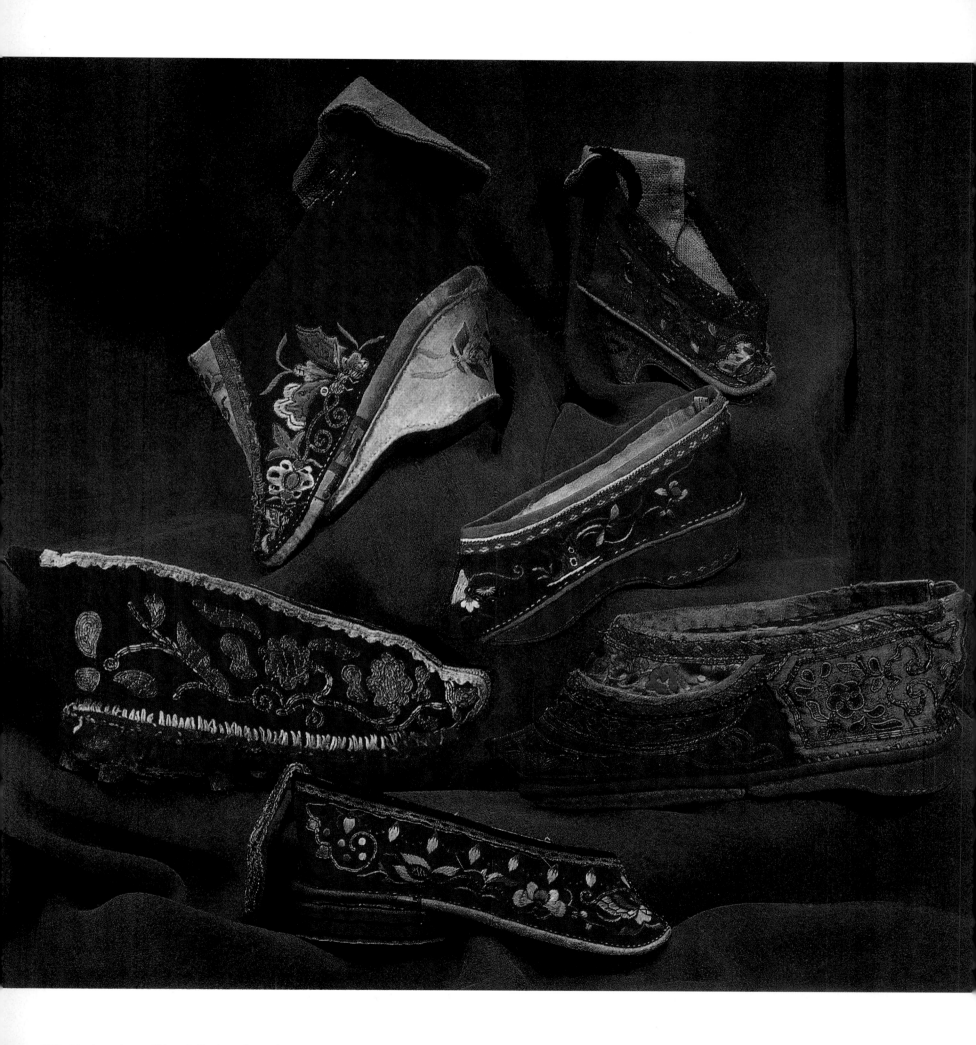

208. Marriage shoes. China. Collection of Beverley Jackson.

During the Ming dynasty (late 16th-mid 17th century), foot deformation was an integral part of Chinese culture; this custom became prevalent, circulating through all levels of society. It was beginning with the Ming dynasty that the practice was adopted for clearly erotic or aphrodisiac purposes in the art of hiding and revealing the foot. A Chinese woman who showed a bare foot in public was committing an indecent assault. This is why Catholic missionaries caused a scandal in the late 19th-century when they spread images of the Virgin with bare feet, Our Lady of Lourdes.

To avoid a clash of civilizations, they had to order more appropriate iconography from the West. In 1664, imperial edicts forbid women of the Manchurian dynasty to deform their feet under penalty of death. The emperor Kangxi (1662-1722) imposed a total ban on foot binding for girls born after 1662. A father or husband who broke this law would be punished by eighty blows with a stick, and then exiled three thousand lilies (about one thousand five hundred kilometers). Nevertheless, the decree was ineffectual and Kangxi had to repeal it. When the same prohibition was reintroduced in 1694, Manchurian women responded by adopting a different shoe style.

Under the soles of their shoes made for normal feet, they attached a two-inch high support covered in silk, a trick barely visible under their pants. In this way they were able to imitate the unsteady, but charming walk of deformed feet, creating the perfect illusion. Foot binding led to a number of private superstitions and beliefs among the Chinese.

Above all, for the wellborn, foot binding was necessary preparation for a good marriage; failure to perform this custom condemned a girl to being single. The initial binding was usually performed with some ceremony. The child's mother would place a pair of embroidered shoes and some strips on an altar to Zaojun, "god of the hearth." An experienced and virtuous woman would be invited to come officiate several days later.

After god's help was invoked, the first wrapping was applied while the young girl held in her hands a small water chestnut or a little brush and recited her prayer. She asked for feet as sweet and as smooth as the water chestnut and as fine as the brush. On her wedding day, the bride wore shoes embroidered with sayings such as "one hundred years of happiness" or "health and wealth until white-haired."

In northern China, husbands were given miniature shoe-shaped cookies symbolizing concord and harmony. Lotus-shaped shoes for the wives meant "a succession of sons." In central China, engaged couples took their vow of "until death do us part" by exchanging their shoes.

Finally, four pairs of embroidered slippers were part of a bride's dowry, a guarantee of a lasting marriage. After the wedding, the young woman carefully put them away. The most surprising beliefs are associated with women's shoes used as treatments by Chinese doctors to cure various illnesses.

For example, an effective cure for tuberculosis consisted of wearing three pairs of a young bride's slippers until they were totally worn out. For a daughter-in-law to offer her slippers to her sick mother-in-law was a very thoughtful gesture; in particular it demonstrated great filial piety, which her husband would never forget if he later wanted to repudiate his wife.

According to Tan Sivy, in his thesis, "The golden lotus, or little Chinese feet," in the late 19th-century there was a doctor in Huang named Song You who healed the sick by using shoes as a remedy. Many students followed his teachings. The writer Yao Lingx affirms it:

"Fevers: apply a small slipper firmly over the patient's navel. The fever will leave the patient through this orifice and go into the shoe. Cholera: boil the sole of a young virgin's slipper until the liquid becomes thick. Have the patient drink the beverage while it is still hot."

At the start of the Ming dynasty, in the late 14th century, the town of Datong in Shanxi carved out a reputation for itself throughout the Empire for having women with beautiful feet.

Under the Qing, a new style of binding was introduced that became standard until the waning of the Empire. Lévy H.S. describes it clearly in his book, Chinese Footbinding, the history of a curious erotic custom: "…smooth and soft at once, tiny and pointed, the very mention of the Datong foot stirred the soul of aesthetes."

Beginning in the 19th-century, the town organized an annual foot beauty contest that quickly spread to most other large towns, usually taking place within Buddhist pagodas. The contest drew several hundred candidates and attracted a crowd of admirers who came from afar. Old Chinese who were eyewitnesses at the beginning of the-century, describe the scene:

"The competitors were seated with their legs extended on small stools. Their shoes were decorated with pearls, little bells, and silk butterflies. Spectators came and went in groups, criticizing, admiring, and making their preferences known out loud, but they weren't allowed to touch the feet or the shoes."

Winners, according to witnesses, merrily joined the harems of wealthy and powerful men. And it is even said that some women over age sixty, with ugly, wrinkled faces, surpassed much younger contestants. Practiced until the end of the Empire, theses contests disappeared after the prohibition of foot binding declared by the republican government in 1913. How was mutilation achieved?

Deliberately induced, irreversible deformation was inflicted upon little girls from childhood. Their feet were bound in a progressive and continuous manner. At first the binding would be rather loose, but then the tension would be gradually increased. The binding was replaced at least every two days, and each time the foot was left bare for a few moments in order to wash it and rub it with sorghum alcohol to prevent infection. To obtain a foot in greater conformity to the fashion's canonical version, a semi-cylindrical metal piece sized in proportion to the foot was placed under the arch before bandaging was applied. The young girl continued to bind her feet with regularity at the risk of loosing the effects of the treatment. When adulthood was reached, each foot measured approximately thirteen to sixteen centimeters.

The term "golden lotus" was reserved for feet less than nine centimeters; feet longer than ten centimeters only rated a "silver lotus."

The deformity achieved by foot binding lead to the creation of special shoes; courtesans especially wore red shoes. Catholic missionaries later helped put an end to foot binding, although in 1900 Chinese women of all social classes still observed the custom, more frequently in the town than in the country. The fashion still lingered in 1948 in spite of prohibitions.

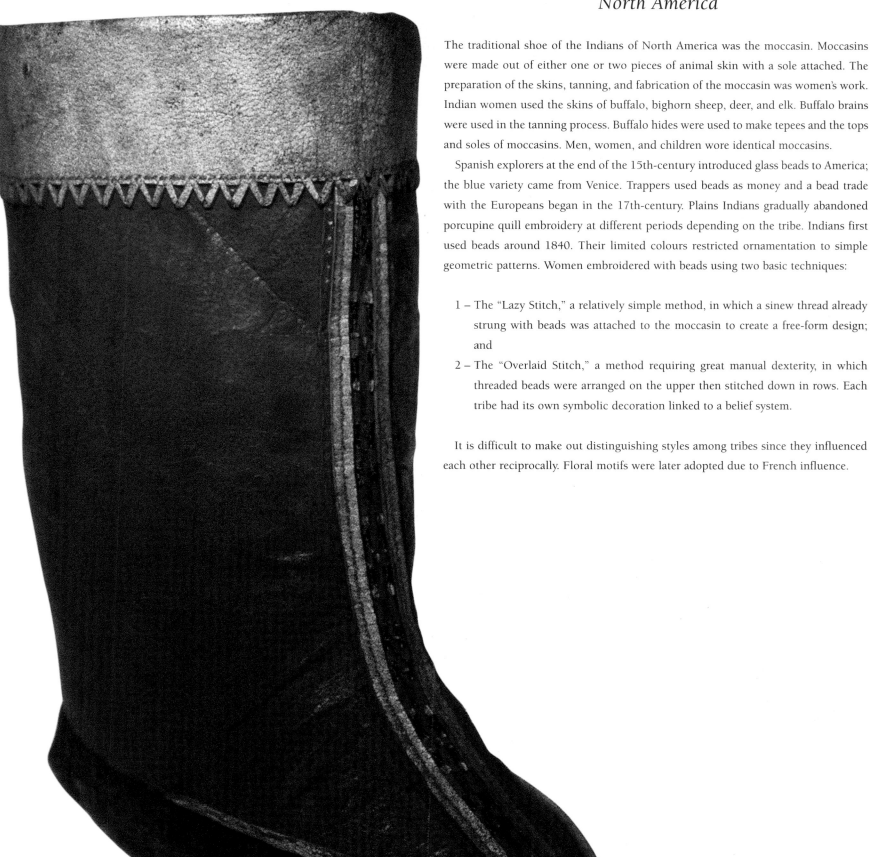

North America

The traditional shoe of the Indians of North America was the moccasin. Moccasins were made out of either one or two pieces of animal skin with a sole attached. The preparation of the skins, tanning, and fabrication of the moccasin was women's work. Indian women used the skins of buffalo, bighorn sheep, deer, and elk. Buffalo brains were used in the tanning process. Buffalo hides were used to make tepees and the tops and soles of moccasins. Men, women, and children wore identical moccasins.

Spanish explorers at the end of the 15th-century introduced glass beads to America; the blue variety came from Venice. Trappers used beads as money and a bead trade with the Europeans began in the 17th-century. Plains Indians gradually abandoned porcupine quill embroidery at different periods depending on the tribe. Indians first used beads around 1840. Their limited colours restricted ornamentation to simple geometric patterns. Women embroidered with beads using two basic techniques:

1 – The "Lazy Stitch," a relatively simple method, in which a sinew thread already strung with beads was attached to the moccasin to create a free-form design; and
2 – The "Overlaid Stitch," a method requiring great manual dexterity, in which threaded beads were arranged on the upper then stitched down in rows. Each tribe had its own symbolic decoration linked to a belief system.

It is difficult to make out distinguishing styles among tribes since they influenced each other reciprocally. Floral motifs were later adopted due to French influence.

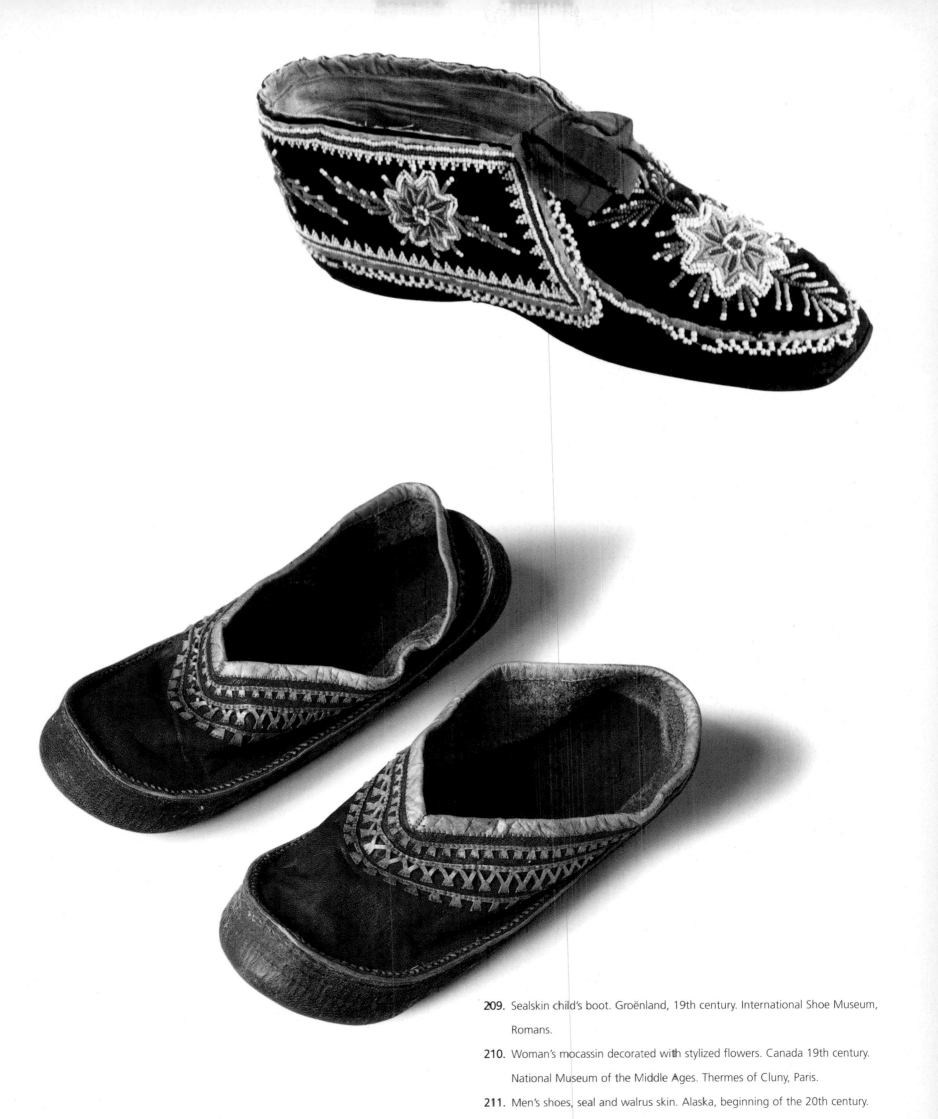

209. Sealskin child's boot. Groënland, 19th century. International Shoe Museum, Romans.

210. Woman's mocassin decorated with stylized flowers. Canada 19th century. National Museum of the Middle Ages. Thermes of Cluny, Paris.

211. Men's shoes, seal and walrus skin. Alaska, beginning of the 20th century.

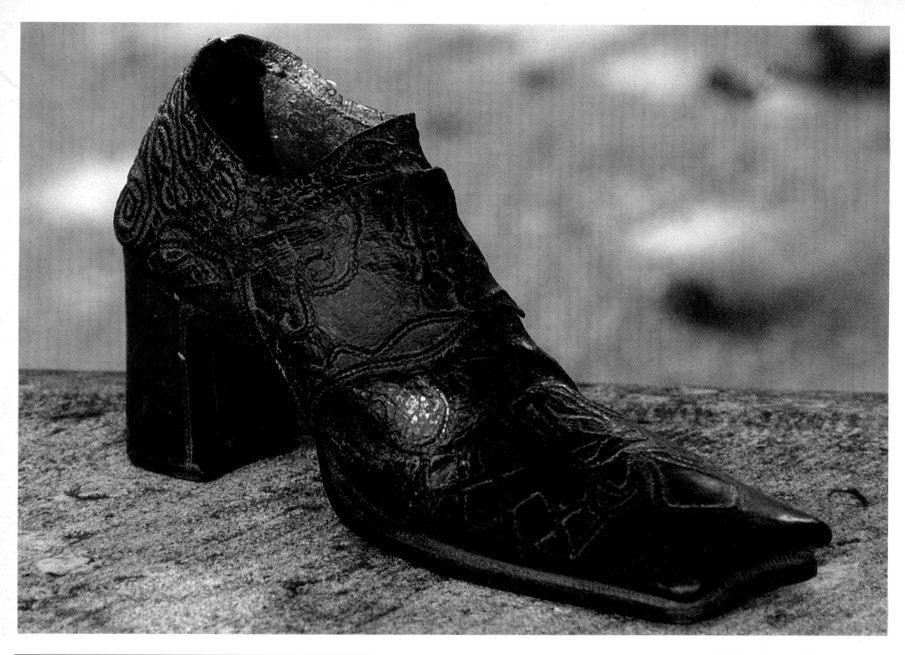

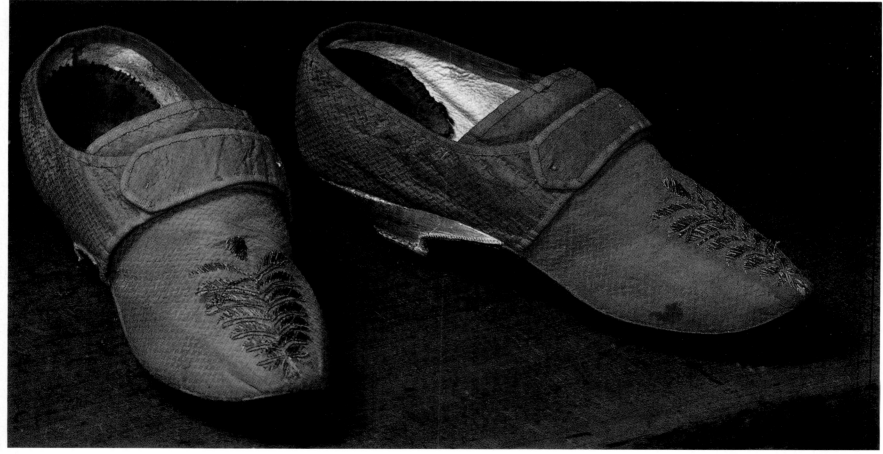

Shoes Worn by Celebrities

Shoe of Henry II de Montmorency

Henry II de Montmorency was the grandson of Anne de Montmorency, supreme commander of the French army, Marshal of France, and advisor to kings Francis I and Henry II. The last representative of this illustrious family's older branch and the nephew of king Henry IV, Henry II de Montmorency added to his family's prestigious appointments: Admiral of France and Brittany, viceroy of New France, and finally, governor of Languedoc after his father's resignation in 1613. The scepter of Marshall awarded his military victories. But Gaston d'Orléans convinced him to rise up against Languedoc; his impudent revolt against Cardinal Richelieu led to his imprisonment at Castelnaudary. Abandoned by Monsieur, the king's brother, as Gaston d'Orléans was called, de Montmorency was condemned to death and beheaded in Toulouse in 1632. His leather shoe, preserved at the International Shoe Museum, is monogrammed and decorated with a fleur-de-lis on top of the upper. It is evidence of the type of virtuoso shoemaking that existed during the first half of the 17th century.

Madame de Pompadour's Shoes
Or the triumph of the heel under Louis XV

These low-heeled shoes in yellow silk embroidered with silver thread and with a slightly raised toe have lost their buckles and show some wear. They come from the estate of Madame de Pompadour who left them to her personal maid.

The seated portrait of Madame de Pompadour, painted by François Boucher in 1758 and now in the Victoria and Albert Museum, shows her crossed feet dressed in new shoes embellished with a substantial buckle, probably of silver. In Boucher's standing portrait of Madame de Pompadour in the Wallace Collection, her right foot is hidden by her yellow dress, but the left foot, dressed in a heeled shoe fastened with a buckle, is similar to the example found in the International Shoe Museum, Romans. A third portrait by Boucher, in the collection of Maurice de Rothschild, highlights Madame de Pompadour's sumptuous pink mules. These shoes have raised tips in the oriental style and are enhanced by elaborate decoration on the upper, which is also trimmed with a meridian coil running lengthwise and bordered with shirred fabric. The high heel covered in white leather is a typical example of a Louis XV heel. These pink shoes create a visual echo of delightful harmony with the pink ornaments on Madame de Pompadour's green dress. Quentin de la Tour's pastel portrait preserved at the Louvre Museum depicts beautiful pink mules that are rather similar, but the ornamentation is simplified.

As she displays her own shoes in these four portraits, Madame de Pompadour, who was famous for her elegance, perfectly illustrates which women's shoes where fashionable during the reign of Louis XV: shoes fastened with a buckle and mules. Mules with Louis XV heels (still a commonly used term) would experience a considerable vogue and are still fashionable in the 21st century. The technical dictionary of the shoe industry written by Louis Rama, an authority in the matter, defines the Louis XV heel as follows: "Louis XV heel: a high heel, much knocked down by a concave profile; the throat is covered by an extension of the sole obtained by splitting called the heel breast flap." Although methods of heel manufacture and styles have definitely evolved over time, the concept of the Louis XV heel, elaborated in the 18th century, remains unchanged. It is still a heel with an evocative name, whose very mention calls forth the symbol of eternal femininity.

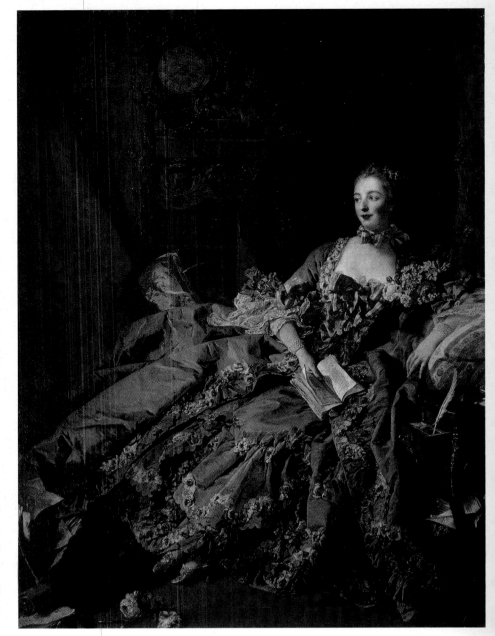

212. Shoe having belonged to Henri II de Montmorency. Leather decorated with a fleur de lis on the vamp. Initials of the duke on the flap. France, 17th century. International Shoe Museum, Romans.

213. Shoe of the Marchioness of Pompadour. International Shoe Museum, Romans, dépôt of the National Museum of the Middle Ages, Thermal Baths of Cluny in Paris.

214. François Boucher. *Portrait of the Marchioness of Pompadour.* Alte Pinakothek, Munich.

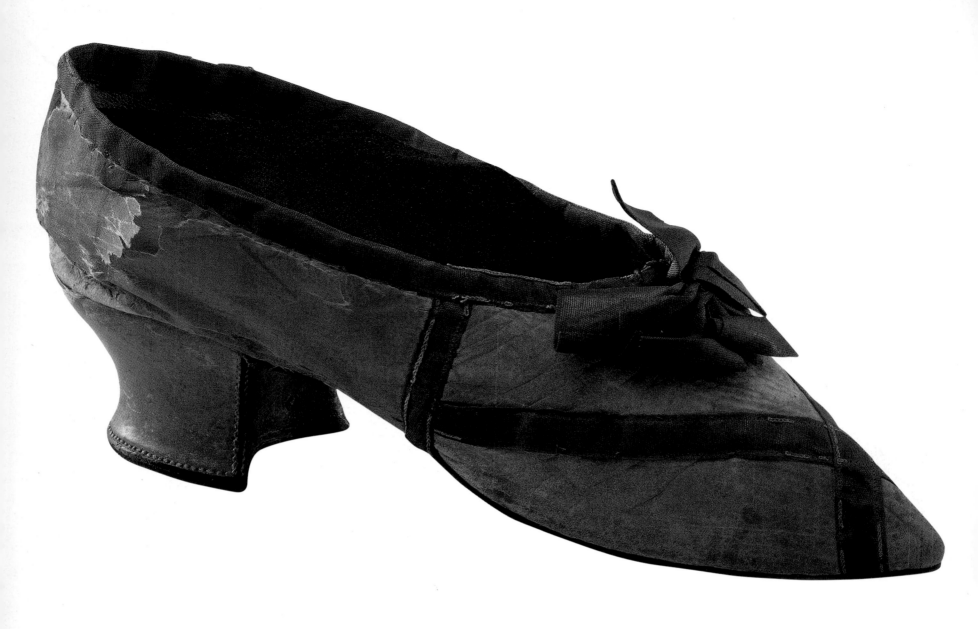

The Shoe of Marie-Antoinette

Attributed to the Queen, this shoe was found at the base of a guillotine at the place de la Révolution in Paris on October 16, 1793. It was sold the same day for one louis to the Count of Guernon-Ranville, who immediately turned it into a relic.

The interior bears a handwritten inscription inserted like an innersole:

"Shoe worn by Queen Marie-Antoinette on that horrible day she mounted the scaffold, this shoe was picked up by an individual the moment the queen died and immediately purchased by Monsieur le Comte de Guernon-Ranville."

As André Castelot writes in his book on Marie-Antoinette (1):

"She hurried and climbed the steep ladder with such haste (with bravado said one witness) that she lost one of her little plum Saint Huberty shoes."

According to the account of Rosalie Lamorlière, the Queen's personal maid at the Temple, Marie-Antoinette went to her execution wearing plum shoes with two-inch heels (they measured two pouces or about six centimeters) in the Saint Huberty style. The style was named after the opera performer who started the trend. This shoe could be of silk or leather.

215. Shoe of Marie-Antoinette collected the 10th of August 1792.

Anonymous, Carnavalet Museum, Paris.

216. Shoe of the parish priest of Ars. International Shoe Museum, Romans.

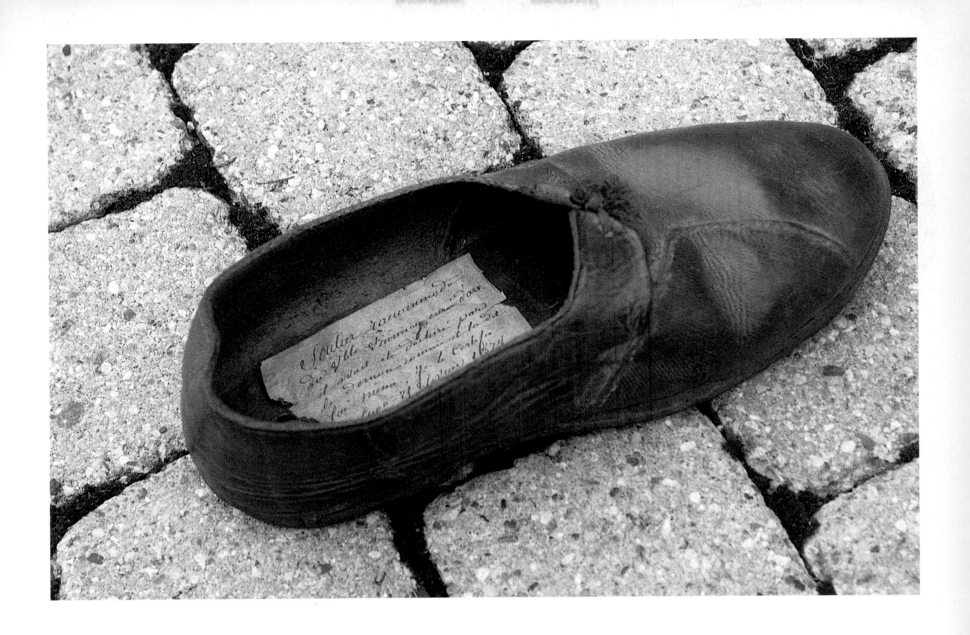

Shoes of Saint-Jean-Marie Vianney,

Parish Priest of Ars

Jean-Marie Vianney, the fourth child in a humble farming family, was born on May 8, 1786, in Dardilly in the vicinity of Lyons. As a child he tended flocks with other peasant children his age, but stood out through his kindness and devotion. Responding to God's call, he entered the seminary. Threatened with being sent back because he lacked an aptitude for study, Jean-Marie Vianney was finally ordained at age twenty-nine.

Appointed parish priest of Ars, a small village located thirty-five kilometers from Lyon, he practiced his ministry there until his death. People came rushing from all over France to confess to Father Vianney and to listen to his catechisms and sermons, which were delivered straightforwardly with examples from everyday life. He often spent sixteen hours a day behind the confessional and said the rosary every evening. His tireless zeal for charity and kindness was coupled with great austerity in living. Sleeping four hours at night, contenting himself with a frugal diet, and wearing a patched cassock, the priest imposed the severest penance upon himself.

Like many saints, he engaged in heroic combat against the Devil, who shook his doors, knocked around his furniture, tried to throw him out of his bed, and even set upon his shoes and tore them apart.

A crude, worn leather shoe preserved in a private collection affirms this, as we read on a document written by the shoe repairman: "Repaired shoe of the actual Priest of Ars. It had been torn apart by the Devil, as he himself said. I certify it in Lyon, February 21, 1875."

This extremely modest cleric, long scorned by his brethren, was promoted against his wishes to the dignity of Canon. Napoleon awarded him the Legion of Honor, again against the priest's wishes.

The Bishop of Belley started the canonical proceedings in 1866. Pius X declared him blessed in 1905. In 1925, Pope Pius XI proclaimed him Saint and Patron of Parish Priests. This humble country priest is now world famous. On October 5, 1986, Pope Jean-Paul II personally visited Ars as a formal tribute to Saint-Jean-Marie Vianney.

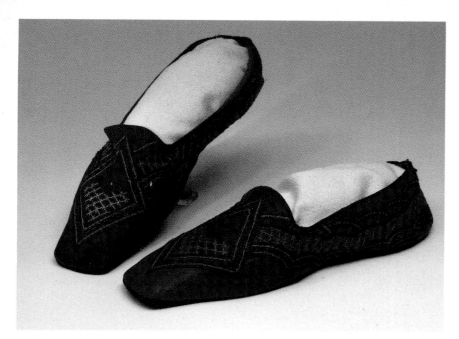

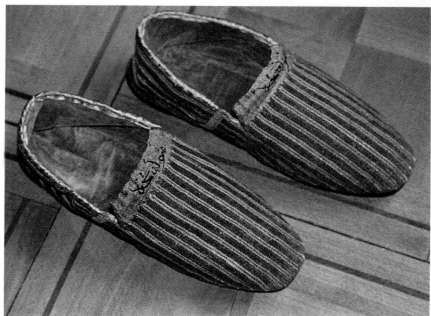

Gœthe's Slippers

Marianne de Willemer secretly prepared a Christmas present that she was saving to give her friend Gœthe on December 25, 1816. Two letters addressed to the writer's son, Auguste, which she signed by the fitting pseudonym, "the baby Jesus," reveal the playful way in which she went about it.

"I intend to send your father a pair of slippers from above. Saint Catherine and Saint Theresa are ready to take on the work, but they must be absolutely sure about his size. Would you kindly have your father's shoemaker cut an exact pattern of the upper and send it to me in Frankfurt where I am attending to business.

If the shoemaker is unskilled and does not know how to draw, a slipper your father doesn't wear anymore or which no longer suits him will do just as well, as long as it still fits him. I will ask Saint Crispin to make a new pair. I hope that you will keep my secret and that you will reveal nothing of my plan to your father or anybody else."

On December 20, 1816, she sent Auguste a package accompanied by another letter. "Thank you for handling my errand so well and best wishes for your birthday, which is the same day as mine. Please open the small box that will probably arrive in Weimar Monday evening or Tuesday morning and give your father the slippers and the little picture it contains on Christmas Eve and light a few candles (because the light is my element)." In a letter dated December 31, Gœthe replied to Marianne de Willemer.

"Admittedly the baby Jesus has been especially well disposed towards me this year, but he couldn't stop himself from making some mischief. Although a man must kiss the Pope's slipper because it bears a cross and caress the feet of his beloved to symbolize his complete abandonment to her will, it is incredible that someone can use magic symbols to make a decent person venerate his own shoes, in this way forcing him into uncommon moral and physical contortions."

The band around the uppers on these famous slippers bore the name Suleika in Persian script, behind which was hidden the name Marianne de Willemer, the poet's muse who inspired his poems in the *West-Eastern Divan*. This literary figure's real attraction to the female foot and its accessory, the shoe, was no secret. As he wrote to one of his girl friends: "Send me your last pair of shoes as soon as possible so that I can have something of yours to press against my heart."

217. Slipper of Emperor Franz-Joseph of Austria. Ledermuseum, Offenbach.

218. Slippers of Goethe. Bally Museum, Schönenwerd, Switzerland.

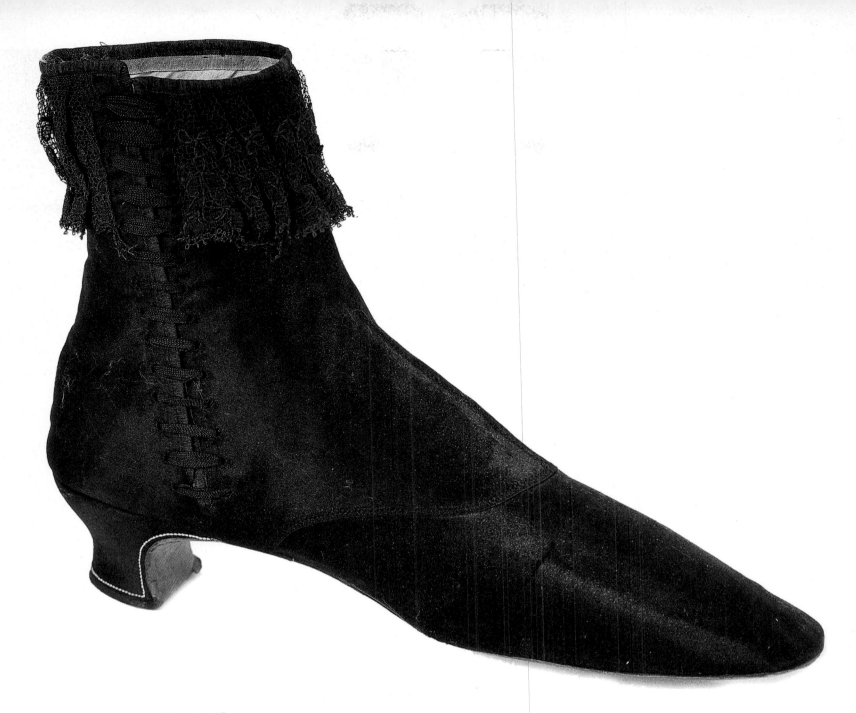

Sissi's Shoes

The life of Elisabeth von Wittelsbach, princess of Bavaria better known by her first name Sissi (immortalized in film by actress Romy Schneider), took on a fairy tale quality the moment she became engaged to her cousin, German Emperor Franz-Joseph of Austria. Almost immediately, the First Lady of the Empire came up against the hostility of her mother-in-law, Archduchess Sophie. Stuck in the restraints of a rigid and old-fashioned protocol dating back to Charles V, Sophie imposed this manner of dress on the princess. This etiquette required the Empress to wear a new pair of shoes everyday. She refused. The domestic supplier was outraged, losing an important revenue source. (Nevertheless, at one time an inventory listed one hundred and thirteen pairs of shoes in the Empress's wardrobe!) Meanwhile, sharp-tongued ladies-in-waiting criticized the Empress for going horseback riding too often, repeating their concerns to the ladies of the court, and even to the despised maids, that grooms and passers-by could not keep their eyes off her Majesty's ankles when she mounted a horse. The Empress's radiant beauty and her agile walk made her one of the most attractive women of her era. It was while walking with a quick step on the quai du Mont Blanc in Geneva on her way to the steam ship line that Sissi met her fate at age sixty-one, struck down by an assassin named Luigi Lucheni, an Italian anarchist.

219. Bottines of Sissi Empress of Austria. 19th century.

Ledermuseum, Offenbach.

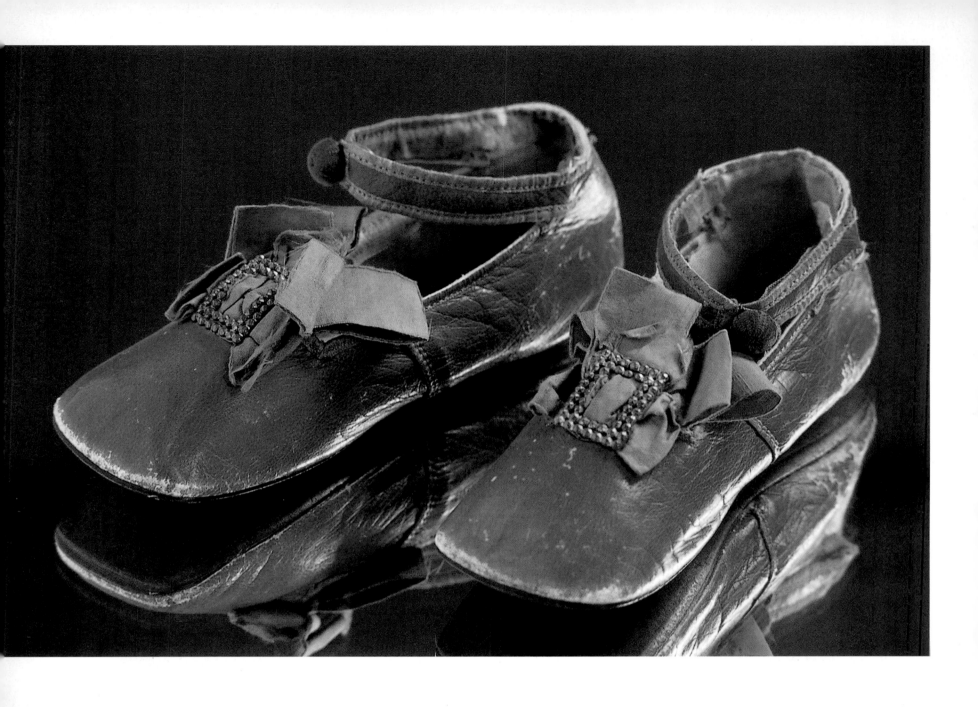

Shoes of the Countess of Castiglione
(Florence 1837-Paris 1899)

Born in Florence in 1837, Virginia Oldani came from an old, noble Genoese family. In 1854 she married Count François Verasis, equerry to the Sardinian King Victor Emmanuel II. Her beauty soon made her Turin's idol. The king's minister Cavour got the idea of using her beauty for diplomatic purposes and sent her the court of Emperor Napoleon. Her mission was to seduce Napoleon into joining the cause of Italian unity and obtain the support of the French government. She became his mistress in 1856 and facilitated the Emperor's decision to form an alliance with the Piedmontese. This beautiful woman, who was also a strange narcissist, sat for the photographers Mayer and Pierson. Both prominent photographers in the capital, they excelled in the art of flattering portraiture through a highly perfected technique, which they used to photograph the Second Empire's political, artistic, and social elite.

The Countess also asked Pierson to photograph her legs and feet. The resulting photograph sent an erotic message in no uncertain terms. It was an image perfectly consistent with the male fantasies of the period, which were fixated on this part of the female anatomy, normally protected from lustful glances under crinoline.

220. Slippers of Prince Imperial Jean-Joseph-Eugene-Louis Napoleon.

International Shoe Museum, Romans.

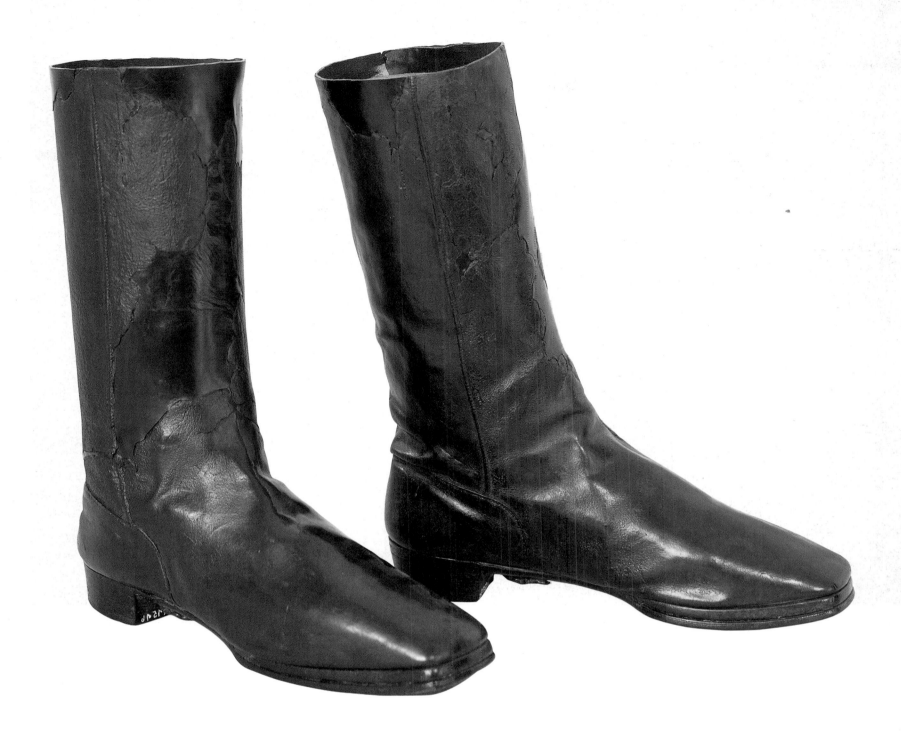

A photograph by Disderi shows her with her legs in clingy white stockings, her right foot dressed in a buttoned ankle boot with a bobbin heel placed on a footstool. Virginia moreover liked to take her shoes off in public and offered her bare feet for her admirers' contemplation. This eccentric figure went so far as having casts made of her feet, of which two examples exist. These terra cottas may be the work of Carrier-Belleuse, a sculptor especially known for his casts.

The International Shoe Museum, Romans, has a pair of sumptuous apartment mules attributed to the Countess. They are of purple velvet embroidered with gold thread and fine pearls with a gold lamé heel; the shoes bear the following label: J.A. Petit women's shoes, 334 rue Saint-Honoré Paris, 134 Regent Street London. These shoes are a good example of Second Empire style, although their excessive decoration brings to mind the embroidery on Ottoman babouches from the same period.

221. Boots of William I of Prussia. 19th century.
Ledermuseum, Offenbach.

Shoes Worn by Louis Pasteur

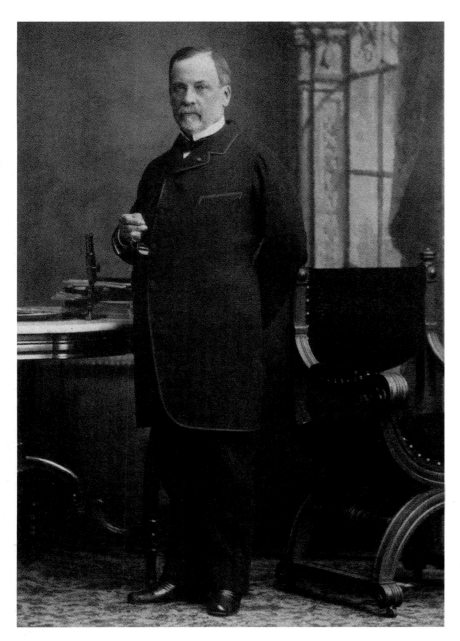

The son of an artisan tanner, Louis Pasteur was born in Dole, the administrative center of the Jura, in 1822. An illustrious French chemist and biologist, this great scientist is internationally known for discovering the rabies vaccine.

As Annick Perrot, Conservator of the Pasteur Museum, explains, Pasteur was a revolutionary in science, but led a conventional private life. His artistic tastes and lifestyle were typical for a 19th-century bourgeois. His clothing habits are telling.

For example, at age eighteen, a boarder at the Collège of Besançon, Louis Pasteur wrote the following to his parents on October 28, 1840:

"Take care of my little case Huguenet made for my boots."

During a trip to Strasbourg, he sent his wife a letter dated October 7, 1852:

"If I have any good shoes bring them to me. My shoes and my gaiters especially. Idem: patent leather shoes and boots…"

Another letter to his father dated January 29, 1856, contains an interesting anecdote:

"I have been very well since the beginning of winter wearing the clogs you sent me in Strasbourg. Apart from this head cold, which should pass in a couple of days or so, I have not been sick at all, especially with the type of stomach upset to which I am so prone; the slightest damp feet gives me a sudden case of diarrhea. I haven't had any attacks since coming back from vacation and I am sure that it's because I am wearing clogs."

Having dry feet will definitely keep you from getting sick, but this statement is amusing coming from the pen of a scientist like Pasteur.

The last seven years of his life Pasteur lived in a huge apartment within the Institute that bore his name. In 1937, it became a museum housing the scientist's furniture, personal possessions, art works, photographs, and even his shoes. The context of his life faithfully preserved in an emotionally charged atmosphere allows us to imagine Pasteur padding back and forth from his room to the bath in slippers made entirely of fine black felt: a testament to his last days? They appear to have been hardly used.

A second pair of solid burgundy, embroidered slippers may be the work of Madame Pasteur, who, like many young girls and women of her era, was an expert in needlework. Needlepoint on canvas in the shape of slippers was moreover very popular in the 19th-century. We can picture Madame Pasteur seated near the fireplace in the small third-floor sitting room pulling her needle, while her husband played cards with his friend Bertin.

The museum also has a pair of black woolen gaiters that fasten with seven small side buttons in addition to three pairs of black leather ankle boots, which Pasteur seems to have worn exclusively at the end of this life, even to the beach.

Two seemingly similar pairs of button ankle boots in black kid actually differ in several details. The first, fastened by six buttons, has the following label in the interior cloth lining near the leg:

"12 boulevard Saint-Michel 12 Marquer. Custom Shoemaker Paris."

These ankle boots match the ones shown in a photograph of Pasteur seated in the garden at the Institute. The second pair, without a label, is noteworthy for its seven-button closure.

222. Photograph of Louis Pasteur.

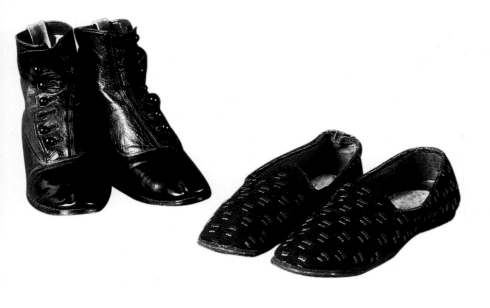

Ankle Boots of La Belle Otéro, a Belle Epoque Beauty

Beautiful women abounded in the decade before 1900 and the one that followed. But three famous courtesans in particular competed for star status during La Belle Epoque: Emilienne d'Alençon, Liane de Pougy, and La Belle Otéro, whose first name was Caroline.

A Spanish beauty, La Belle Otéro debuted at age twelve on the ramblas of Barcelona and then conquered Marseille where she danced at the Palais de Cristal. Her beauty caused a sensation provoking fights between audience members. Her career continued in Paris where her charms earned her a multitude of passionate admirers who ruined themselves to obtain her favors. Rather like a grasshopper among men, she gambled at the roulette table and recovered her losses by spending the night with old casino stooges who were as rich as they were ugly. She returned from one amorous escapade in Saint Petersburg with the necklaces of two empresses and one queen as souvenirs.

At her peak, she walked into Maxim's dressed to kill, while her rival Liane de Pougy, to mock her ostentation, arrived at the fashionable establishment, where it was tasteful to dine after the show, without a speck of jewelry, escorted by her personal maid bending under the weight of a cushion they all carried.

La Belle Otéro slummed at the Bal Mabille (a dance hall), lunched at Armenonville, paraded the Bois de Boulogne, and counted her conquests. Among the vanquished were William II, whom she fascinated, and other admirers who squandered fortunes on her beautiful eyes. Some men killed themselves after being ruined or rejected which led to the unfortunate honour of her being called the "suicide siren."

Yet, this woman from Andalusia who led the dumbest and most consuming lifestyle of all the Belles could actually sing and dance with talent. Mindful of maintaining her artistic reputation, before each opening she would run to light a candle in Notre-Dame-des-Victoires. After a triumphant music-hall version of Carmen, she turned down a contract with the Opéra Comique and retired while still beautiful at age forty-five.

Her fortune, estimated at five million in 1922, melted like snow on a summer day from gambling, putting an end to her expensive lifestyle. From her small mansion built in Nice, she downsized to average rooms in luxury hotels, sold off her "surplus" (for which she received almost nothing), and finally retired to a small room where she lived on a meager pension from the casino.

At age ninety-three, the elderly La Belle Otéro was still courted by a few old men who would come to dine in her room, bringing with them champagne and caviar.

Caroline Otéro died penniless in April 1965, despite several articles in the press that had attempted to bring her out of the shadows of anonymity. Today her ankle boots preserved in the International Shoe Museum, Romans, have rescued her from oblivion. They are fine examples of the art of the shoe during La Belle Epoque.

Additionally, these ankle boots have two five-centimeter pull-tabs in the front and rear of the opening so they could be pulled on with ease. Hemiplegic since the age of forty-six, it was difficult for Pasteur to dress and put his shoes on. A last pair of ankle boots, closed on both sides of the ankle by panels of elastic fabric, clearly represents the tone of fashion at the time and was certainly easier to get on than button ankle boots. As one approaches the stairs in the apartment often climbed by Pasteur, one notices the double handrails that were needed because of the scientist's paralysis and one can almost sense the echo of a slow-footed silhouette moving with difficulty. Carefully placed inside an armoire, his shoes are there to remind us of the "steps" taken by a great man at various moments in his life.

Having died in 1895, Pasteur now rests in the Institute's specially constructed funeral chapel on the first floor designed in the characteristic Byzantine style of the Symbolist period. A cartouche in the center of the vault contains a sentence extracted from Pasteur's acceptance speech to the Académie Française:

"Happy are they who carry God and an ideal of beauty within themselves and who live up to the ideals of art, science, country, and the teachings of the Gospel."

223. Shoes and slippers of Louis Pasteur.

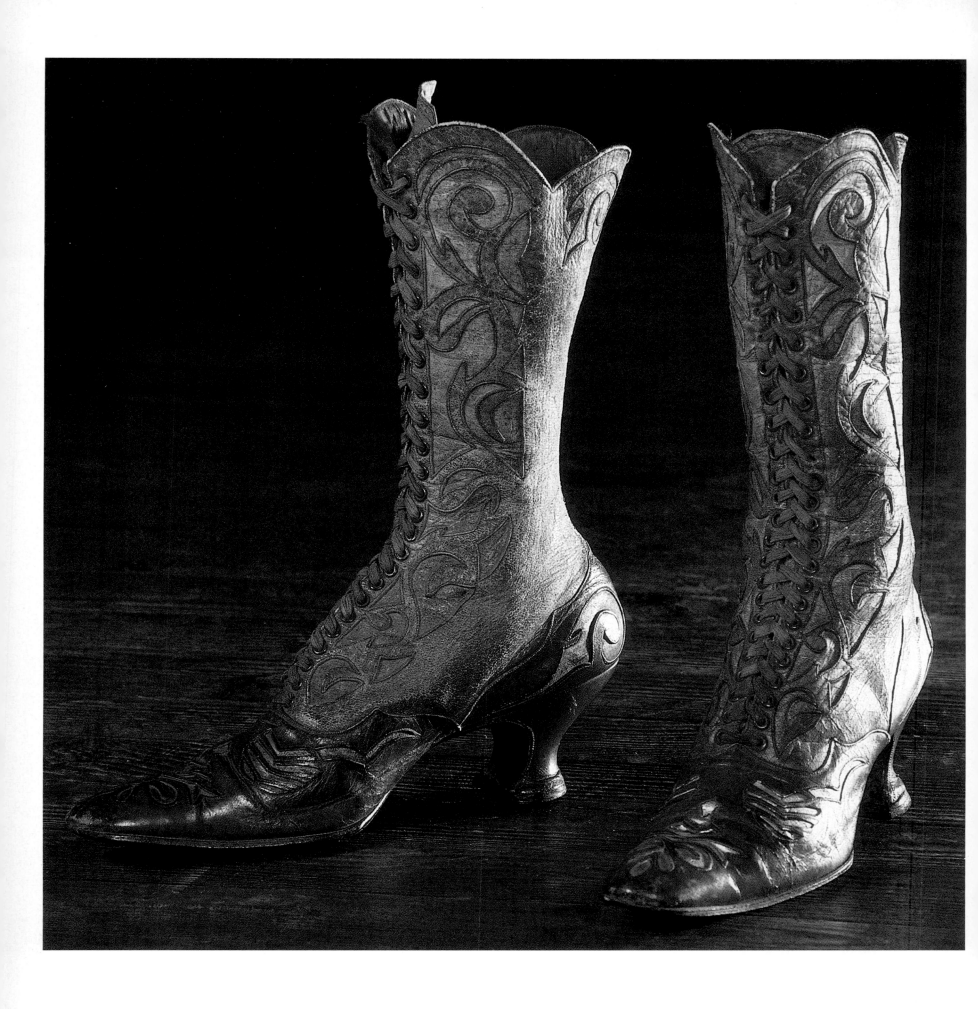

224. Bottines of the Belle Otéro. Brown and beige kidskin, silver kidskin inlays. Paris,

around 1900. International Shoe Museum, Romans.

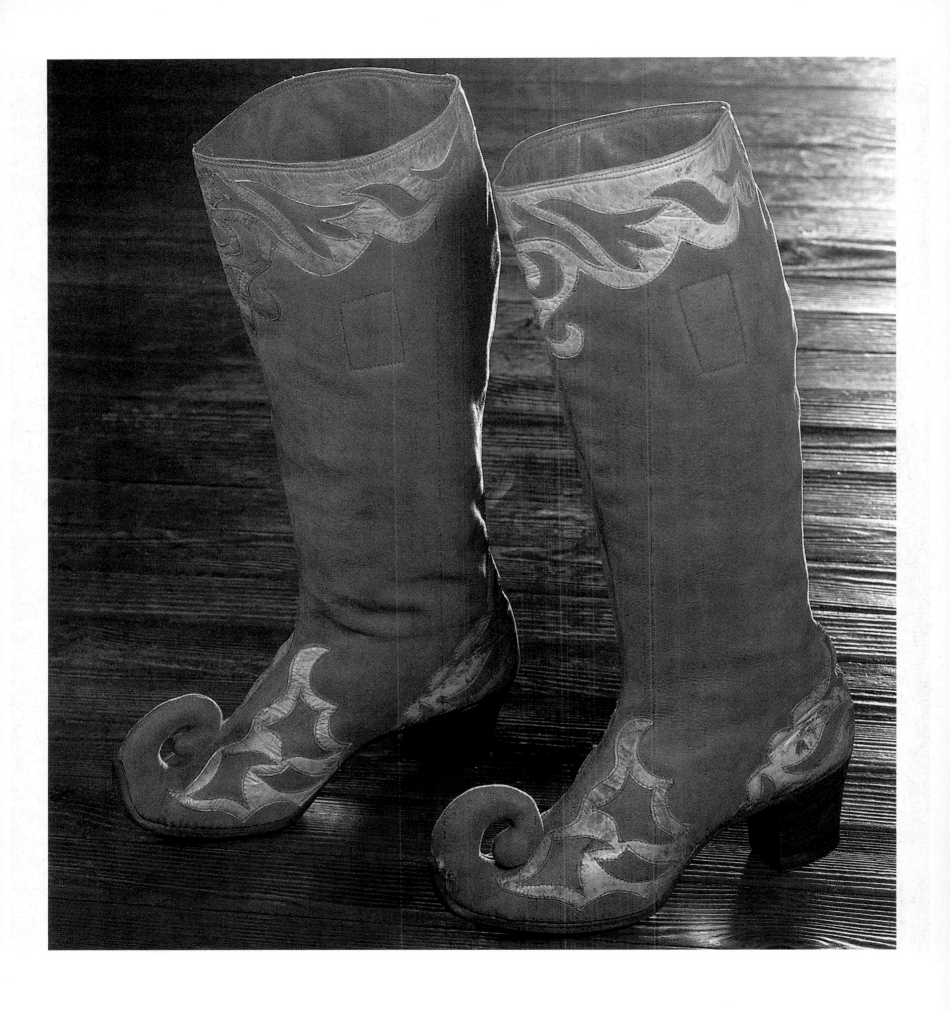

225. Boots of Ninon Vallin worn in *Marouf, the Shoemaker of Cairo*. Brown suede, applications of turquoise kidskin, eastern style roll at the end of the vamp. Around 1917. International Shoe Museum, Romans.

Boots Worn by Opera Singer Ninon Vallin

Once upon a time, there was a voice: "Mârouf, the Shoemaker of Cairo"

Born in 1886, in Montalieu, a village in the Dauphiné, Eugénie Vallin devoted herself to singing from a very young age. The child's talent quickly revealed itself in the choir of the parish church in the small community of Grand-Serre, located in the territorial division of the Drôme, where her father, a notary-lawyer, had just acquired an office in 1906. The Conservatory of Music in Lyon awarded her four prizes in 1910. Her soprano voice of exceptional range permitted her to have a spectacular and triumphant international career performing on the world's most prestigious stages. The International Shoe Museum, Romans, has a pair of oriental style boots worn by the famous opera singer at la Scala in Milan, 1917, in the opera "Mârouf, the Shoemaker of Cairo," by Henri Rabaud; she sang the role of Princess Saamcheddine.

Created by the Opéra Comique in Paris on May 15, 1914, this opera in five acts takes us to Cairo, to Khaïtan, and to the desert. It is the tale of the legendary adventures of a shoemaker practicing his craft in Egypt's capital.

Mârouf, predisposed to laziness, is unhappy at home. His wife, Fatimah, is unattractive, ill natured, and beats him, so Mârouf decides to take off. He gets in a shipwreck, but escapes unharmed. His friend, Ali, picks him up from the shore and takes him to Khaïtan, a big city legend places somewhere between China and Morocco. The humble shoemaker passes himself off as the world's richest merchant expecting a caravan full of marvels.

The Sultan himself invites him to the Palace and, in spite of the suspicions of the vizier, offers him the hand of his daughter, Princess Saamcheddine. Mârouf is living in luxury, frittering away his brother-in-law's money, when he confesses his hoax to his wife. The two lovers decide to flee and take refuge with a poor peasant at an oasis. As a way of thanking him for his hospitality, Mârouf then starts to work, helping the peasant with his field labour.

While pushing the plow, Mârouf strikes an iron ring, which raises up a trap door giving access to an underground chamber. What's more, the ring has magic powers; when the princess strokes it, the peasant turns into a genie who immediately places himself at the young couple's service and introduces them to an incredible treasure. When the Sultan and his guards catch up with the fugitives, the noise of an approaching caravan can be heard in the distance. Mârouf and the princess triumph, whereas the vizier is condemned to one hundred blows with a stick.

Hailed in the world's major capitals, Ninon Vallin was nothing like a diva. She regularly visited her native region and participated in the festivals of her village with a total lack of pretension.

This princess of singing died in Millery on November 22, 1961, on the feast of Saint Cecilia, patroness of musicians.

226. Shoes of Maurice Chevalier. Derby in navy blue suede, worn at the Théâtre des Champs-Elysées at the time of his farewell to the stage. International Shoe Museum, Romans.

Shoes Worn by Maurice Chevalier

"The Symphony of the Wooden Soles"

Maurice Chevalier's famous boater may have been an integral part of his character and repertoire (in the joyful refrain "with my boater hat"), but his shoes mostly went unnoticed. Nevertheless, his heirs donated a pair to the International Shoe Museum, Romans, in 1984 through the intermediary, photographer Jacques-Henri Lartigue. Derbies of navy blue suede labeled Bally Suisse, the artist last wore these shoes on stage; a photograph confirms this, showing Maurice Chevalier taking a bow on the stage of the Théâtre des Champs Elysées, on October 1, 1968, in the same shoes.

Born in Paris in 1888, the screen actor and popular singer was Mistinguett's partner at the Folies Bergères and triumphed at the Casino of Paris. A great boardwalk and music hall professional, he successfully interpreted many songs, such as the Symphony of the Wooden Soles, from 1945:

"I love the tap tap of wooden soles
It makes me gay, it makes me oh how can I say
When I hear this rhythm so strong
Into my heart comes a song
Tap tap says good morning
Little shoes from fir trees
Tap tap tap time to wake up, get out of bed, and go to work,
Romantic young things seem to tap dance as they walk
And all day long we hear the eloquent sound
What a charming racket thousands of little shoes make
Now women are charming
To the tip of their toes
I love the tam tam of the wooden soles
It makes me happy it makes me so oh how can I say
When I hear this rhythm so strong
Into my heart comes a song
Tap tap tap is the refrain
Of the busy street
Tap tap tap the symphony
Of beautiful days with less patent-leather
It clacks, it vibrates, and it sounds more joy than a honking horn
It's the Parisian rhythm of the happy shoe
Its sings of life full of vigor and fun
It's euphoria gets under your skin
I love the tap tap of the wooden soles
It makes me happy, it makes me so oh how can I say
When I hear this rhythm so strong
Into my heart comes a song
It's wonderful! How wonderful!
It's really wonderful!"

Through his carefully chosen vocabulary the songwriter recreates the echo of the very specific noise made by the wooden-heeled shoes worn during the Second World War. Maurice Chevalier's gift for rhythmic cadences makes the song amusing and playful. It's a big tip of the hat to the ingenuity of shoemakers; they substituted raw materials in the face of a leather shortage during this period of our history and in the process launched a new style adapted to the circumstances.

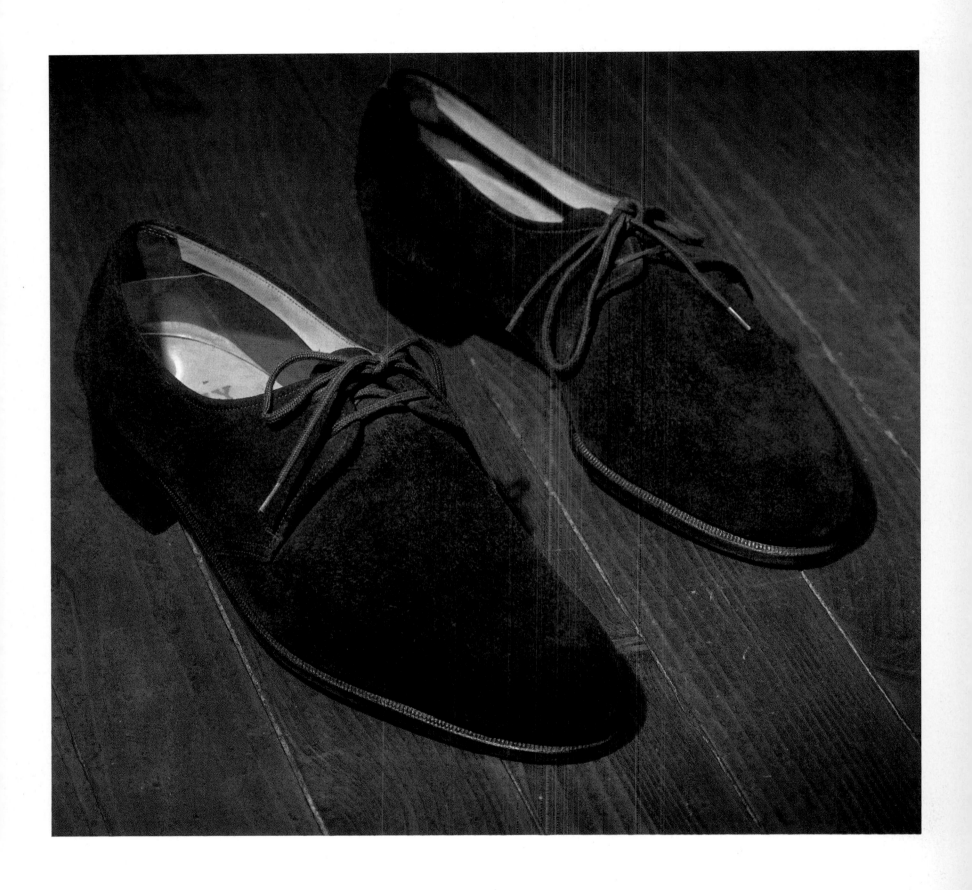

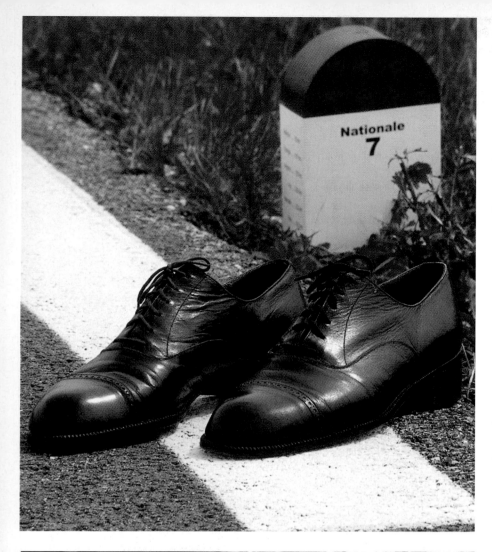

Shoes Worn by Charles Trenet
"Y a d'la joi!" ("Life is good!")

When Charles Trenet gave a recital in Romans on October 7, 1990, he promised to donate his stage shoes to the International Shoe Museum, Romans. After his death on June 21, 2001, the executors of his estate made the official presentation the day of the music festival.

They are unlabeled, comfortable shoes that aided and supported his sensitive feet, concealing the scar from a wound to his right foot dating to the Second World War. A Richelieu model with a black box, the style has a classic elegance that brings back memories when we look at it; the shoes seem to hum his songs, such as *La mer* (Beyond the Sea), *Douce France* (Sweet France), *Que reste-t-il de nos amours?* (What's Left of Our Love?), *Route Nationale 7* (Highway 7), *Revoir Paris* (To See Paris Again), *Le jardin extraordinaire* (The Amazing Garden), *Boum Boum* (Bang Bang), *Y a d'la joie!* (Life is Good) and others.

Now museum pieces, these shoes are back on stage as physical evidence of an immensely talented artist's career. They remind visitors that Charles Trenet, giant of the French chanson and immortal genius of international renown, created a hymn of life out of happiness.

Studio Shoes Worn by César (1921–1998)
Donated to the International Shoe Museum, Romans, by the artist.

The sculptor called "the Vulcan of modern times" by Edmonde Charles Roux, César Baldaccini was a member of Picasso's circle at a very young age. He wore clogs with wooden soles in his studio to weld and assemble the pieces of junk metal he found.

A private visit to the International Shoe Museum, Romans, captivated the sculptor, who marveled at shoe machines built from all different kinds of metal. The artist signed the visitor's book in a manner commensurate with his talent and his art: first, with a vigorous and rapid stroke of the pencil he drew a structure, then he drew the pump that appears on the ground behind a metal gate. The overall drawing has a sense of space and form.

In the adjoining office to his studio, on shelves next to his art books and mementos, the sculptor kept women's shoes. When a journalist who had come to interview him noticed the shoes, César explained, "I've just discovered a wonderful thing: the International Shoe Museum in Romans."

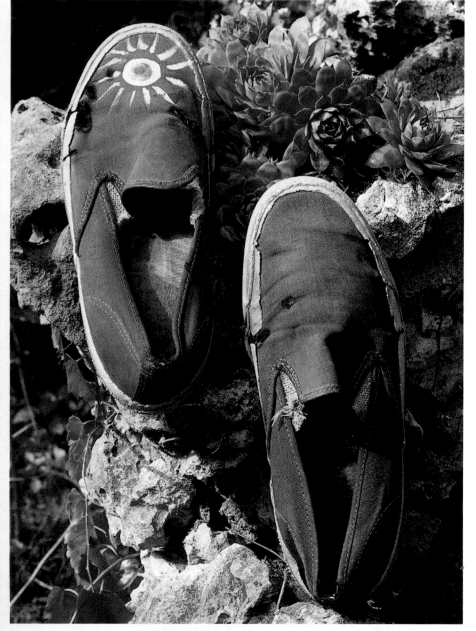

Shoes Worn by Jacques-Henri Lartigue
Painter and photographer (1894-1986)

The photographer who took Valéry Giscard d'Estaing's official portrait as President of the Republic, Jacques-Henri Lartigue was involved in photography at a very young age and exhibited as a painter from 1918. He illuminated his paintings with the sign of a painted sun in addition to his signature.

The same sun is reproduced on his rubber-soled canvas studio shoes donated to the International Shoe Museum, Romans, in 1983.

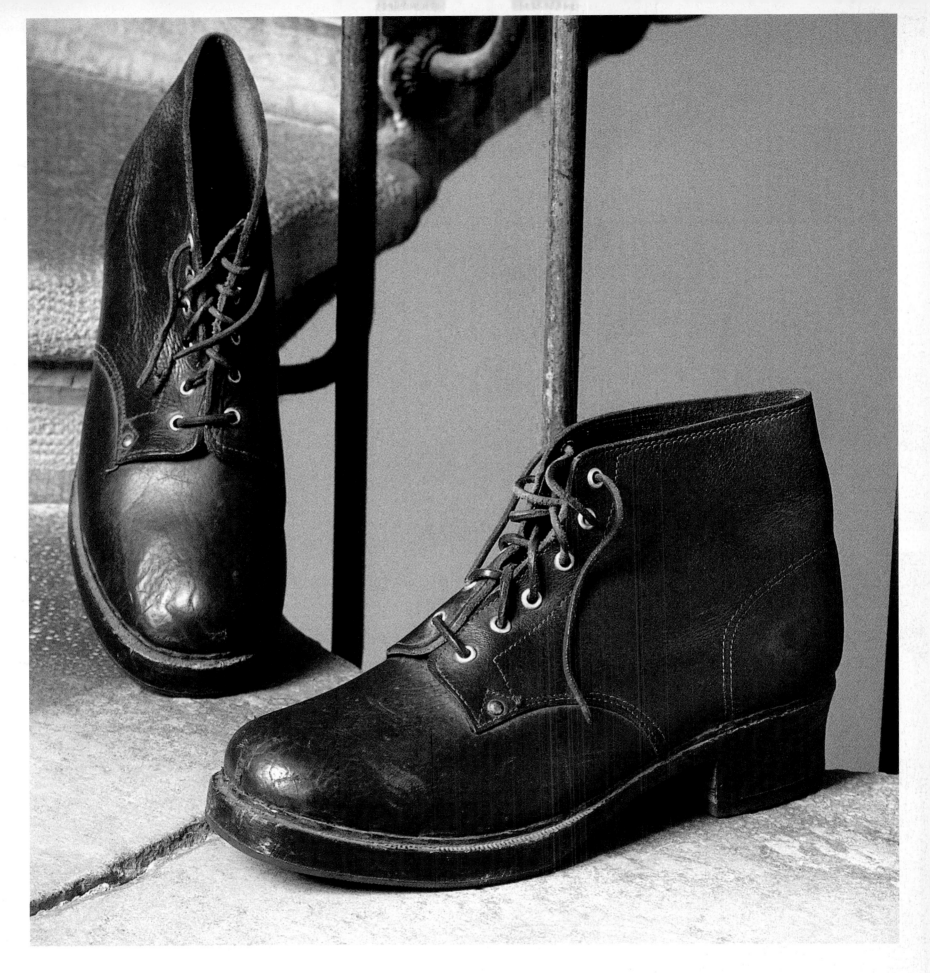

227. Shoes of Charles Trenet. International Shoe Museum, Romans.

Photo by Joël Garnier.

228. Shoes of Jacques-Henri Lartigue, photographer, 1980.

International Shoe Museum, Romans.

229. Shoes from the César workshop, clog in thick brown leather.

International Shoe Museum, Romans.

Mouna Ayoub:
The journey of a Haute Couture collector

Born in the Lebanese mountains, Mouna Ayoub became interested in the world of fashion at a very young age. As a child, she accompanied her mother to "Madame Juliette," a French couturier established in Sid El Bauchrié. Flipping through magazines at this design studio, she discovered the most beautiful styles of Dior, Paquin, Schiaparelli, Vionnet, and Saint Laurent.

At Madame Juliette's, Mouna also learned how to make clothes for her doll. It wasn't long before she shared her mother's unconditional admiration for Coco Chanel and began to dream of Paris, the international capital of elegance that set the tone for fashion and good taste.

After being educated by the Sisters of the Sacred Heart of Bikfaya, where she perfected her French, her studies lead her to Aix-en-Provence, Marseille, and Paris. She quickly developed an eye for fashion before the shop windows of avenue Montaigne and rue Cambon.

On February 1, 1978, she married a rich Saudi. For the occasion she wore a wedding gown designed by Jean-Louis Scherrer. Thenceforth she became a regular attendee of Haute Couture showings. Faithful to the most prestigious Paris firms, her watchful and expert eye also followed the young designers showing on Haute Couture's runways. Her significant and intelligent purchasing policy has made Mouna Ayoub the greatest private collector of Haute Couture. The sumptuous clothes she has collected with wonderful enthusiasm for over twenty years illustrate couture's superb craft traditions.

This extraordinary, ever expanding legacy also includes over one thousand pairs of shoes. During the 2001 autumn/winter season, a selection of her collection was the subject of an exhibition at the International Shoe Museum, Romans; mules, sandals, Charles IX, boots, bootees, ankle boots, Louis XV pumps, all entirely hand-made, represented ten years (1990 to 2000) of Raymond Massaro's work for Chanel. These shoes were shown to the cultural and sensory delight of visitors.

The exemplary patron, Mouna Ayoub, a true supporter of artistic creativity, facilitates the transfer of know-how from one generation to the next. As the talented embroiderer François Lesage explains: "If there were fifteen others like her, the future of Haute Couture would be absolutely assured."

230. Shoe of Mouna Ayoub,

International Shoe Museum, Romans.

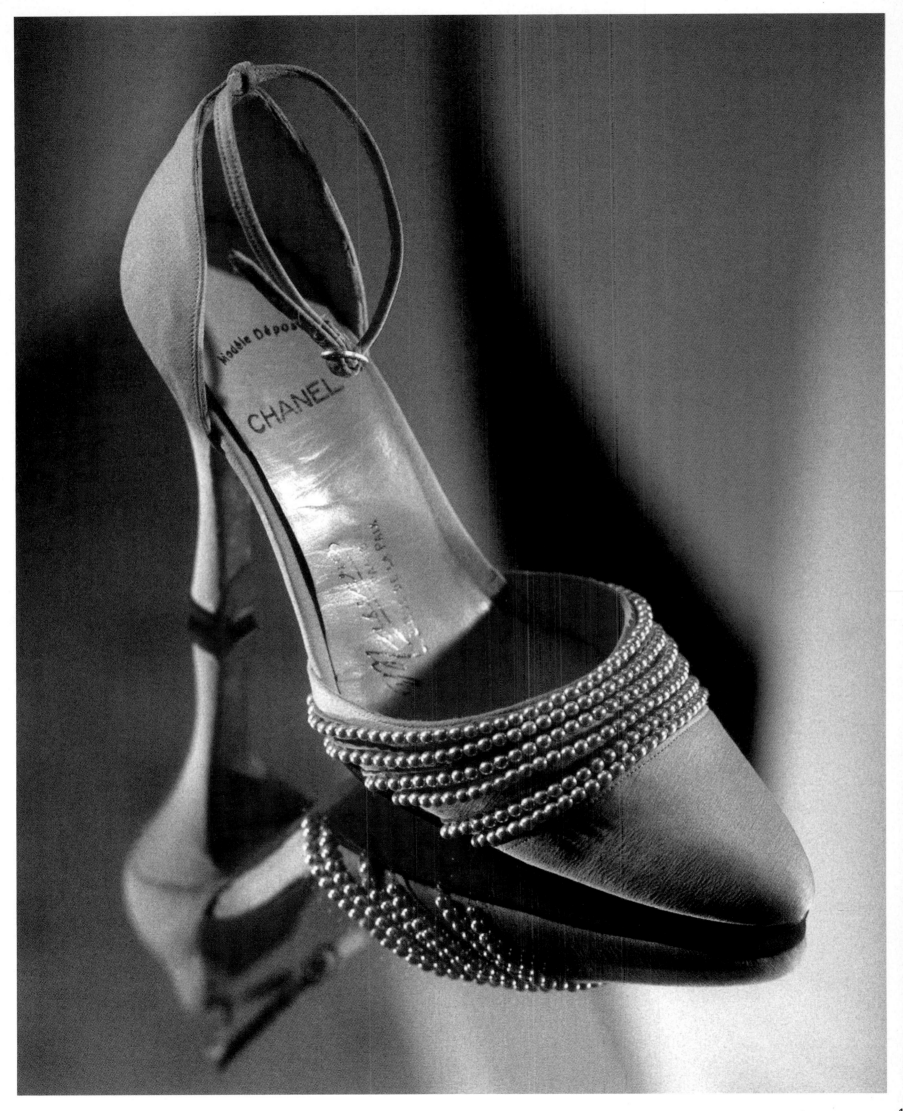

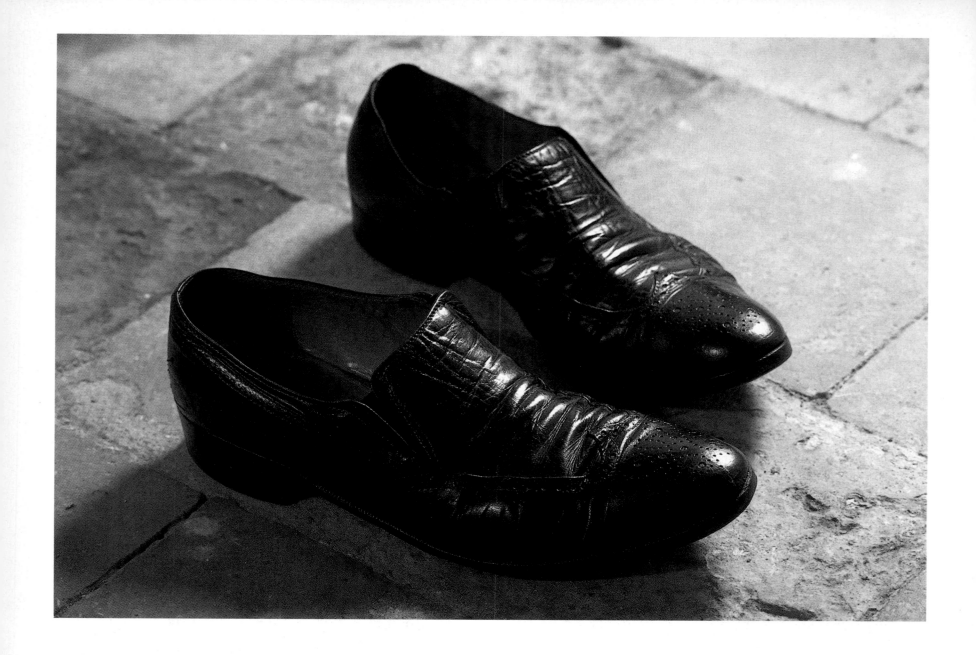

Shoes Worn by Paul Bocuse and Pierre Troisgros

1) Shoes of Paul Bocuse
2) Clogs of Pierre Troisgros

These two ambassadors of world-renown French gastronomy never cease innovating within their great culinary tradition.

Paul Bocuse wore black kid moccasins to chair the jury for the 1961 Meilleur Ouvrier de France (Best Worker in France) award. He decided to keep wearing them in his famous restaurant in Collonges-Au-Mont-d'Or where he warmly greets customers who come to savor his Bresse fowl cooked in a pig's bladder, one of his many famous dishes.

Pierre Troisgros, however, when not in front of the stove in his Roanne restaurant preparing sorrel salmon, slips on his wooden clogs and surveys the vineyards at his estate in Blondins in the Loire.

Several years ago these two great chefs gave these shoes to the International Shoe Museum, Romans. Visitors discover a feast for the eyes!

231. Shoes of Paul Bocuse worn for the competition for the Best Worker in France in 1961. Moccasin style in black kidskin. International Shoe Museum, Romans.

232. Clogs of Pierre Troisgros in wood and leather. Executed by Daniel Drigeard, clog maker in Renaison. Worn in the vineyard, "Les Blondins," that the chef in the kitchen cultivates.

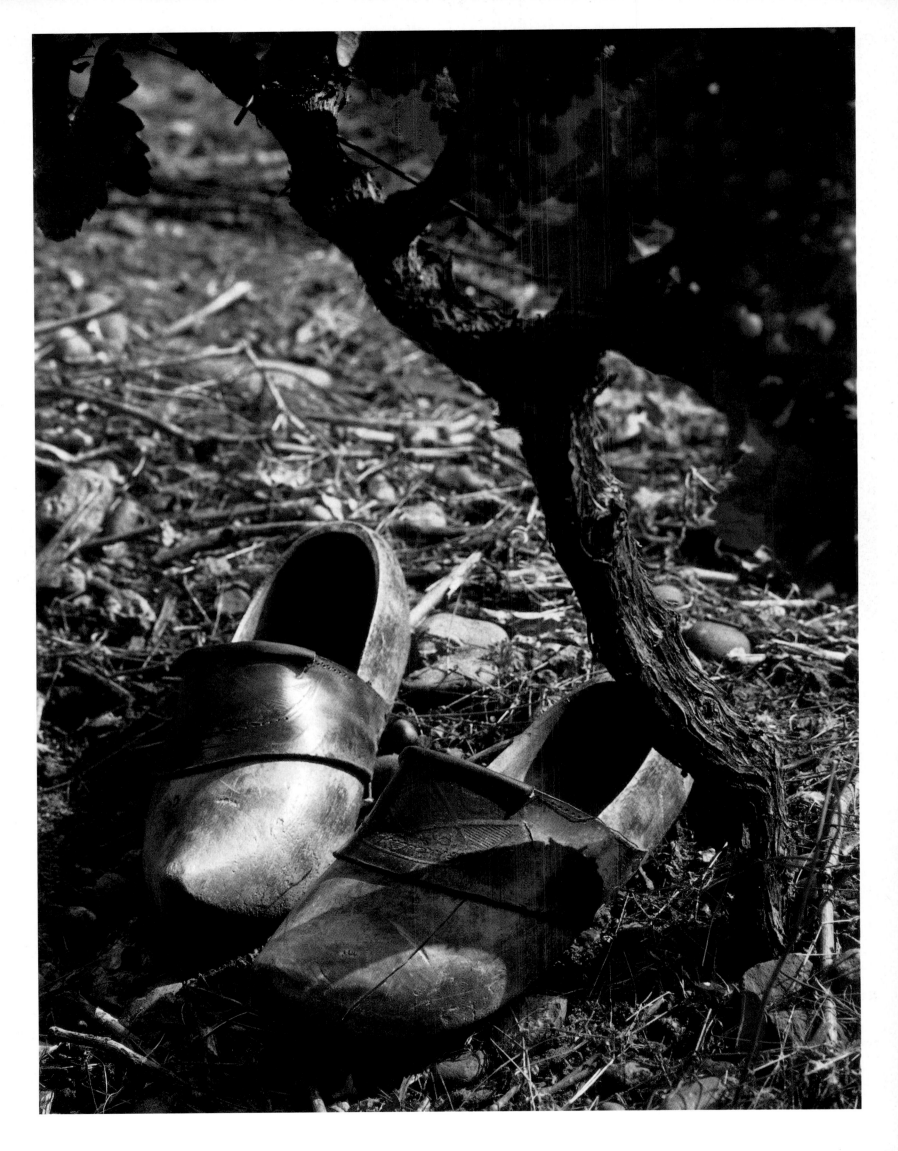

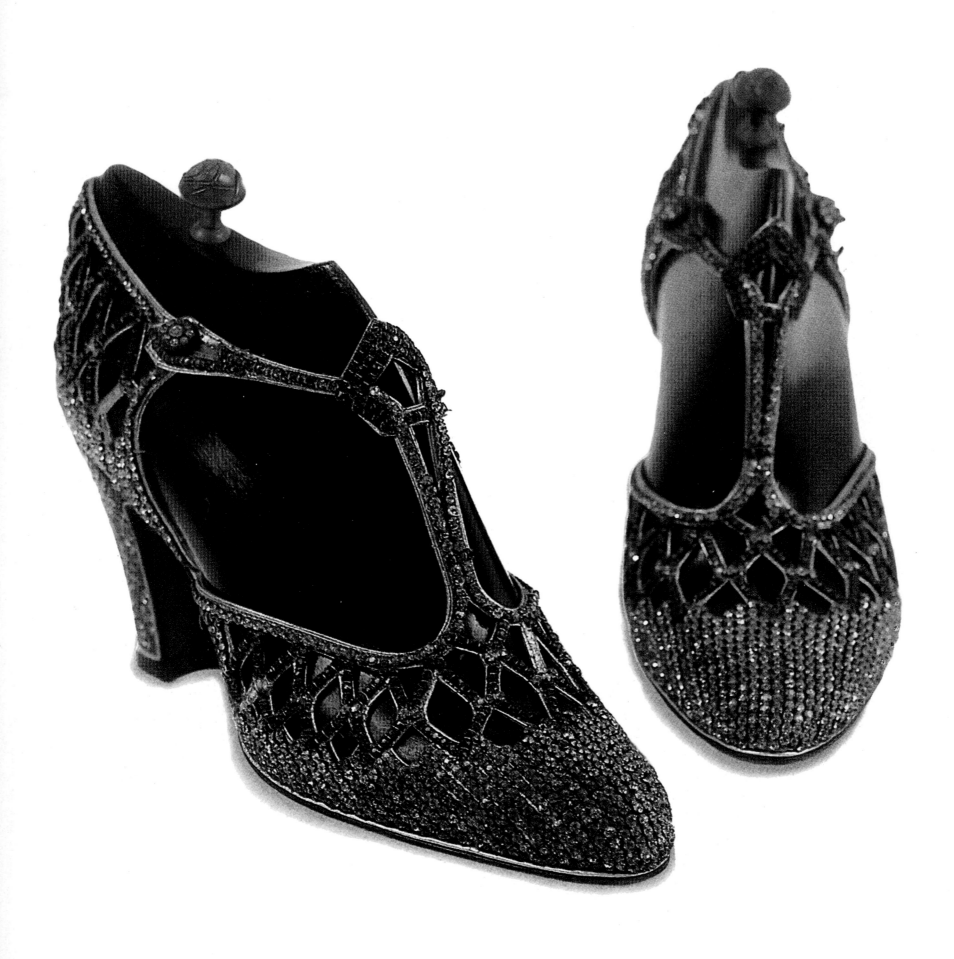

233. Salomé, Shoes of Mistinguett. Galliera Museum, Paris

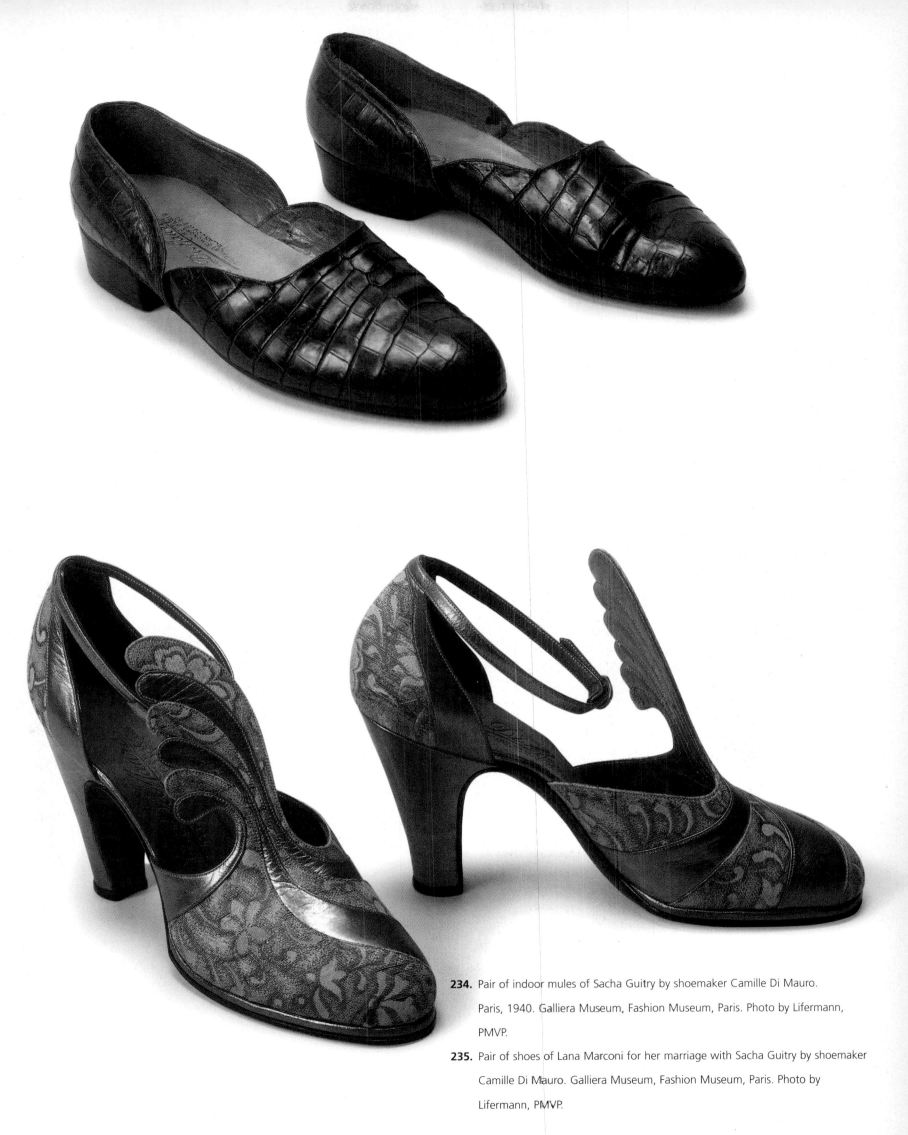

234. Pair of indoor mules of Sacha Guitry by shoemaker Camille Di Mauro.
Paris, 1940. Galliera Museum, Fashion Museum, Paris. Photo by Lifermann,
PMVP.

235. Pair of shoes of Lana Marconi for her marriage with Sacha Guitry by shoemaker
Camille Di Mauro. Galliera Museum, Fashion Museum, Paris. Photo by
Lifermann, PMVP.

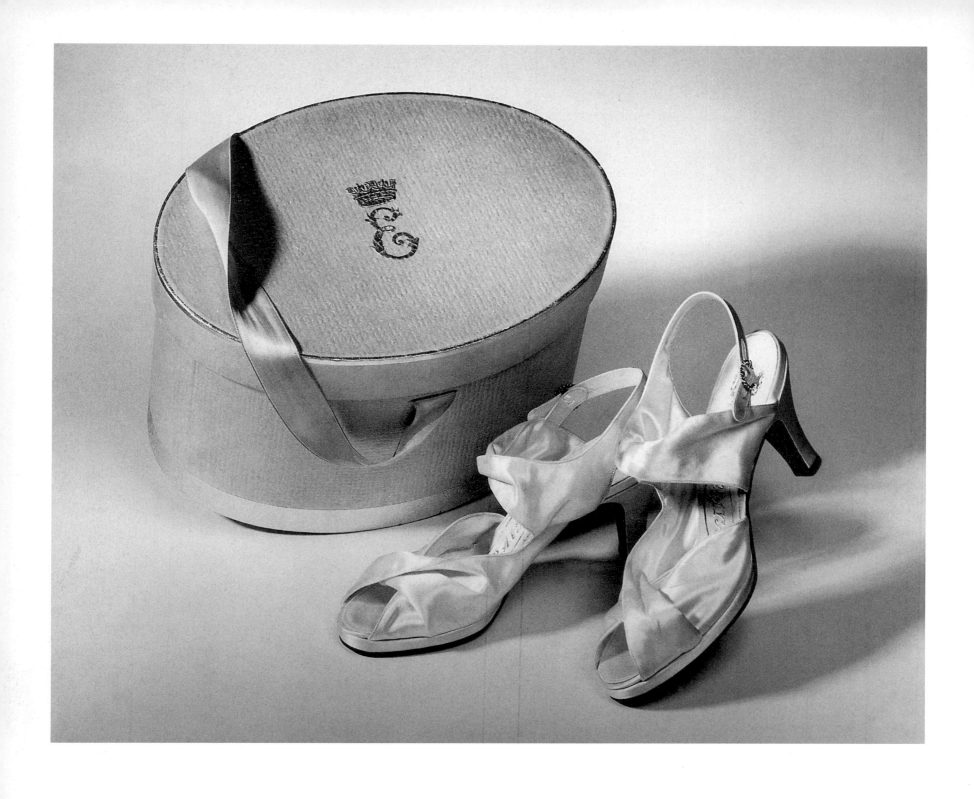

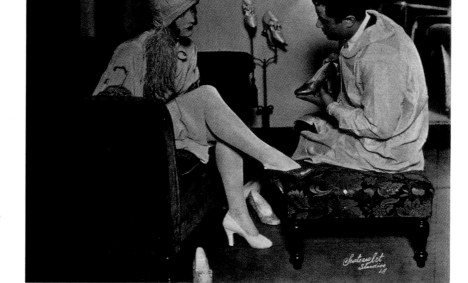

236. Marriage shoes of Queen Elizabeth II. Bally Museum, Schönenwerd, Switzerland.

237. Joan Crawford in the "Hollywood Boot Shop" that Ferragamo opened in 1923. Ferragamo Museum, Florence.

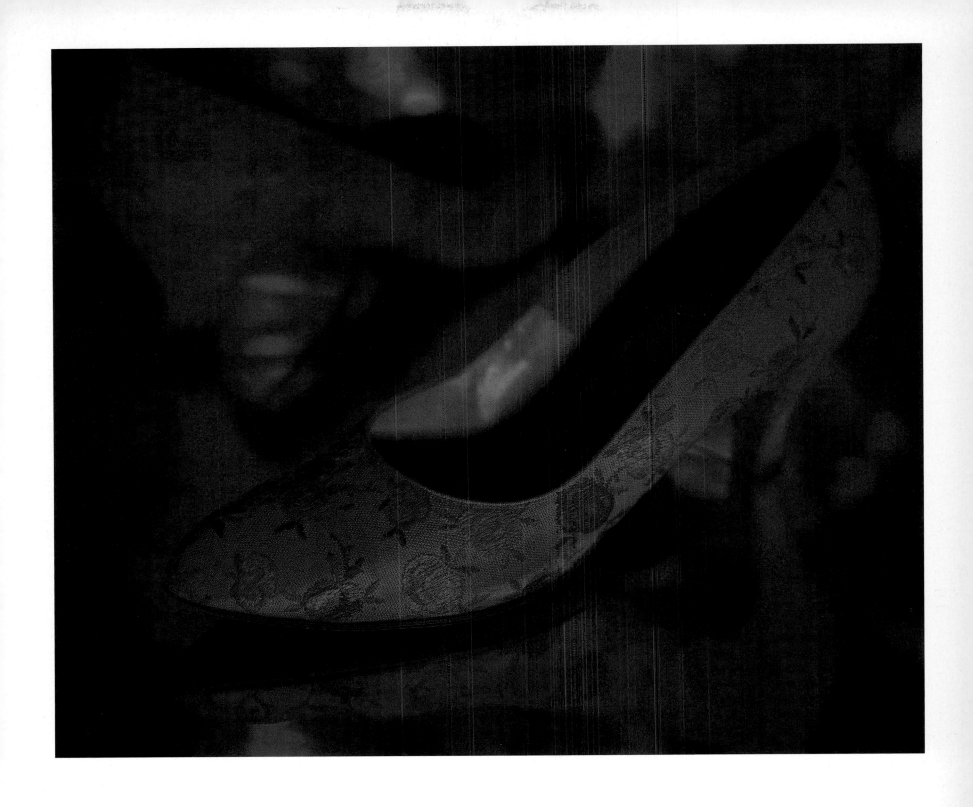

238. Shoes of Princess Grace of Monaco. Beige cloth embroidered with multicoloured flowers, Louis XV heel. Exclusive model conceived by Evins and realized by Miller. International Shoe Museum, Romans.

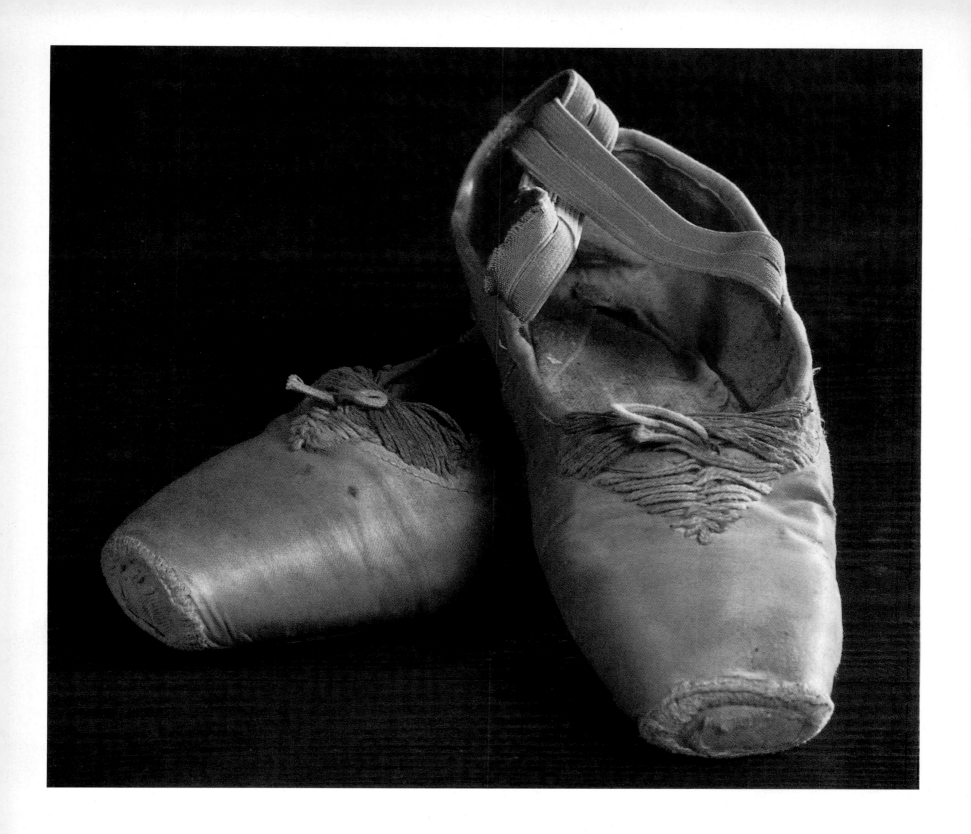

239. Dance slippers of Wilfride Piollet. 1998-1999.

International Shoe Museum, Romans. Photo by Joël Garnier.

240. Boots worn by Meryl Streep in the role of Karen Blixen and aviator boots worn

by Robert Redford in the role of Denys Finch Hatton in Sydney Pollack's

Out of Africa in 1986, Created by Pompei Companie

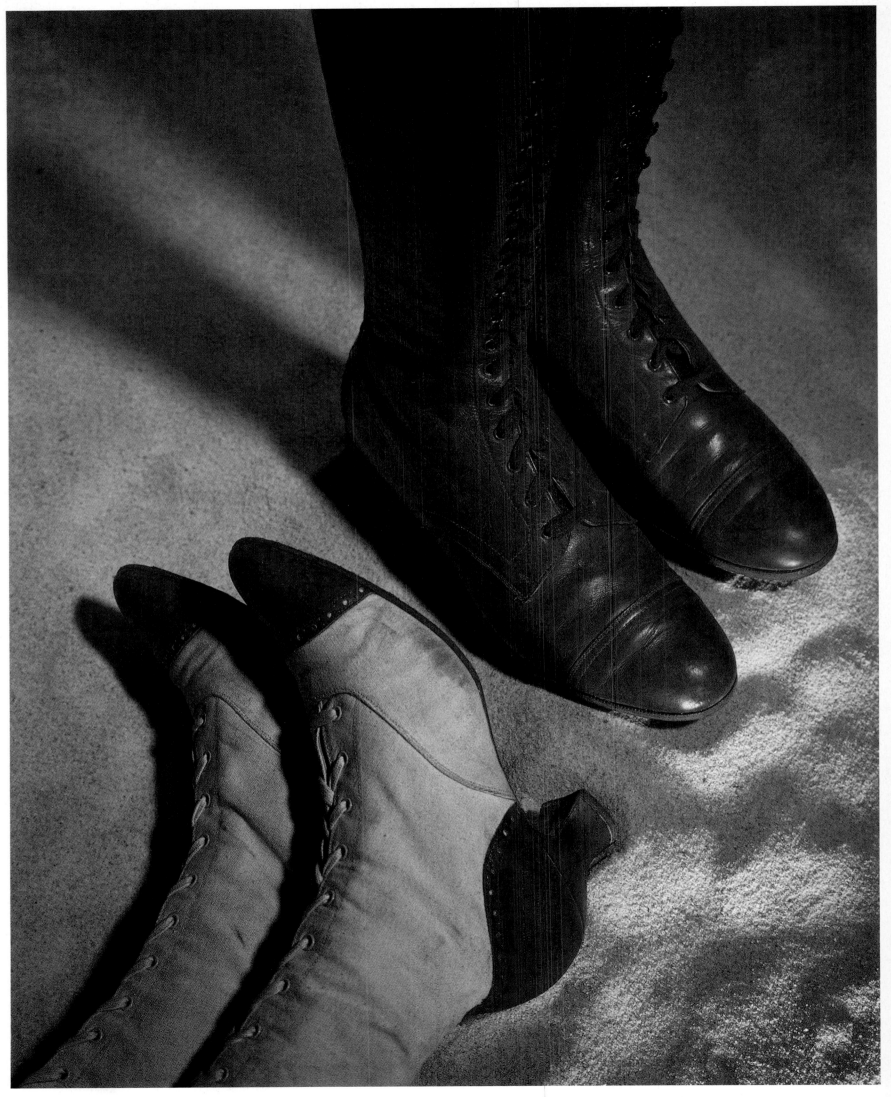

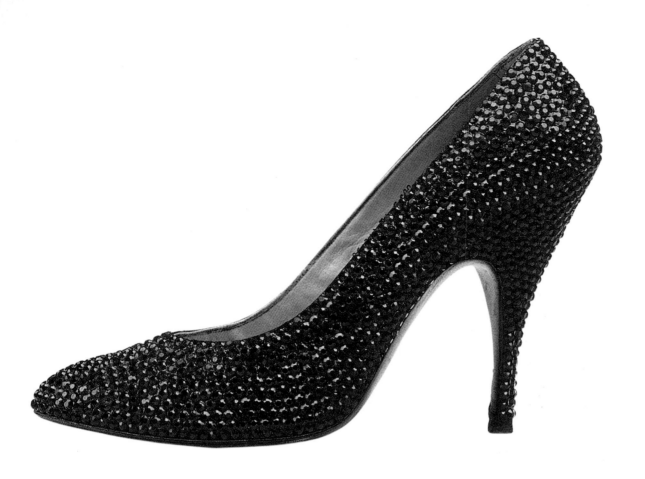

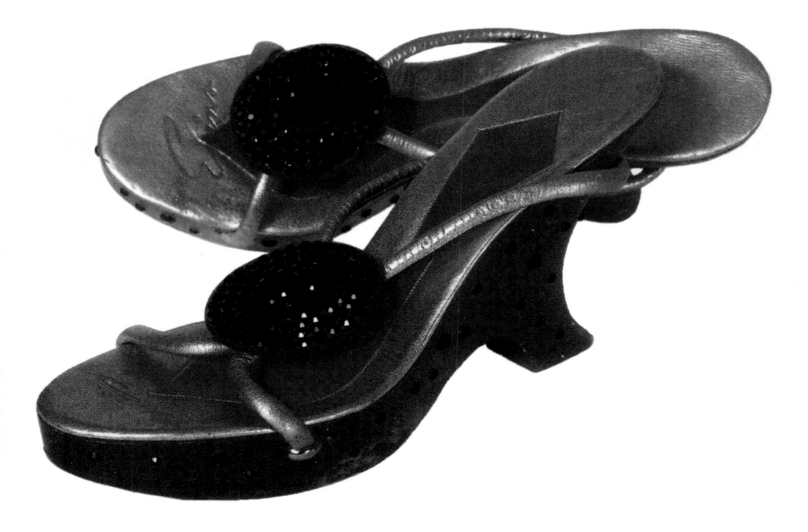

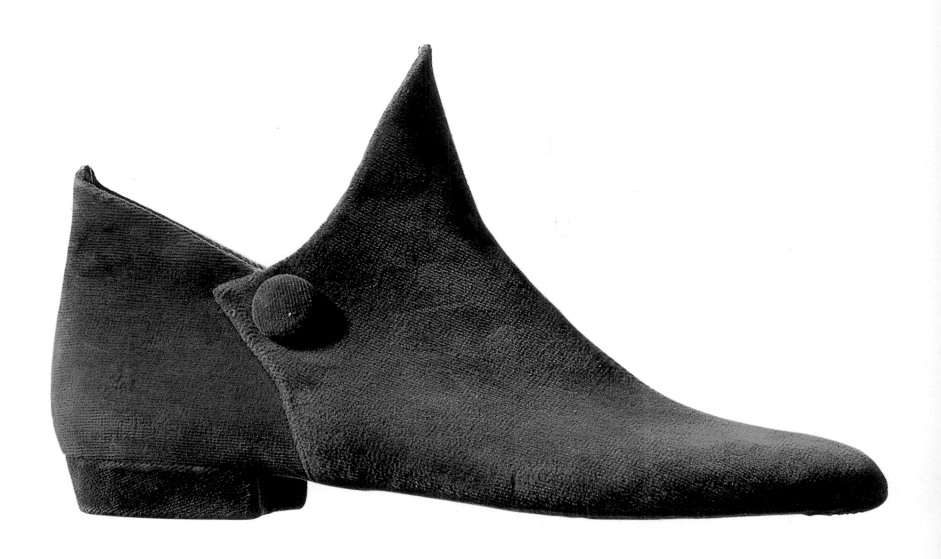

241. "Low-cut" pumps of Marilyn Monroe decorated entirely with red Swarovski strass, strass covered heel. Created by S. Ferragamo for the film *Let's Make Love*, directed by George Cukor in 1960. Ferragamo Museum, Florence.

242. Sandals of Elizabeth Taylor in *Cleopatra*, 1963.

243. "Pull-Over" style created for Brigitte Bardot in 1966. Bottine covered in velvet. Ferragamo Museum, Florence.

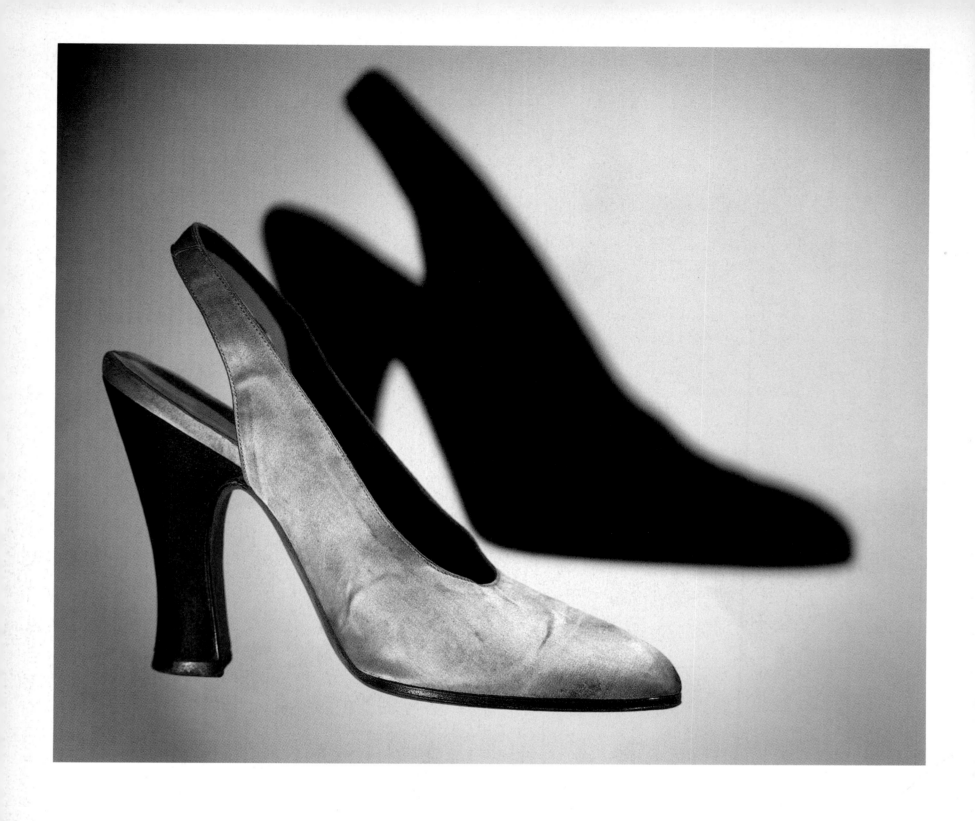

244. Shoes worn by Romy Schneider in the role of Marthe Hanau in Francis Girod's

The Banker, 1980.

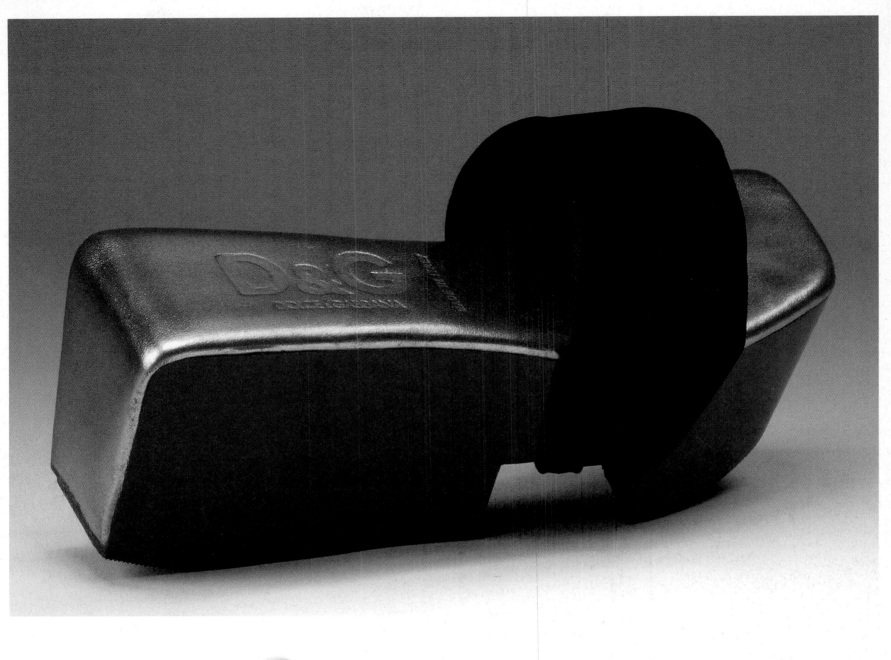

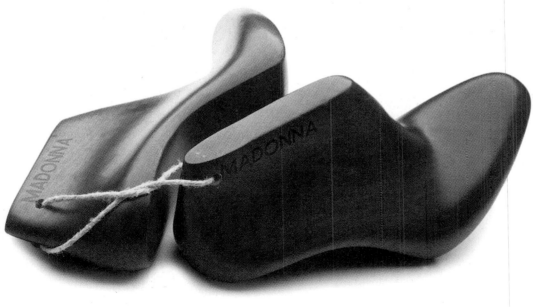

245. Mule of Madonna by Dolce and Gabanna. Ledermuseum, Offenbach.

246. Wooden lasts of Madonna's feet preserved at the Spini Feroni Palace.

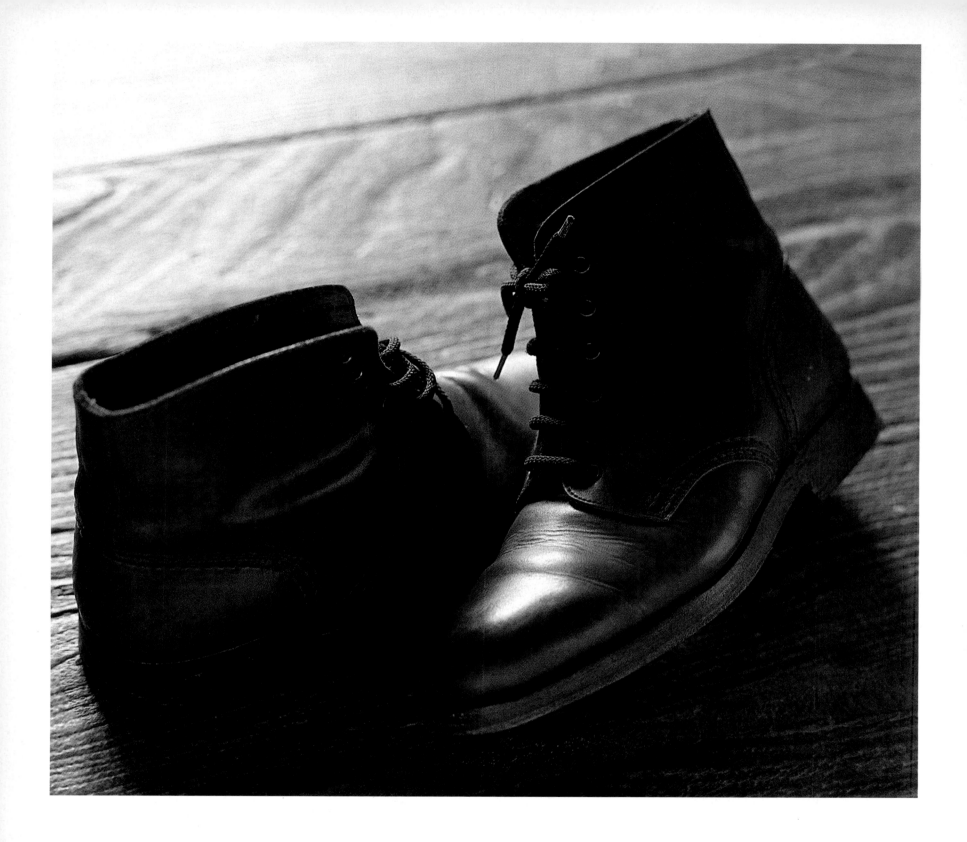

247. Ankle boots worn by Leonardo DiCaprio as Jack in *Titanic*.

Ankle boots created by the House of Pompéi. 1996.

248. Charles IX style shoe worn by Kate Winslet as Rose in the film *Titanic*.

Shoe created by the House of Pompéi. 1996. Vamp varnished black,

quarters and attachments in violet velvet calfskin.

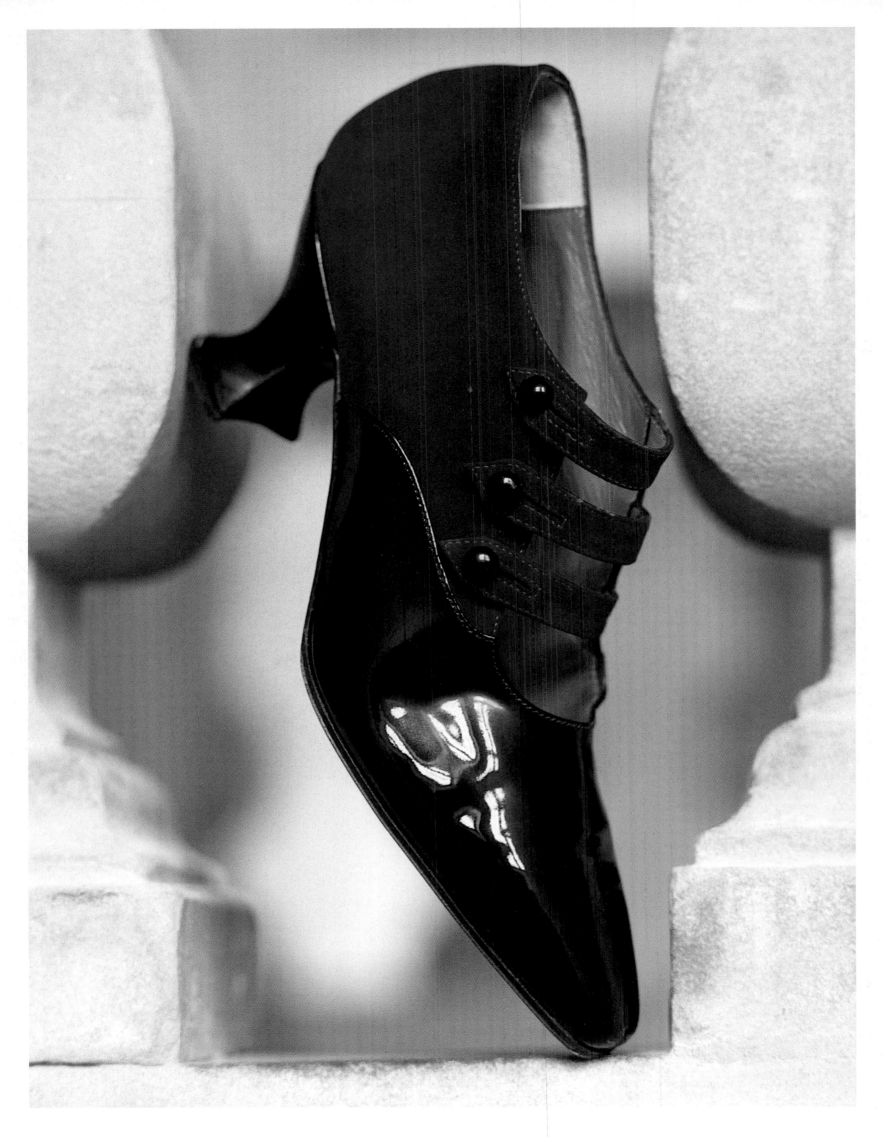

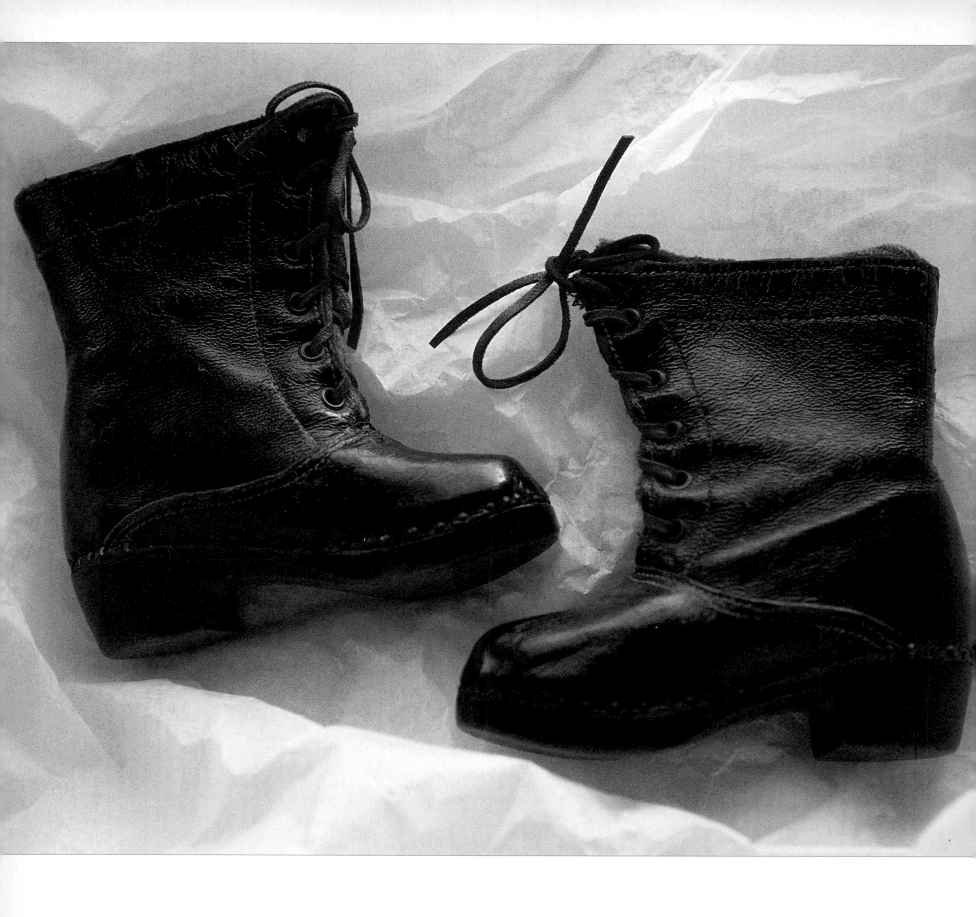

249. Bottines for the doll Rosalie in black leatherware. Around 1889.

Given by a grandfather shoemaker to his granddaughter for Christmas.

International Shoe Museum, Romans.

The Stories Shoes Tell

On the surface, most shoes appear extraordinarily banal, even trivial. Some shoes, however, have transcended their everyday reality through the human story they tell and the themes they embody.

Theresa's Doll Shoes

At age eight Theresa played with a doll just like other little girls her age. Theresa's doll wore a gathered blue dress and had porcelain eyes, but she lacked shoes. This was a serious omission because Theresa was the granddaughter of a master shoemaker.

On her way home from school, Theresa never forgot to stop at her grandfather's workshop to give him a kiss. There, with the help of a few workers, shoes were custom made and "hand sewn." On Thursdays, when there was no school, the little girl often spent the afternoon in the workshop where a mingled scent of leather, glue, and polish emanated. Theresa nosed about every nook and cranny, between the workbench and the shelves full of wooden forms and boxes of nails, while the steady sounds of the workshop resounded around her; the sound of the lasting pliers pushing in nails to fit the leather on the last and the sound of the hammer pounding out the leather.

One cold and gloomy November afternoon in 1889, the little girl, with doll in arms, pushed open the door, as was her custom, and entered the shop like a stream of sunlight, filling the place with joy. In that same instant, the grandfather's eyes fell upon the doll's bare feet. Now Theresa, who could not stop herself from thoroughly exploring the world of the shoemaker's workshop, placed her "daughter" on a stool. Taking advantage of the moment, her grandfather rapidly measured the doll's feet. When his workday was done, and with the utmost secrecy, the master craftsman put his heart into skillfully crafting miniature ankle boots for the doll. On Christmas Eve, he wrapped them in tissue paper and, while the child lay asleep, placed the doll shoes inside her own shoes left in front of the fireplace.

Christmas morning, Theresa discovered her shoes stuffed with the little doll shoes. Her eyes blazed with delight as she turned to her grandfather and said, "Look Grandfather what Father Christmas brought me. He knows how to make shoes just like you and you did not even teach him how."

Theresa carefully preserved the little ankle boots as a memento of the deep affection she shared with her beloved grandfather. Years passed. It was Christmas season when Theresa decided to donate the shoes to the International Shoe Museum, Romans. She was age ninety-five. In offering them, the elderly woman said, "Grandfather is watching from above. How happy he must be to see his ankle boots join the thousands of pairs gathered here and made by men practicing his craft from over four thousand years ago to the present day."

As the holidays approached, the Museum could not have asked for a more wonderful gift than Theresa's doll shoes.

The Well-Digger's Boots

In 1880, many dwellings, farms in particular, only had one source of water: the well, a source of life in the broadest sense. Jules was a well digger in the northern region of the Drôme in Dauphiné. It was arduous and dangerous work. To descend forty or fifty meters under ground, this digger, a specialist in sinking wells with small diameters,

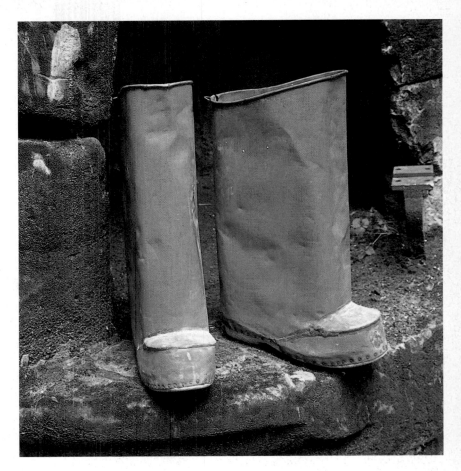

wore protective boots of his own design crafted by an artisan in his village. Made of a thick wooden sole with cut zinc encasing the foot and the leg, each boot weighed two kilos.

As his grandson explains: "When my grandfather performed maintenance on a well, he had to descend to the bottom and splash about in icy water. So the thick wool socks knit by my grandmother and these big boots pulled on over them protected him from the cold. And then to sink a well, he had to go at the wall before he reached the water layer, using an iron pick on the marl or clay; there was always the risk of being hit by a rock."

The primary function of these boots was therefore to protect Jules's feet and legs in his struggle against a hostile environment. They foreshadow the work shoes that became standard for many high-risk professions after 1950. The industrialization of work shoes owes its development to public health and safety committees, which led to the appearance of protective shoes in civil engineering, firemen's fireproof boots and the clogs worn in food chains and hospitals. The wearing of clogs in hospitals arose as an antiseptic measure in the operating room, instead of covering their town shoes with cloth boots, it is now mandatory for surgeons to wear clogs with surgical scrubs.

250. The boots of the well-digger. International Shoe Museum, Romans. Photograph: Joël Garnier.

Following pages:

251. Shoes of Zoya. Pumps in beige kidskin, heel and buckle in amber. Russia, around 1920-1925. The heels are exceptional and highly representative of the country's resources. Zoya played the piano in the concert circle.

252. Bottines of Mathilde, winter 1920. International Shoe Museum, Romans.

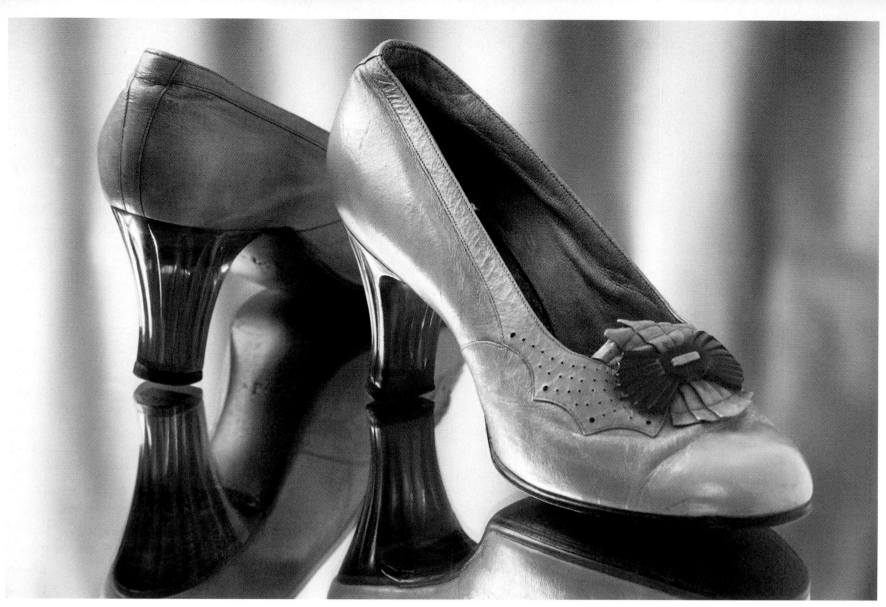

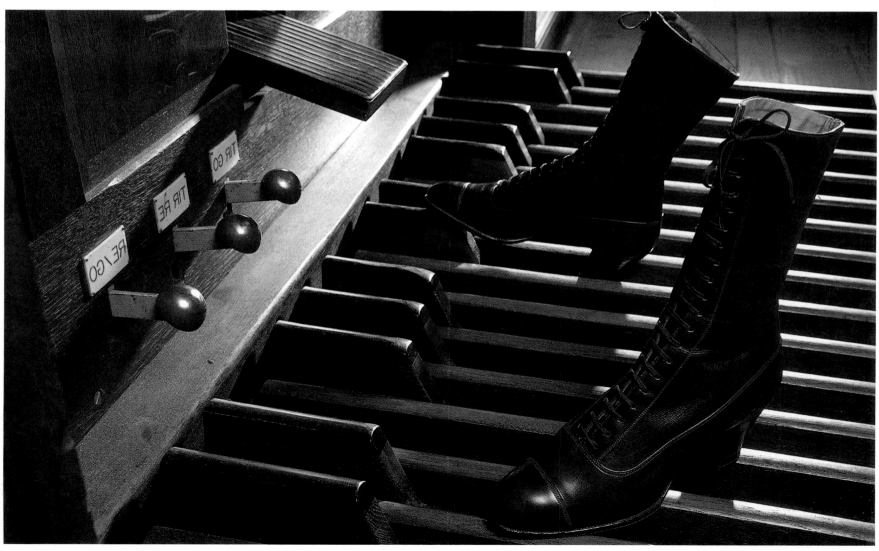

Zoya's Shoes

Zoya came from a noble family of Russian landowners. Born in Crimea around 1900, she learned to play the piano as a child, like many girls her age in her social class. An exceptionally gifted student, she continued her training at the conservatory in Simferopol. Despite her country's major social and artistic upheavals, Zoya kept up her studies at the Petrograd conservatory. While historical events lead many of her fellow countrymen to emigrate abroad, Zoya refused to leave, deeply attached to her Russian roots and her friends with whom she shared a love of music.

Exiled to the interior, her talent made her an appreciated and recognized concert pianist, while her charm, elegance, and sublime beauty caught the attention of filmmakers who offered her a screen test and implored her to take up acting. Zoya, nevertheless, declined the offer. The irresistible call of music, her happiness interpreting it, and the immaterial, almost supernatural joy it gave her and those who listened to her play, was much stronger.

Thenceforth, Zoya devoted herself completely to her art with an audience of Leningrad's upper classes. It was the 1920s and her country was anemic, devoid of vitality in the aftermath of the war of 1914 and the Bolshevik revolution of October 1917. Lenin then launched his New Economic Policy (NEP) that allowed private enterprise, deeming that the country needed to take a breather. During this period, Zoya wore a fabulous pair of beige kid pumps made by a Petrograd shoemaker. What elevated these shoes to the category of masterwork were the buckles and heels cut from single pieces of amber, evidence of the imagination and know-how of Russian craftsmen during a difficult period of scant luxury. Her talent in full bloom, terrible experiences awaited Zoya who was taken prisoner in 1937; she died in the Gulag.

For many years Zoya's niece lived in France. In the 1960s, during a trip to Russia, the niece met her cousins and they offered her the gift of their most precious possession: Zoya's shoes. In 2000, the family heirloom's new owner donated the shoes to the International Shoe Museum, Romans, where they are preserved on display. For all that they embody, these shoes invite silence, reverence, and meditation.

Mathilde's Ankle Boots

It was 1920 and Mathilde was twenty years old when she boarded a train one winter morning with her cousin. The two young women were going on vacation to visit their grandparents. Thin and elegant, Mathilde was a charming brunette. This morning, she wore laced ankle boots in glazed brown calfskin, showing off her shapely legs. Georges was already seated by the window when the two cousins settled into the compartment. Mathilde's arrival struck him like a bolt of lightening. For a split second, he saw nothing but the young woman's ankle boots and legs because the conductor stood in front of her like a screen, but her figure quickly emerged in its full glory, blinding Georges who could not take his eyes off her appearance. Mathilde sensed she was the subject of intense observation, but her upbringing did not permit her to give the slightest regard to the stranger, whom she noticed was quite distinguished, all the same. While the landscape rolled by like pictures of happiness, the two cousins chatted softly. Georges strained his ears to take in all he could of the conversation, which was sometimes muted by the locomotive's loud cries, revolving around the work of Johan Sebastian Bach and a church rehearsal of "Jesus Joy of Man's Desiring." Arriving at her destination, Mathilde exited the compartment leaving Georges two clues with which to undertake a proper investigation to find the unknown women: her first name and, better yet, the name of the town where she played organ for a collegiate church at Sunday mass.

Days passed, but Georges' memory of the encounter refused to recede into the impenetrable fog of oblivion. On the contrary, Mathilde's image was permanently etched on his mind; the image of her pretty legs in ankle boots was foremost among his thoughts while her silhouette marked by a combination of elegance and vulnerability occupied the rest. Georges ended up confiding the wonderful secret in his heart to his mother who was offended by this unexpected revelation, especially in the way it went against the accepted behavior of his milieu. Yet, his heart, a little later, filled with a strange joy he had never felt before, when he decided to travel the five hundred kilometers that separated him from Mathilde. When he entered the church to attend eleven o'clock high mass, the organ resounding at full volume matched his own emotions. The sonorous rush of the music sustained his feelings and touched his innermost soul, transporting him to another realm where he had a momentary glimpse of eternity. When the service was over, Georges was as much in contemplation as he was on the look out. He hid behind a pillar by the small wooden spiral staircase that connected the organ gallery to the nave. Suddenly, as if a signal, he heard the sound of Mathilde's footsteps coming down the steps. It echoed in his ears, regulating his heartbeat like a metronome. Finally he caught sight of her. Wearing the famous ankle boots he had so admired on the train, she was surrounded by friends and acquaintances, radiating an inner beauty that exalted her.

The memory of love at first sight on the train and future plans leapt into his head; his heart beat in double-time. A silent lover observing from afar, Georges came and went for three consecutive Sundays, traveling a total of four thousand kilometers in an era when slow transportation methods made traveling difficult. Unable to get his mind off Mathilde, the young man located the parish priest, who spoke of his organist in the most laudatory terms. And so it happened that in this church, a few months later, the priest united them before God and man in the sacrament of marriage.

The love the couple shared steadily grew as a result of the countless attentions they paid each other and, from these daily little nothings which amount to so much, the ordinary was transformed into the extraordinary; it was the art of producing happiness, but also a way to overcome trials. The rest was chemistry; the union produced four children.

Near the end of his life, after forty-five years of marriage, Georges still had the strength to tell Mathilde what an exceptional wife she had been and how deeply he had loved her with unparalleled devotion. He said it was because she knew how to be all the different women he needed at different times over the course of their lives. He told her again how, on that winter morning in 1920 on the train, he had instantly known that this person, as beautiful as a spring day, would change his life. Mathilde replied that she too, at the very same moment, was affected by an inexplicable feeling before the stranger and had expected nothing but happiness. Georges had always had a weakness for women's legs in lovely shoes and bought his wife beautiful ones. However, it was the ankle boots of their first meeting that were carefully preserved like relics, protected in their original brown and beige canvas bag and stored on the top shelf of the closet in the couple's bedroom.

One day, shortly before Georges died, Mathilde had a premonition as to how she would like to remember him after his passing into eternal life; she decided to present her ankle boots to the International Shoe Museum, Romans, sharing the story attached to them with great candor and emotion. Today, in this vault of preserved memory, the ankle boots represent mutual love shared between a man and a woman elevated to the sublime, expressed through the reciprocal gift of oneself.

Toine's clogs

Toine owned a small family farm he inherited from his father. At the break of dawn, he would put on his clogs and start such daily chores as opening the hen house door, climbing the hayloft to empty hay into the manger with the two mules, milking the goats, giving an alfalfa ration to the rabbits in their hutch and cleaning the pig pen.

Constantly coming and going from the well (sole source of water for the house) to the kitchen garden, to the cellar (where large vats for the grape harvest were lined up), and passing through the kitchen (where the food the land produced was prepared and eaten), Toine needed to wear sturdy shoes.

As the seasons changed, he wore the same shoes across the fields to harvest the corn, and in high summer, to harvest the peaches. During the period of heavy labour that followed, Toine plowed the fields behind a mule named Negro.

His clogs lefts tracks in the furrows of loose earth he sank his feet into as the village church bell chimed the hours and signaled when it was time to return to the farmhouse. And when autumn's wind bared the trees along the road near the stables, Toine's clogs made the leaves crackle underneath.

There was a boot scrapper, a thin, timeworn iron strip supported by two segments of weather-beaten vine stakes and raised fifteen centimeters off the ground, near Toine's main door. Its only purpose was to remove the mud still stuck on his wooden soles.

Toine's "all terrain" clogs are a good illustration of agricultural practice between the wars in the small rural community of Génissieux located in the Drôme des Collines. Donated to the International Shoe Museum, Romans, by his nephew in 1978, their presence memorializes the bond between man and his land.

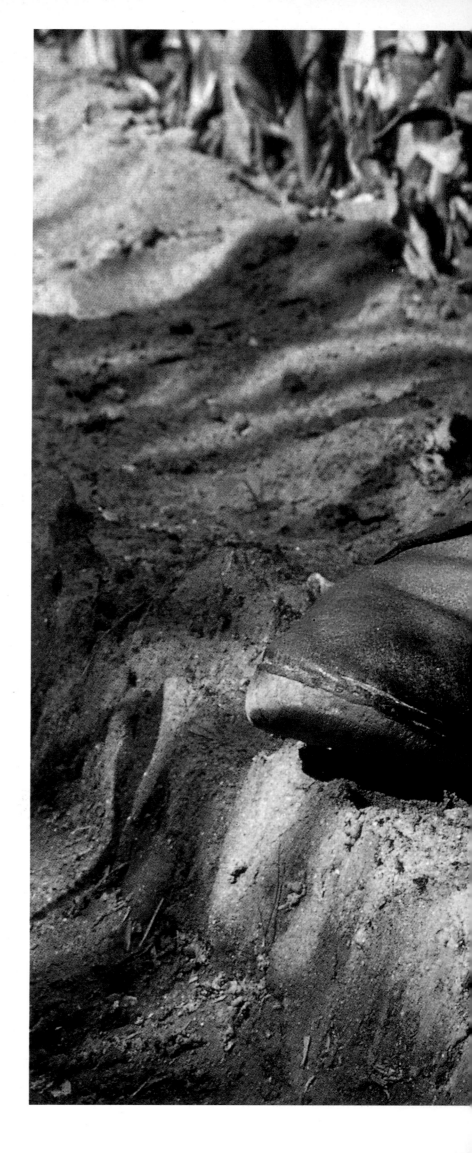

253. Clogs of Toine, farmer. 1950. International Shoe Museum, Romans.

Photograph: Joël Garnier.

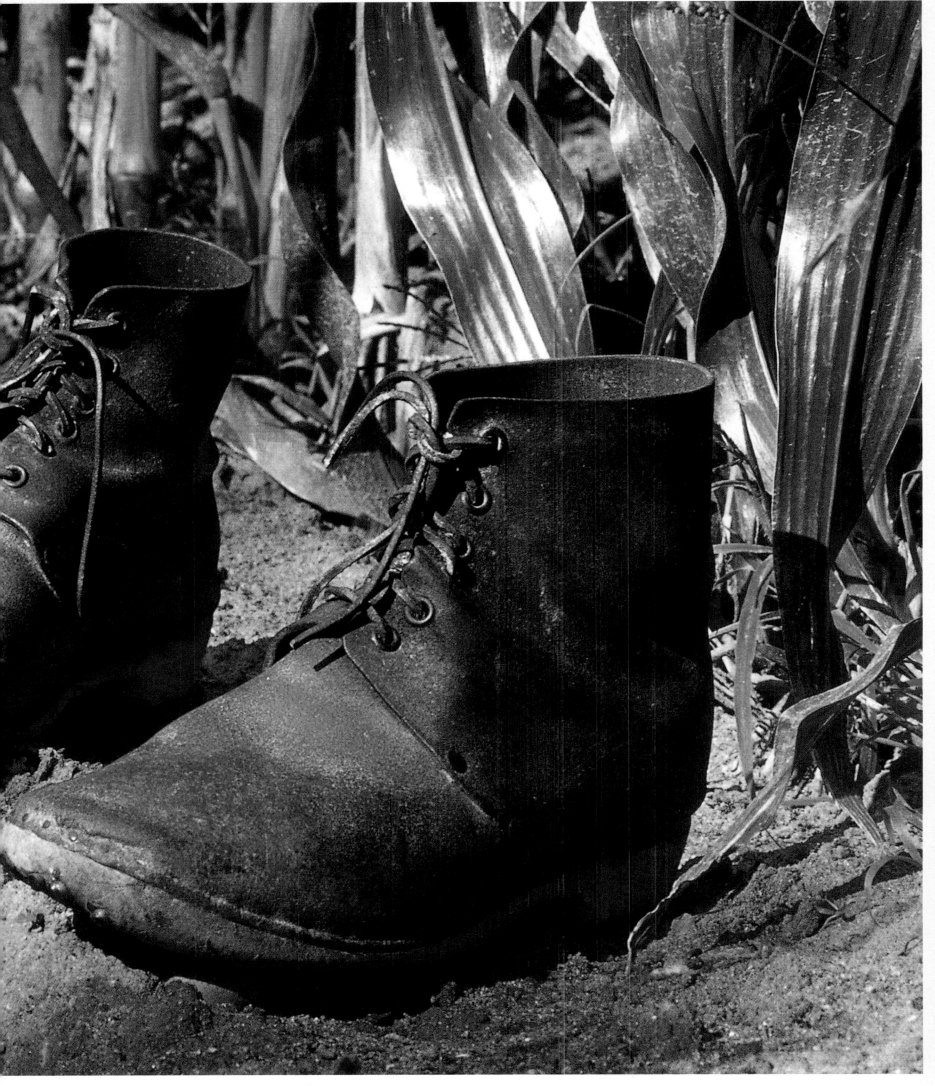

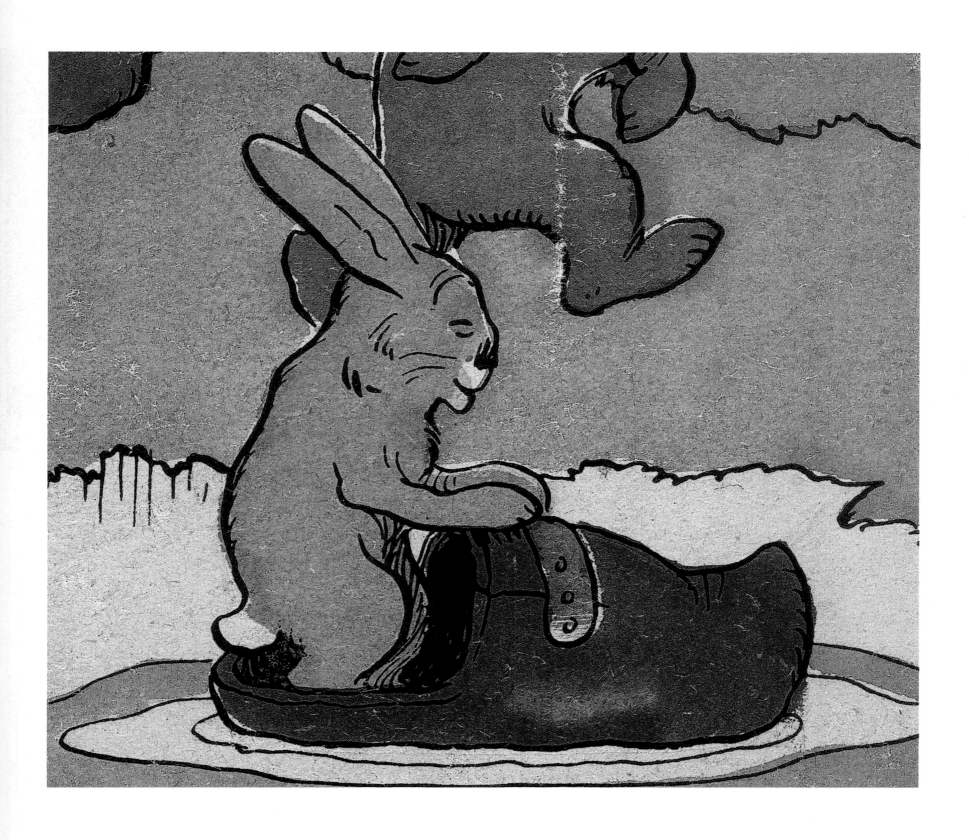

The Shoe in Literature

Literary descriptions of shoes have abounded since Antiquity. Valuable backups to iconographic sources, often the only meaningful reference for lost shoes and archaeological fragments of ancient shoes, literary descriptions are also an indispensable source for dating shoes before the advent of fashion journalism.

Additionally, literature is a source of reference for shoe manufacture (the most famous example being Jean de la Fontaine's fable, The Cobbler and the Financier), and even for the world of the shoe business, as portrayed by the mimes of the ancient Greek poet Herodas. However, among literary images of the shoe, the most sublime, symbolic and poetic image is indisputably that evoked in Paul Claudel's masterpiece, "The Satin Slipper." It tells the story of Doña Prouhèze who is guilty of an illicit love for Don Rodrigue. After removing her shoes and entrusting her satin slipper to the Virgin Mary as a symbol of a solemn vow, she offers the following prayer:

Take my heart in one hand and my slipper in the other while there's still time. I put myself in your hands! Virgin Mother, I give you my slipper! Virgin Mother, hold my miserable little shoe in your hand! I warn you, soon I won't be seeing you anymore; I'm about to completely turn from you! But when I try to leap into sin, let it be with a crippled foot! When I desire to clear the barrier you've set up, clip my wings! I've done what I could; it's up to you to protect my poor little shoe, hold it against your heart…

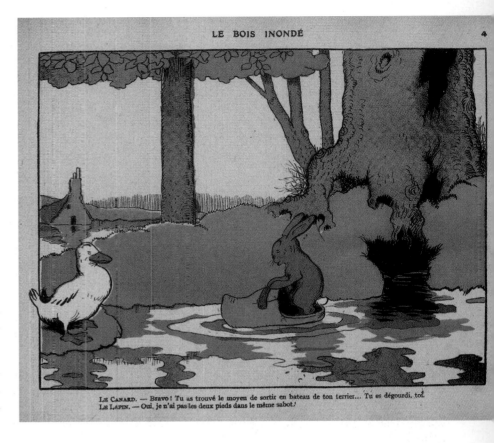

LE BOIS INONDÉ

LE CANARD. — Bravo! Tu as trouvé le moyen de sortir en bateau de ton terrier… Tu es dégourdi, toi.
LE LAPIN. — Oui, je n'ai pas les deux pieds dans le même sabot!

The Papyrus of Herodas Mimes

Although severely damaged and with portions missing, we can still get the general idea of the text.

The scene unfolds in the shop of Kerdon, an upscale shoemaker. Metro brings in a female client and Kerdon makes a pitch for his shoes. The female client takes the floor and negotiates the price with Kerdon – a price comparable with that of other custom shoemakers. Kerdon finalizes the sale, agrees to a small discount, and performs a fitting. He promises Metro that a pair of shoes previously dropped off for repair will be ready on a specific date. The discussion is a central part of the mime.

METRO – KERDON – A FEMALE CUSTOMER

Metro: Kerdon, I've brought you these ladies to see if you have some ingenious piece of handiwork worthy of being shown to them.

Kerdon: Ah! I'm not your friend for nothing. Aren't you going to get the large seat for these ladies? I'm talking, Drimylos. Still sleeping? Pistos, slap his face and really wake him up. Or rather, attach the backbone … to his neck … rapidly loosen his legs … louder than these … Then … shine … I am going to dust the seat … Sit down, Metro. Pistos, open the shelf above, not that one, the one above, and quickly take down the items that are ready to use … Ah! Dear Metro, what things you shall see. Careful … open the box of shoes. Look at this one first Metro: the shape … well done; ladies look too; see how the heel is attached, decorated with …

254-257. Comic Scenes in the Forest by Benjamin Rabier. 20th century.

Following pages:

258. *The Cobbler and the Banker,* fable by Jean de la Fontaine illustrated by Gustave Doré. 19th century.

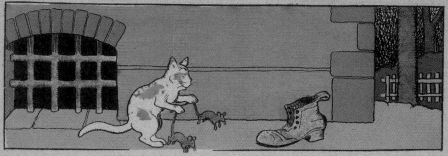

LE CHAT. — C'est sans doute pour que je lui trouve un lacet que le garde-chasse a déposé cette bottine devant son pavillon.

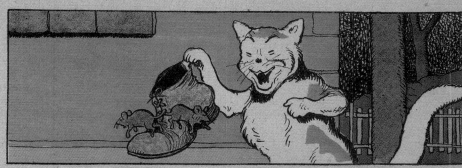

LE CHAT. — Le voilà satisfait !

and it doesn't have some good places and some bad: it's all by the same hand. As for the polished leather, I wish that … you must agree you couldn't ask for anything better, you won't find a better-polished leather than this … nor a brighter wax. It's three gold staters that K … gave to Kandas … this one and another polished, … all that is sacred, … to tell the truth, … no bigger lie than that … that Kerdon has no longer … any happiness in this world. As for my recognition, … they still want … to earn more … the products of our art … cobbler, a form of poverty. … keeping warm night and day … of us don't take a bite before evening … to dawn; I don't believe Mikion's candles … And I'm not talking anymore (I have thirteen slaves to feed), but all, ladies, laziness personified and Zeus turns a beautiful day into rain, and they've but one refrain: "Give what you can"; and for the rest … like fish for warming the backside. But, as they say, words don't make the sale; money does; if this pair pleases you, Metro, it would certainly be well to take out one pair after another until you are absolutely sure that Kerdon doesn't lie. Bring all the shoeboxes Pistos; it is necessary that … you will return home ladies. Examine all these different styles: Sikyonians, Amrakians, canary yellow, plain colours, parrot green, espadrilles, mules, slippers, Ionians, heels, sauts-de-lit, low cut, crayfish-red, sandals, Argives, scarlets for the young man for walking. Say which ones your hearts desire, and ask yourself, who consumes more leather, a woman or a dog.

Female Customer: This pair that you just took, how much are you asking for it? Don't shock us too much and scare us off.

Kerdon: Figure it out yourself if you wish and name your own price … the bald fox has come home to roost, name a price that will provide bread for those who handle the tools. – Dear Hermes, god of profit, winning Eloquence, yes, if I don't catch something in my net today, I don't know how I will be able to improve my boiled dinner.

Female Customer: What are you muttering about, can't you honestly name a price, what is it?

Kerdon: Madame, this pair costs one mina, you can look it over up and down; if Athene wanted to buy it in person I couldn't knock a penny off.

Female Customer: I see why, Kerdon, your boutique is full of beautiful and costly items; look at them…; it's the twentieth in the month of the Bull, Hekate is marrying Artakene, and she will need shoes. Too bad! Perhaps, although with any luck they are going to run to you, actually it is certain, but you'll have to close your purse so the cats don't carry away your minas.

Kerdon: Hekate, if she comes, will not have one less mina, nor Artakene either; so if you like, think about it.

Metro: Hasn't Fortune already granted you Kerdon the joy of caressing little feet made for the caresses of Desires and Loves? But you are nothing but a nasty scoundrel, so that on our part… And this other pair, what are you asking for it? A little louder, as you normally speak.

Kerdon: That's five staters, yes, by gods, but the zither player Eueteris comes in everyday and begs me to let her take it, but I dislike her, when she promised me four Darics, because she made fun of my wife with ugly insults; if you need it too, go on, watch out … give … And this one and that one, look, I'll give it to you for seven Darics, because of Metro but here, because you have nothing to complain about … would make me ascend in flight, me the shoemaker, as heavy as a stone, up to the sky. Because that is not a language that you have, it's a sieve of delicacies. Ah! That one there … not far from the gods, for whom your lips open night and day. Place your little foot here so that I can put it in the form. There, nothing to add; nothing to take away. Beautiful things fit beautiful ladies, always. One might think Athene cut this sole. And you, give me your foot as well; an ox did that to you kicking with his scabby hoof. But one could sharpen his leather knife on the contour of the upper, because in the house of Kerdon, it doesn't leave the shop unless it's perfect. You over there, that will be seven Darics for you, the one neighing by the door as strong as a horse. Ladies, if you ever need anything else, such as sandals or something you like to shuffle in around the house, all you have to do is send over your little servant. For you Metro, come back on the ninth; in any case you will have your crayfish-red shoes. Even a fur-lined coat has to be mended in order to keep out the cold if one has any sense at all.

This text has a dual interest: Herondas gives details about the ancient Greek shoe trade and lists a wide variety of shoe types, confirming the richness of the shoemaker's craft. Often brightly coloured, Greek shoes were adapted to various circumstances, for example, the young man's scarlet Argives for walking.

Mainard – La Bruyère – La Fontaine

A disciple of Malherbe with a taste for epigrams, François Mainard satirized a nouveau riche former cobbler: Pierre, who was a famous cobbler during his youth, is filthy rich and ashamed of his old job. The author's lively form heralds La Bruyère:

Iphis noticed a new shoe style at church; he looked down at his own and blushed; he felt underdressed. He had come to mass to show himself, but hid himself instead; and so for the remainder of the day, he was held captive in his room by his shoes.

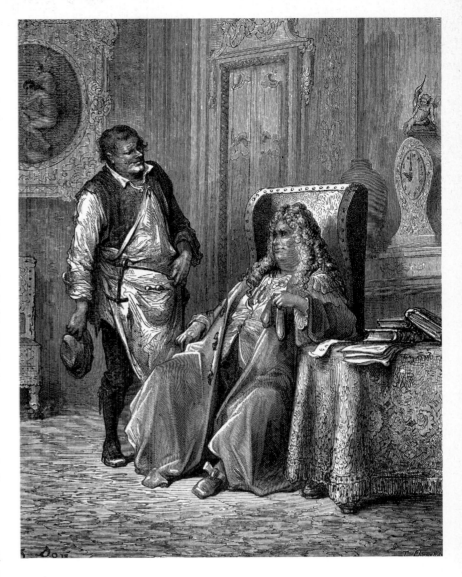

This picture of morals by a contemporary of La Bruyère, leaves the last word to La Fontaine's fable, *The Cobbler and the Financier*, in which wisdom and common sense prevail:

"There once was a Cobbler who sang from morning to night. He was a sight to be seen and heard, phrasing more contentedly than seven sages. His neighbor, on the other hand, who was rolling in money, sang little and slept even less: he was a man of finance. If he were occasionally sleeping at daybreak, the Cobbler would start singing and wake him up. The financier complained that God had neglected to make a market where he could buy sleep, like he could buy food and drink. So he invited the singer to his townhouse and said to him,

'Mr. Grégoire, what do you make a year doing that?'

'Per year? Good grief my lordship,' the strapping Cobbler grinned,

'I don't really think of it like that. I don't make that much from one day to the next, which is fine as long as I come out all right at the end of the year. There's food on the table everyday.' The financier continued,

'What then do you make per day?'

'Sometimes more, sometimes less,' the cobbler replied.

'The bad thing is – and if it weren't for this we'd make a reasonable profit – the bad thing is we have to take so many days off. The holidays are killing us. Profits and holidays don't mix. And the Priest is always extolling the virtues of some new Saint to us.'

The financier smiled at the cobbler's naiveté and told him, 'I'd like to extol your virtues for a day. Take these one hundred crowns and hold onto them in case you need them.'

The Cobbler felt as though he were holding in his hand the sum of the entire world's wealth produced over the last hundred years for the use of mankind. He returned home and buried the money in his cellar and along with it his joy. There would be no more singing; he lost his voice the moment he acquired the root of all evil. Restful sleep departed his lodgings, which were now host to anxiety, suspicion, and undue alarm. The Cobbler was on the lookout all day long and if at night some cat made a sound, he thought someone was taking the money. Finally the poor man ran to the house of his neighbor, whom he could not wake up!

'Give me back my songs and my sleep,' he told him, 'and take back your hundred crowns.'"

As for Perette, in La Fontaine's fable of *The Milkmaid and the Pot of Milk*, when she dreams of getting rich, she does not have her "shoes on the ground." She wears her shoes her own way, as La Fontaine chose to dress her in flats:

"Sporting light and short clothes she moved with big steps, this particular day having put on a simple petticoat and flat shoes, in order to be more nimble"

(La Fontaine, *Fables,* p.198, France Loisirs, Paris, 1983).

In this instance, the issues of concern at the farm are worlds away from the fashion concerns of Iphis in the art of looking one's best.

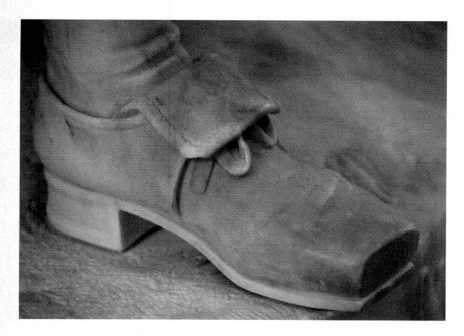

Restif de La Bretonne

Restif de La Bretonne had a gift for glorifying the foot and the shoe in his literary works. He leaves no doubt as to his predilection through the thoughts of the "anti-Justine": "More than anything else I have a weakness for pretty feet and pretty shoes."

In his "contemporary" novel, the hero Saintepallaire is a young husband with a foot fetish. As the author writes: "Nothing imaginable was more distinguished and valuable than his young wife's shoes. They were covered up to the heel with pearls and brilliant diamonds. They had cost over ten thousand crowns and had been a gift from Saintepallaire. At night, when they were alone in their bedroom, the young husband knelt down and with a trembling hand removed the beautiful shoes from her pretty feet. Then he dressed them in slippers, which were no less beautiful, although less expensive. The shoes were placed in a small glass temple made up of a round base atop crystal ionic columns with gold capitals. The shoes were kept in this box as the evidence and guarantee of an immortal love. Ten years had passed since then with the young wife never forgetting on each wedding anniversary to wear the shoes. The husband's erotic passion did not diminish. Perhaps this ritual always renewed his love. Or perhaps his wife, under the advice of her admirable mother-in-law, used methods unknown to other women. Or perhaps men like Saintepallaire are more loving and more sensitive to many and often repeated stimuli…"

During the first year of marriage, the shoemaker delivered a new pair of shoes everyday to Saintepallaire, who did the ordering and selected the colours and ornaments himself.

His wife only wore them for one day and then put them away in a wall cabinet. During the second year, he only ordered white shoes. His wife successively wore all the shoes she had but once, including a few pairs that he had bought her before the marriage. Thanks to this activity, he was always occupied with his wife and her charms.

In novels such as *Le pied de Fanchette* (The Foot of Fanchette) and *Monsieur Nicolas*, to name only the most famous, the shoe is much more than a discrete accessory. In these books, clogs, pumps, slippers, and mules are described in detail worthy of a whole catalogue of 18th-century women's shoe styles.

It should be noted that, although the symbolism of these shoes harks back to the 17th century through their resemblance to Cinderella's slipper, they also announce the foot and shoe fetishism examined by Octave Mirbeau in his *Diary of a Chambermaid*.

Chateaubriand, *Atala*
"The Mocassins of Chactas"

Chateaubriand set sail for America in 1791. The story of Atala, published in 1801, tells of the love between Chactas and Atala.

This swamp idyll plunges the reader into the exoticism of America. As Chateaubriand writes: "Atala made me a coat from the inner bark of an ash tree, because I was almost naked. With porcupine quills she embroidered moccasins for me made out of muskrat skin." The author's description of the moccasins demonstrates his gift for meticulous observation that he exercised when in contact with the Indians.

For example, that moccasin production was in fact women's work and porcupine quill embroidery was commonplace in the 18th-century. It is interesting to note that the author does not put shoes on Atala for her funeral, whereas the painter Girodet's discrete brush depicts her feet covered by a shroud. "Atala was laid upon a bed of mimosa; her feet, her head, her shoulders, and part of her breast were uncovered. A wilted magnolia was visible in her hair… Her lips like a pink bud picked two mornings ago seemed to languish and smile. In her astonishingly white cheek one could make out a few blue veins. Her beautiful eyes were closed; her humble feet were together."

Gustave Flaubert, *Salammbo*

Gustave Flaubert spent five years writing the historical novel *Salammbo* based on an episode of the first Punic war in the 3rd century BC. He traveled to Tunisia and dug up everything he could read on Mediterranean antiquity in order to accurately blend fact and fiction. When his great pictorial and poetic masterwork appeared in 1862, it was the result of much research.

Carthage had called upon barbarian mercenaries to fight the Romans, but when they did not receive their due, the mercenaries threaten revolt. To appease them, the Senate offers a festival. The Libyan Matho allies himself with the mercenaries and makes himself their leader. He succeeds in removing the sacred veil, called the "zaimph" from the goddess Tanith, Carthage's talisman. But Matho is passionately in love with Salammbo, the daughter of the suffet Hamilcar and a Tanith worshipper. She gives herself to Matho, but faithful to her own, makes him restore the veil. Meanwhile, Hamilcar manages to block the rebel army on the warpath where they die of hunger and thirst. Captured and tortured, Matho dies at Salammbo's feet. Salammbo then declares her own love for him and emits her last breath by the will of Tanith.

In reconstructing history, Flaubert successfully evokes the atmosphere of an African town at the crossroads of civilization and barbarism with its contrasting wealth and poverty. The shoes worn by Roman characters over the course of the book are depicted in functional contexts. Sandals, cothurni, leg armor, slippers, and ankle boots abound. The author also remembers those who, because of their social status, are unable to wear shoes, and walk barefoot: priests and slaves. In addition, complementing these descriptions are the highly variable sounds of footsteps in different circumstances that echo in the reader's ear through the evocative power of Flaubert's carefully chosen vocabulary.

Here are a few examples from among the many shoes mentioned. First, the sandal makes a noteworthy entrance with the theatrical appearance of Salammbo: "She wore a small gold chain between her ankles to regulate her steps and her great dark purple cloak, cut from an unknown fabric, dragged behind her, following each of her steps like a large wave. Now and then the priests plucked nearly muffled chords from their lyres and in the pauses between the music one heard the sound of the gold chain with the regular clatter of her papyrus sandals" (Ch. I, The Festival, pages 21 and 22).

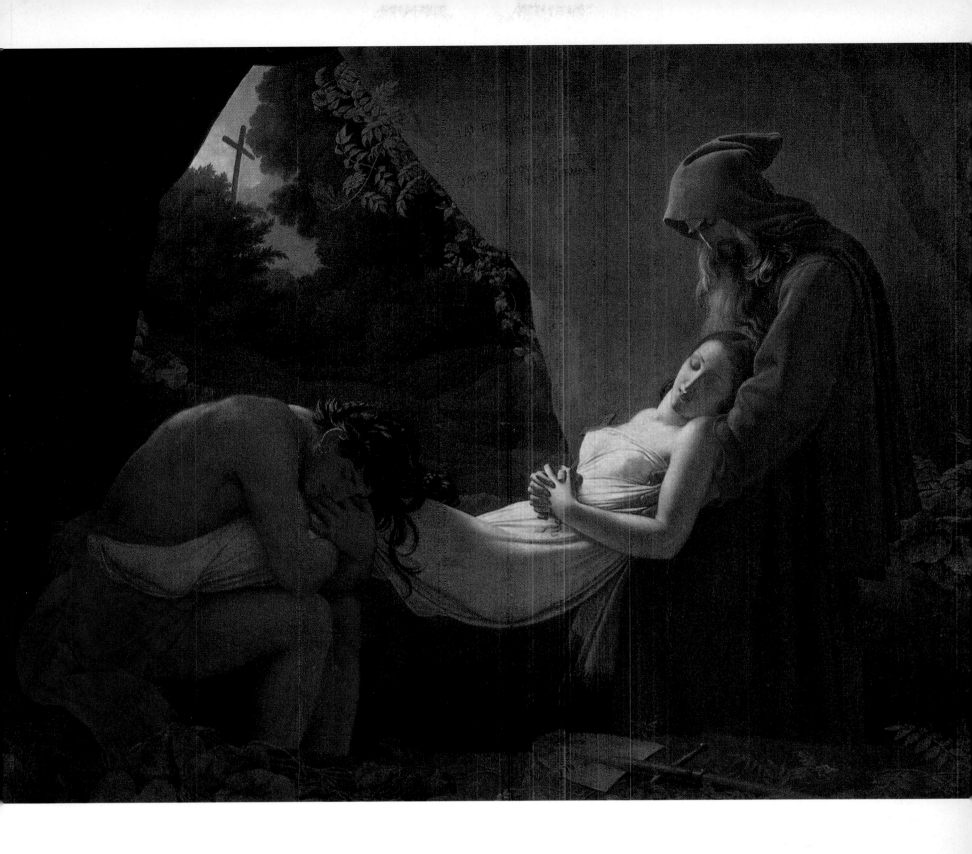

259. Detail by Julien. *La Fontaine*. Marble. Height: 1.73 m. Louvre Museum, Paris.

260. Anne-Louis Girodet de Roucy-Trioson. *The Entombment of Atala*.

Louvre Museum, Paris.

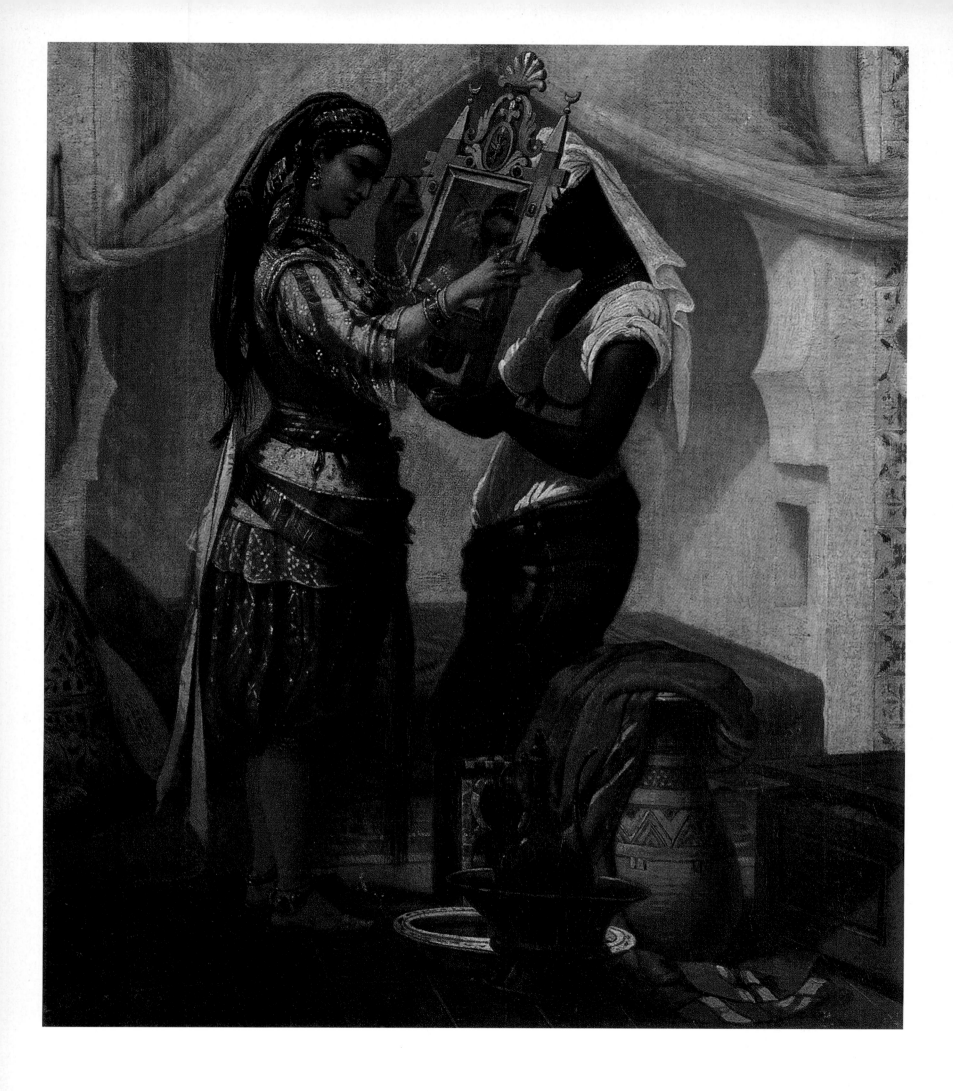

The sandals make Matho yearn for her love when he remembers them:

"Doesn't she go up to her palace terrace every night? Ah! How the stones must quiver under her sandals…" (Ch. II, A. Sicca). Salammbo's shoes are over the top in the variety of materials used and the richness of their ornamentation: "Her sandals with curved ends disappeared under a mass of emeralds" (Ch. III, Salammbo, p.56). "An onyx step went around an oval pool: fine snakeskin slippers were left on the edge…" (Ch. V, Tanith, page 93). "Salammbo, however, continued to walk… and her outfit had all the trappings of the goddess's… Her sandals, cut from bird feathers, had very high heels…" (Ch. VII, Hamilcar Barca, p.143). The heel, which was unknown in Antiquity, is understandable here because of Salammbo's association with a goddess. It is reminiscent of the Greek theater's high-soled cothurni reserved for actors playing heroes and Gods.

To seize the veil of Tanith, Matho and Spendius must scale the wall of the Carthage aqueduct during a nocturnal mission that requires special shoes: " 'Master!' Said the old slave,' if you're an intrepid soul I will lead you into Carthage… Bring along an iron pick, a helmet without a plume, and leather sandals' " (Chap. IV, Under the Walls of Carthage). Before going to Matho's tent to retrieve the sacred veil, Salammbo puts on a pair of blue leather ankle boots. The situation is reminiscent of the departure scene in the Book of Judith when the Biblical heroine Judith undertakes a mission to the enemy camp to seduce General Holophernes (The Book of Judith, 10:4). But Salammbo does not resist Matho: "Matho seized her by the heels, the little gold chain broke and the two ends came flying and struck the fabric like two springing vipers…. She put one foot to the ground and realized that her chain had broken. Virgins in prominent families were expected to treat these fetters with an almost religious respect and Salammbo, blushing, wrapped the two sections of the gold chain around her legs" (Ch. XI, Under the Tent, pages 225-226). Additionally, her shoes gave her away to prying eyes of old Gisco: "Salammbo recognized old Gisco… this is how Gisco saw it was Salammbo. He had guessed a Carthaginian woman, by the little balls of sandastrum that knocked against her cothurn" (Ch. XI, Under the Tent, p.228).

The reference is to an ornament of precious oriental stone with gold markings in the form of a star. A little later Hamilcar and his father are quick to surmise what happened: "He noticed that her little chain was broken. He shuddered, seized by a terrible suspicion" (Ch. XI, Under the Tent, p.233).

Moloch's servants pick Hamilcar's little brother Hannibal to be sacrificed to the gods. To save his son's life, his father substitutes a slave's child. He hastily prepares him for the ghastly ceremony: "…and he dressed him in sandals with pearl heels – the sandals of his own daughter!" (Ch. XIII, Moloch, p.284).As for the Suffete Hanno, he wore shoes typical of his vocation: "… the litter stopped and Hanno, followed by two slaves, put his feet on the ground, wavering. He wore black felt ankle boots, strewn with silver moons. His legs were wrapped in bands like a mummy with his flesh showing between the crossed bands" (Ch. II, A Sicca, p.46).

Although different, Hanno's shoes were similar to those reserved for patrician Roman Senators, who wore closed black leather shoes with a crescent referred to as a moon concealing the opening. Plebian Senators were barred from wearing the crescent.

While soldiers usually wore sandals, the men of Narr'Havas wore hyena-skin shoes: "Narr'Havas entered followed by about twenty men. They wore white wool cloaks, long daggers, leather collars, hanging wooden earrings, and shoes of hyena skin" (Ch. VI, Hanno, p.101). Leaders generally wore cothurni: "The captains, wearing bronze cothurni, were positioned on the middle path…" (Ch. I, The Celebrations, p.11).

"Matho sank into sorrow: his legs hung to the ground and the grass whistled continuously as it whipped against his cothurni" (Ch. II, A. Sicca, p.36).

But he put on sandals when he went to Carthage to boldly steal the veil of Tanith, encourage by Spendius, who told him: "One day you will enter Carthage, and walk among the colleges of pontiffs who will kiss your sandals" (Ch. V, Tanith, p.84).

And he used sandals to show his anger when he left the town and thrust himself against a closed door: "The people jumped up and down with joy, seeing the impotence of his rage; he took his sandal, spit on it, and slapped the rigid boards" (Ch. V, Tanith, p.98).

And shoes were among Hamilcar's bad memories of war: "'And when my situation was desperate – we drank the mules' urine and ate the straps of our sandals'" (Ch. VII, Hamilcar Barca, p.134).

The preparations for the battle of the Macaras highlight the important status granted to shoes. Hamilcar concerned himself with them: "…he ordered shorter swords, the stronger laced boots…" Among the troops: "Two thousand young men had slings, a dagger, and sandals" (Ch. VIII, The Battle of the Macaras, pages 164-165). This amounts to a total of two thousand pairs of sandals! Once again bulk is observed: "…bronze knemids (soldiers' leather or metal leg coverings) covered all their right legs" (Ch. VII, The Battle of the Macaras, p.174). Shoes were subject to daily inspection: "Everyday the captains inspected clothing and shoes… and to protect the hoofs of the horse, ankle boots out of woven vegetable fibers were made for them" (Ch. IX, On Campaign, p.187).

We have to look to Rome for an explanation of these strange ankle boots. The Romans dressed their horses and mules with loose shoes that could be put on and taken off easily. Usually made of simple materials such as rush or iron, they sometimes were made of silver or even gold.

But during the dark hours of battle there still remained nearly seven thousand men facing a shoe shortage: "They had plugged the holes in their cuirasses with the shoulder blades of quadrupeds and exchanged their bronze cothurni for sandals made of rags" (Ch. XIV, The Warpath, p.329). Flaubert also deals with the world of shoe fabrication when Matho and Spendius move about Carthage on foot: "They went by the tanners' street, Muthumbal square, the herb market, and the Cynasyn crossroads" (Ch. V, Tanith, p.92).

Spendius, the former slave, turns out to be a man with manual dexterity:

"Spendius told him about his travels, about the people and the temples he had visited. He had knowledge of many things: he knew how to make sandals, spears, and nets, how to tame wild animals, and how to cook fish" (Ch. II, A. Sicca, p.36).

Wealthy Hamilcar visits his stockrooms that give off an odor of leather and he oversees the artisan activity within his walls: "He came from the other side of the gardens to inspect the domestic artisans who sold products in their stalls. Tailors were embroidering cloaks; others were weaving nets, combing cushions, or cutting sandals" (Ch. VII, Hamilcar Barca, pages 155-156).

In a succession of spectacular scenes of truly mosaic detail, Flaubert offers the reader a colorful account full of imagery of the shoe in Antiquity. Salammbo's final appearance in the story exemplifies this and therefore must be emphasized; this moment, occurring on the day she is to wed the Numidian prince Narr'Havas, which becomes the day of both her and Matho's death, appears in the novel's the epilogue. With a marvelous profusion of descriptive prose, Flaubert dresses Salammbo in sumptuous clothes, but refrains from putting her in shoes. He only writes: "She was led forth on an ivory-coloured stool with three steps" (Ch. XV, Mathopage, p.342). Was this an intentional omen on Flaubert's part meant to contrast with to the Cinderella myth already known to Antiquity in the legendary story of Rhodopis told by Strabo? It appears to be a veiled allusion to the fact that, unlike Cinderella, Salammbo failed to find the shoe that fit her foot.

261. Léopold de Moulignon. *La Toilette de l'Odalisque*. 19th century.
Orsay Museum, Paris.

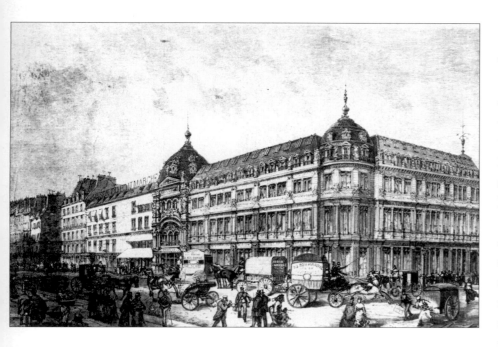

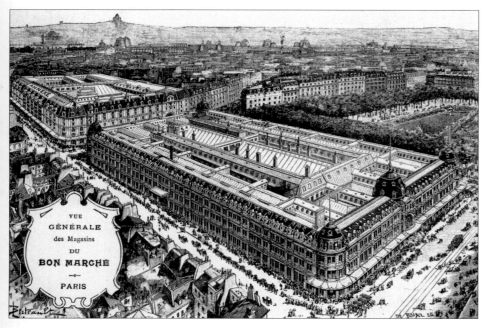

VUE
GÉNÉRALE
des Magasins
DU
BON MARCHÉ
—◦—
PARIS

Emile Zola, *Au bonheur des dames*
(Ladies' Delight)

The advent of large department stores during the Second Empire changed domestic trade in France. The concept was to present departments, carrying all kinds of everyday items, to hundreds of customers. The terms of sale were also new; the store would take only a small profit on each item sold at a fixed price, but would make up the difference through volume. When Aristide Boucicaut came to seek his fortune in Paris, he started out as a humble employee before heading a department in a general store. In 1852 he bought a small boutique of thirty meters called Le Bon Marché located in a popular neighborhood.

From 1863 the store's sales reached seven million; by 1877 Le Bon Marché comprised of a variety of shops. The store inspired Émile Zola to write Au Bonheur des dames (Ladies' Delight), which was published in 1883. The novel recounts how Octave Mouret successfully reinvents modern commerce when artisan boutiques are replaced by large department stores. The department store inspires Mouret to exanimate feminine vanity. Among the store's various departments, a position of privilege was accorded the shoe department:

"But Madame Marty became especially feverish over new departments; a new department could not be opened without her inaugurating it. She rushed in and bought something all the same… Then she went down to the shoe department in the back of a ground floor gallery, behind neckwear, to a counter opened just that day, where she wrecked havoc on the cases, swooning before the white silk mules decorated with swan feathers, shoes, and white satin ankle boots with high Louis XV heels."

" 'Oh! Dear,' she stammered, 'make no mistake. They have an incredible selection of great coats. I picked out one for myself and one for my daughter… And Valentine, what about the shoes?' " " 'It's unprecedented!' added the young girl, with her feminine bravado. 'There are boots for twenty francs fifty. Oh! The boots!' "

Gérard de Nerval, *Sylvie*
Alain Fournier, *Le Grand Meaulnes*
(The Wanderer)

"Shoes of Yesterday"

Sylvie and *Le Grand Meaulnes* (The Wanderer) were published sixty years apart, but the two writers are united by two descriptions of shoes. The 1853 novel *Sylvie* evokes the author's cherished memories of the Valais. Nerval is torn between his feelings for his childhood friend Sylvie and Adrienne's mysterious seductiveness; Adrienne's magical attraction is the stronger.

Searching for an old style of lace, Sylvie rummages in her aunt's drawers: "She rummaged again in the drawers. Oh! What riches! How wonderful this item felt; how that one shined, how another shimmered with bright colours and modest beading! Two slightly broken pearl fans, tins with Chinese motifs, an amber necklace, and tons of frills and flounces, among which shone forth two little shoes of white drugget with buckles incrusted with Irish diamonds! 'Oh! I want to put them on if I can find the embroidered stockings!'"

"Just then we unfolded silk stockings of pale pink with green patches; but the Aunt's voice accompanied by the chattering stove suddenly brought us back to reality."

262. Illustration of the Bon Marché.

263. Illustration of the Bon Marché.

"'Go downstairs quick!' said Sylvie, and regardless of what I said, she would not allow me to help her with her shoes."

Like Gérard de Nerval, Alain Fournier places his novel in the beloved landscapes of his childhood. Meaulnes mysteriously disappears for three days and gets lost in the most isolated corner of the Sologne. He comes upon an estate, goes inside an abandoned room, and falls asleep. In the morning he wakes to find old-fashioned clothes nearby that seem to have been left for him.

"They were outfits worn by young men a long time ago, frock coats with high velvet collars, fine, very open vests, countless white ties and patent leather shoes from the turn of the century. He dared not touch anything with this fingertips, but after cleaning himself up as he shivered, he put one of the great coats on over his schoolboy's blouse, turning up the pleated collar, exchanged his steel-tipped shoes for the fine patent leather pumps, and prepared to go downstairs bareheaded" (*Le Grand Meaulnes* (The Wanderer), Ch. XIII, "La fête étrange" (The Strange Celebration) p.67, Le Livre de poche Brodard et Taupin).

What these two writers have in common is a continuous back and forth movement from dream to reality. Both delightfully conjugate the past with the present; the surprise and pleasure of discovering old-fashioned shoes experienced by both Sylvie and the Great Meaulnes highlights this. Gérard de Nerval and Alain Fournier revive the worlds of childhood and adolescence, which reappear even today in the joyful and playful art of dress up, by allowing the reader to plunge into fantasy for a moment's pleasure.

Pierre Loti, *Madame Chrysanthème*
"In Japan: Introductions…"

"I could make out the rear view of a beautiful young thing all fixed up, who was finishing being rigged out in the empty street: there was a final maternal glance at the waistband's enormous shells and at the pleating around the waist. Her dress was of pearl gray silk; her obi (1) in mauve satin; a sprig of silver flowers trembled in her black hair; she was lit by one last melancholy ray of the setting sun; five or six people were with her…"

"Yes, it was definitively her, Miss Jasmine… my fiancé that was being brought to me! … I hurried downstairs where my landlord, the old Mrs. Prune lived with her husband. They were praying before the altar of their ancestors."

"'They're here, Mrs. Prune,' I said in Japanese, 'they're here! Quick, the tea, the stove, the embers, the small pipes for the women, the little bamboo spitting pots! Bring all the items necessary for the reception with haste!' I heard the door being opened and I went back upstairs. Wooden clogs were left on the floor; the stairs creaked under bare feet…"

Pierre Loti's travels took him to countries that were poorly understood during his time. His literary work reflected his attraction to exotic countries. He visited Japan in 1886 and published *Madame Chrysanthème* a year later. The novel transports the reader to the country of the rising sun where the author is introduced to a fiancée. The author faithfully observes the ancestral custom of taking off one's wooden clogs before entering the house and uses the staircase to recreate the sound of bare feet.

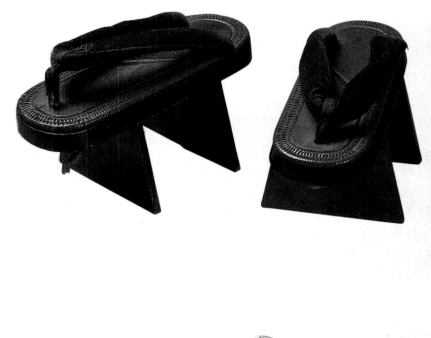

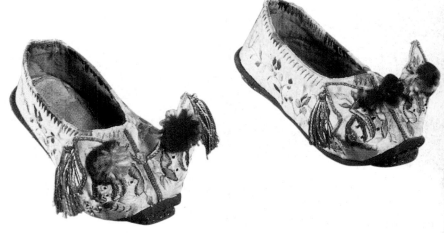

264. "Getta," wood and straw core. Japan, 19th century. Traditional shoes whose shape remains unchanged for several centuries. International Shoe Museum, Romans.

265. Child's shoes resembling a cat's head, embroidered silk. China, 19th century. Guillen Collection, International Shoe Museum, Romans.

(1) A large waistband of Japanese costume.

219

André Chamson, *Les hommes de la route*
(The Road Workers)
"Shoes and Work"

Les hommes de la route (The Road Workers) was published in 1927. In this novel, André Chamson observes the men hired to build a road in the Cévennes region at their worksite. The heavy labour on steep granite soil required sturdy shoes: "A long strip of land lay flattened and stretched out as if in submission before the dark-skinned men in black felt hats smoothed by rain and the traces of their sweaty fingers; thickset men in shirtsleeves with open collars and no tie; dark-chested, agile men in heavy corduroy breeches held up by a red or black tayole (1); sturdy men wearing big leather cleats stronger than the granite, course-grained with shiny steel – real men like those who built the jambs of the cathedrals, swung scythes at harvest, and shoved loaves into ovens, men who lived with the seasons and years – men in timeless garb made for heavy labour, intimate with sun and rain, walking tough over hard stones in the middle of a procession of lights."

(1) Term used for belt in the Cévennes region.

Margaret Mitchell, *Gone with the Wind*

Margaret Mitchell's 1936 novel, adapted for the screen by Victor Fleming in 1939 featuring such unforgettable actors as Vivien Leigh and Clark Gable, is based on the American Civil War (1861-65) that pit the North (the Union) against the South (the Confederacy).

The novel repeatedly describes the character's shoes, but it is interesting to note that they are never mentioned at the beginning of the novel, when all the characters are enjoying prosperity. The first mention of shoes occurs when Scarlett arrives in Atlanta during the war: "Scarlett stood on the lower step of the train, a pale pretty figure in her black mourning dress, her crêpe veil fluttering almost to her heels. She hesitated, unwilling to soil her slippers and hems, and looked about in the shouting tangle of wagons, buggies and carriages for Miss Pittypat" (p.131).

From this point on, the novel frequently touches upon shoes, which are always portrayed as a sign of decline or wealth. A person's social status is indicated by the condition of their shoes: "How can we endure these scavengers in our midst with their varnished boots when our boys are tramping barefoot into battle?" (p.216).

Rhett Butler's elegance is always complete with new boots, in contrast to everyone else's bare footedness:

"How dare he sit there on that fine horse, in shining boots and handsome white linen suit, so sleek and well fed, smoking an expensive cigar, when Ashley and all the other boys were fighting the Yankees, barefooted, sweltering in the heat, hungry, their bellies rotten with disease?" (p.234).

The shoe scarcity among Confederate soldiers is also a primary indicator of the condition of their army. This observation is repeated in many passages. For example, when Melanie notes the appearance of Ashley's military uniform he responds:

"'And as for looking like a ragamuffin, you should thank your lucky stars your husband didn't come home barefooted. Last week my old boots wore completely out, and I would have come home with sacks tied on my feet if we hadn't had the good luck to shoot two Yankee scouts. The boots of one of them fitted me perfectly.' He stretched out his long legs in their scarred high boots for them to admire.

'And the boots of the other scout didn't fit me,' said Cade. 'They're two sizes too small and they're killing me this minute. But I'm going home in style just the same.'

'And the selfish swine won't give them to either of us,' said Tony. 'And they'd fit our small, aristocratic Fontaine feet perfectly.

Hell's afire, I'm ashamed to face Mother in these brogans. Before the war she wouldn't have let one of our darkies wear them.'

'Don't worry,' said Alex, eyeing Cade's boots. 'We'll take them off of him on the train going home. I don't mind facing Mother but I'm da – I mean I don't intend for Dimity Munroe to see my toes sticking out'" (p.243).

The most poignant extract is undoubtedly the letter Darcey Meade sends to his parents from the front, asking them to find him a pair of boots, because he was recently promoted and needs to wear appropriate footwear:

"Pa, could you manage to get me a pair of boots? I've been barefooted for two weeks now and I don't see any prospects of getting another pair. If I didn't have such big feet I could get them off dead Yankees like the other boys, but I've never yet found a Yankee whose feet were near as big as mine. If you can get me some, don't mail them. Somebody would steal them on the way and I wouldn't blame them. Put Phil on the train and send him up with them. (…) Pa, do try to manage some boots for me. I'm a captain now and a captain ought to have boots, even if he hasn't got a new uniform or epaulets" (p.231).

"'Yes, Scarlett, I think the Yankees have us. Gettysburg was the beginning of the end. The people back home don't know it yet. They can't realize how things stand with us, but – Scarlett, some of my men are barefooted now and the snow is deep in Virginia. And when I see their poor frozen feet, wrapped in rags and old sacks, and see the blood prints they leave in the snow, and know that I've got a whole pair of boots – well, I feel like I should give mine away and be barefooted too.'

'Oh, Ashley, promise me you won't give them away!'" (p.250).

Once again, shoes indicate one's circumstances. As money depreciated during the war, prices rose and shoes became scarce. Atlanta women therefore had to use a lot of imagination to shod themselves: "Shoes cost from two hundred to eight hundred dollars a pair, depending on whether they were made of 'cardboard' or real leather. Ladies now wore gaiters made of their old wool shawls and cut-up carpets. The soles were made of wood" (p.255).

Scarlett's difficulty climbing back up the social ladder is always indicated by her shoes: "The soles of her slippers were practically gone and were reinforced with pieces of carpet" (Chapter 31, p.473).

And when Scarlett thinks back to the past, to the luxury of the old days, she remembers her delicate mules of green Moroccan leather.

After the war ends Ashley is late returning to Tara and no one has any news; anxiety is at its peak: "'But don't cry Melly! Ashley'll come home. It's a long walk and maybe – maybe he hasn't got any boots.'

Then at the thought of Ashley barefooted, Scarlett could have cried. Let other soldiers limp by in rags with their feet tied up in sacks and strips of carpet, but not Ashley. He should come home on a prancing horse, dressed in fine clothes and shining boots, a plume in his hat. It was the final degradation for her to think of Ashley reduced to the state of these other soldiers" (p.458).

Then there is the character of Aunt Pittypat, who provides a bit of humor alongside the seriousness of war. Named after her little feet, although a large woman, her caricature includes a pair of overly narrow shoes that make her feet swell.

However, in *Gone With the Wind*, Margaret Mitchell observes the shoe from a primarily military perspective. Her analysis of the army's shoe shortage is thought provoking and recalls the words of Emperor Napoleon I: "A well-equipped soldier requires three things: a good rifle, a military coat and good shoes."

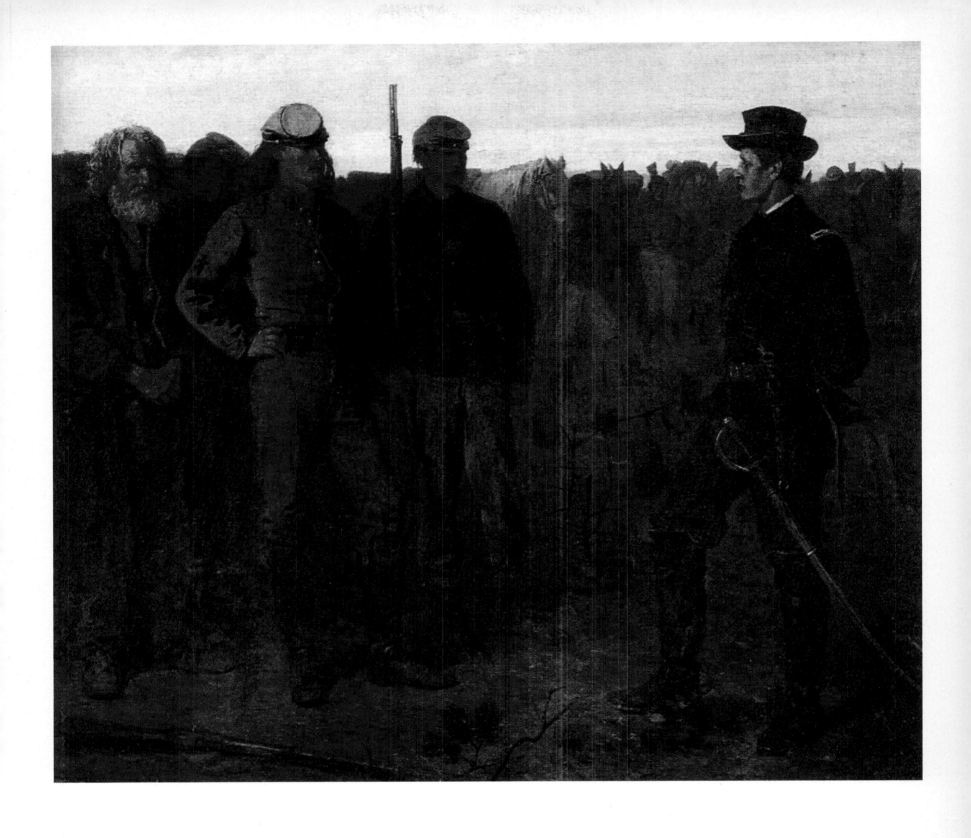

266. Winslow Homer. Detail from *Prisoners from the Front*, 1866.

The Metropolitan Museum of Art, New York.

Pearl S. Buck, *East Wind, West Wind*,
"Peony"

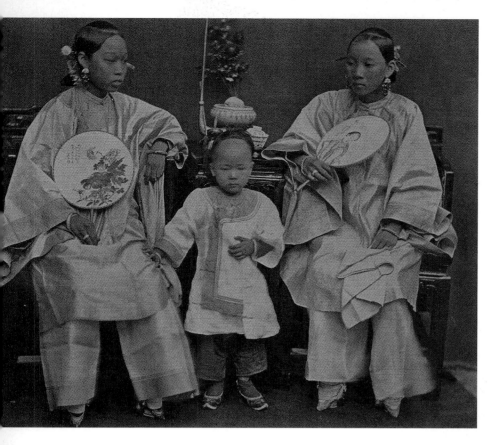

Pearl S. Buck lived in Northern China from 1923. As the setting for her novels, East Wind: West Wind and Peony document various aspects of Chinese life, giving the reader the illusion of entering the everyday reality of characters such as Peony, the protagonist of the novel bearing her name. In these two novels, the shoe is treated from a cultural perspective, including the frequent evocation of small, banded feet.

In her first novel, East Wind: West Wind, published in 1929, Pearl S. Buck shows how important foot banding was to Chinese women and the pride they took in this custom. However, by showing noless respect for the West, Buck denounces the cruelty of such a tradition though defended by the torturers themselves.

On the verge of marrying the man to whom she was promised even before she was born, Kwei-Lan listens to her mother's advice: "'The manners and etiquette of aristocratic life… these things you know… the cunning of shoes upon your little feet – ah, me, those feet of yours and all the tears they have cost! But I know of none so small in your generation. My own were scarcely more tiny at your age. I only hope that the family of Li have paid heed to my messages and have bound as closely the feet of their daughter, the betrothed of your brother, my son'" (*East Wind: West Wind*, pages 10-11, Moyer Bell, 1993). At the dawn of the Communist Revolution, Kwei-Lan remains attached to her parents' traditions and authority, but her husband, a young doctor, persuades her to renounce foot binding.

"'I have wished ever since our marriage to ask you if you will not unbind your feet. It is unhealthful for your whole body. See, your bones look like this.' He took a pencil and sketched hastily upon the leaf of his book a dreadful, bare, cramped foot.

How did he know? I had never dressed my feet in his presence. We Chinese women never expose our feet to the sight of others. Even at night we wear stockings of white cloth.

'How do you know?' I gasped.

'Because I am a doctor trained in the West,' he replied. 'And then, I wish you to unbind them because they are not beautiful. Besides, foot-binding is no longer in fashion. Does that move you?' He smiled slightly and looked at me not unkindly.

But I drew my feet hastily under my chair. I was stricken at his words. Not beautiful? I had always been proud of my tiny feet! All during my childhood my mother herself had superintended the soaking in hot water and the wrapping of the bandages – tight and more tight each day. When I wept in anguish she bid me remember that some day my husband would praise the beauty of my feet.

I bowed my head to hide my tears. I thought of all those restless nights and the days when I could not eat and had no desire to play – when I sat on the edge of my bed and let my poor feet swing to ease them of their weight of blood. And now after enduring until the pain had ceased for only a short year, to know he thought them ugly!

'I cannot,' I said, choking as I rose, and, unable to keep back my weeping, I left the room.

It was not that I cared over-much about my feet. But if even my feet in their cunningly embroidered shoes did not find favor in his sight, how could I hope to win his love?

Two weeks later I left for my first visit to my mother's home, according to our Chinese custom. My husband had not spoken of unbinding my feet again. Neither had he addressed me by my name" (*East Wind: West Wind*, pages 55-57, Moyer Bell, 1993).

Kwei-Lan's husband, through his medical studies in Europe, has abandoned the law of the ancestors and does not respect his country's customs or rituals. The poor little

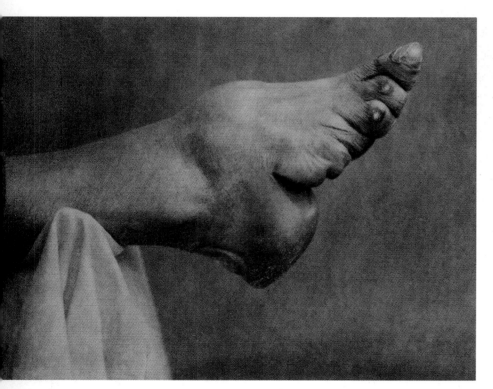

267. Photo of women and a little girl with bound feet. China. The Peabody & Essex Museum, Salem, Massachusetts.

268. Photo of a mutilated foot. The Peabody & Essex Museum, Salem, Massachusetts.

269. Shoe cloisonné, gift offered between spouses. China. Collection of Gérard Lévy. 18th century.

270. Shoes for bound feet. China. International Shoe Museum, Romans.

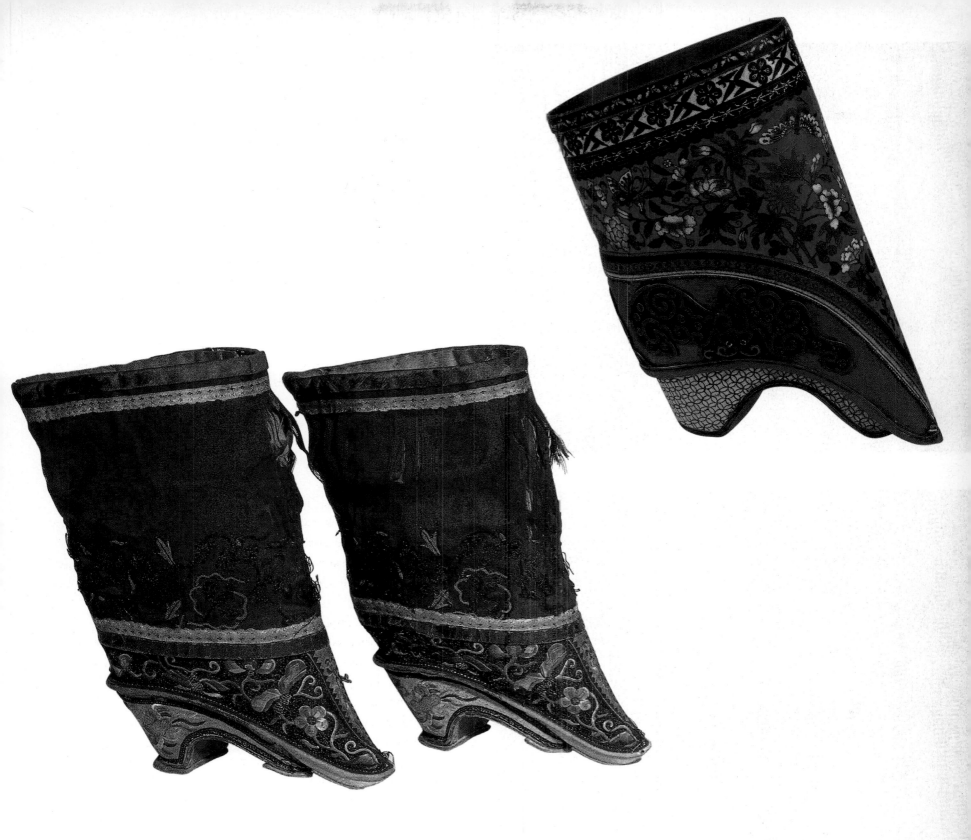

wife tries in vain to seduce her husband using all the resources of her meticulous and refined education, but the young doctor responds with indifference to all these attentions, making the young woman an exile in her own country.

The husband's point of view reappears in Peony in a passage describing how Peony, a young slave, is happy with her condition of servitude, because it allows her to escape foot binding, giving her the ability to run:

"How she loved to run! It was her luck to be bondmaid in this house of foreigners. Had she been in a Chinese house her feet would have been bound small as soon as it was sure she was to be pretty, so that if a son of the house were to love her and want her for a concubine, she would not shame the family by having feet like a servant's" (Peony, pages 28-29). Kwei-Lan's opinion of a Western woman's feet says a lot about the persistent attachment Chinese women had to foot mutilation: "I looked at her feet and saw that they were like rice-flails for size."

(East Wind: West Wind, p. 105, Moyer Bell, 1993). This issue marks a cultural divide between East and West. On the other hand, Buck often mentions shoes furtively in descriptions of costume or uses shoes to describe movement. These indications are always under the sign of lightness and silence, because the shoes were made of black satin or velvet:

"So saying she tripped away, her satin-shod feet silent upon the stones of the court" (Peony, p.65). The descriptions always emphasize the simplicity of Chinese shoes, slippers, and sandals, but the author also lingers over children's shoes adorned with animal heads that were embroidered by mothers for their sons:

"I have made him a pair of shoes with tiger faces" (East Wind: West Wind, p.110, Moyer Bell, 1993).

With this description of pretty shoes for little boys, Pearl S. Buck juxtaposes the sad privilege reserved for young girls in great Chinese families who have little feet.

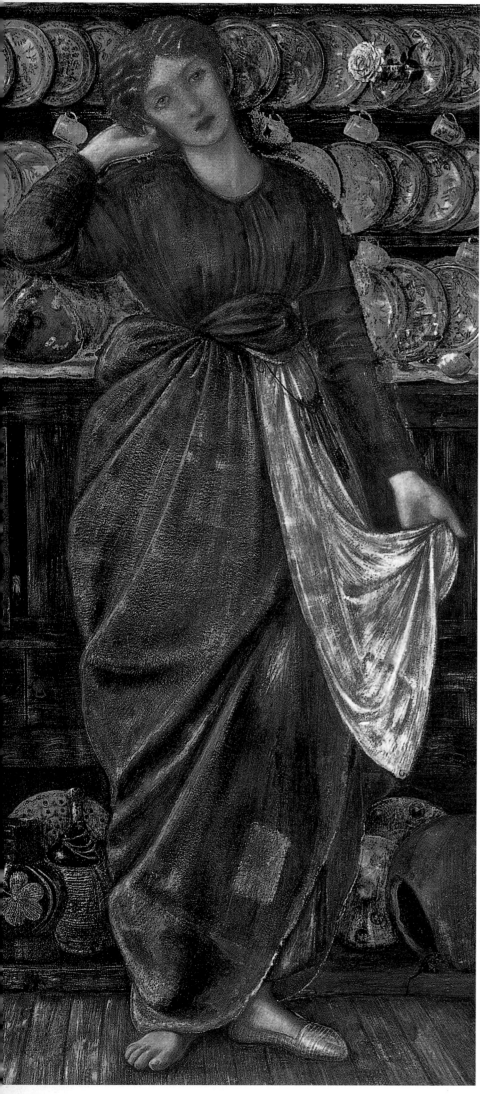

Charles Perrault

The countless adaptations of these three fairytales for children have overshadowed Charles Perrault's original works intended for adults. A trilogy of the shoe, the stories offer the following perspectives: Cinderella, or the slipper of seduction; Puss in Boots, or the boots of appearances and rediscovered dignity; and Little Thumb, or the boots of power. One has only to return to the originals to be convinced.

Cinderella

Cinderella's glass slipper is the story's centerpiece:

"Her fairy godmother merely tapped her with her wand … then she gave here a pair of glass slippers, the most beautiful in the world."

At the ball, "The young lady was having so much fun she forgot her fairy godmother's advice; as a result, she was surprised when she heard the first stroke of midnight, having thought it was only eleven o'clock: she stood up and ran out as nimbly as a doe. The prince followed her but was unable to catch her. She dropped one of her glass slippers, which the prince picked up with great care. Cinderella arrived home completely out of breath without a coach and footman and wearing her old clothes: nothing remained of her former magnificence except for one of her little slippers, which matched the one she had allowed to fall off." This scene recalls the story of Rhodopis told by Strabo in the 1st century BC (which Perrault probably knew), as well as the Chinese tale of Sheh Hsien mentioned previously. As for Cinderella's lightness of foot, compared to that of a doe, the image has its source in a number of Biblical passages, such as in Habaquq III:19 (… he makes my feet like doe feet and makes me walk on my high places…), the Psalms, and the Book of Samuel. One also thinks of the Buddhist story of Padmavati, daughter of a Brahmin and a doe whose hooves are hidden in silk wrappings, which leads us to the Séducta label created by Charles Jourdan, its lively mark shows a doe-like creature in a leaping pose. Returning to Cinderella's lost slipper:

"When her two sisters returned from the ball, Cinderella asked them if they had fun and if the beautiful lady had been there; they replied yes, but that she had fled at the stroke of midnight and so hastily that she had dropped one of her little glass slippers, the most beautiful in the world; that the prince had picked it up and did nothing but stare at it for the remainder of the ball and that he had definitely fallen in love with the beauty to whom the little slipper belonged. They were right, because a little later the prince announced through his herald that he would marry the woman whose foot fit the little slipper.

Fittings started with princesses, followed by duchesses, then the entire court, but it was a waste of time. The prince was taken to the home of the two sisters, who did everything they could to get their feet into the slipper, but they were unable to pull it off. Cinderella, who was watching, recognized the slipper and said, while smiling:

"I can tell it wouldn't look bad on me!" (…) The gentleman who was doing the fitting regarded Cinderella attentively and found her to be very beautiful, and said that it would be fair, as he had been ordered to try it on every young woman. He made Cinderella sit down and, as soon as he brought the slipper to her little foot, he could tell that it would naturally fit and it slid right on like wax. The two sisters were dumbfounded, but they were even more shocked when Cinderella drew from her pocket the matching little slipper, which she put on her other foot."

And we all know the happy ending:

"She was taken to the young prince dressed just as she was. He found her more beautiful than ever and a short time later he married her" (Extracts from Charles Perrault's original text published in Paris in 1697).

These large extracts from Charles Perrault's original text, published in Paris in 1697, are explicit enough for us to catch the allusion to the sexual act. The symbolism of Cinderella's "glass" slipper in this way makes clear the popular expression "to find a shoe for one's foot." In the early 19th-century, Jackob Ludwig Grimm offered a variation on this tale:

Cinderella had two very ugly sisters. Their mother ordered the eldest to cut off her big toe so she could wear the prince's slipper; the other sister cut off half of her heel.

"The next morning the prince went to see his father the king and told him, 'The only one who can be my wife is the one who can wear this beautiful slipper.' The two sisters rejoiced then, because they had pretty feet. The eldest took the slipper into another room to try it on. But the slipper was too small and she couldn't get her big toe in. Her mother who was nearby said, 'Take the knife and cut off your big toe. You won't be walking on foot when you're queen.' The young girl cut off her big toe, forced her foot into the slipper, overcame her pain, and returned to the prince and the king. He then mounted her on his horse and took off with her as his fiancé."

The prince discovered the deception when he saw blood flowing across the shoe. He returned the girl to her mother who gave him her second daughter. Yet, once again, blood put an end to the ploy. Finally enters Cinderella with her slender foot formed exactly in the shape of the slipper, allowing her to reign in the prince's court happily ever after.

Puss in Boots
"From the Mill to the Castle"

In this fairytale, Perrault puts words in the mouth of a talking cat in the manner of Jean de la Fontaine:

"Don't worry master, all you have to do is give me a sac and make me a pair of boots for going into the brush and you'll see that you're not as bad off as you think you are."

The sole inheritance of the miller's youngest son, this mouse and rat eater assumes the appearance of a man by dressing in boots.

"When the cat received what he had asked for, he bravely put the boots on, threw his sac over his shoulder, grabbed the strings with his two front paws, and set off for a hunting ground where there were a large number of rabbits."

The boots were intended for the cat's hunting expeditions and to protect him from the brush, but proved to be a hindrance when climbing roofs to escape an ogre who turned himself into a lion.

"The cat was so terrified to see a lion in front of him that he immediately jumped into the gutters, which was a difficult and dangerous thing to do on account of his boots, which were not suited for walking on roof tiles."

Unlike Little Thumb's functional seven-league boots, designed for leaving at a moment's notice to cover great distances, the clever cat's boots were instead suited for to his role as a skilled strategist, which resulted in his impoverished master becoming the Marquis of Carabas, a rich landowner, lord, and moreover, the king's son-in-law.

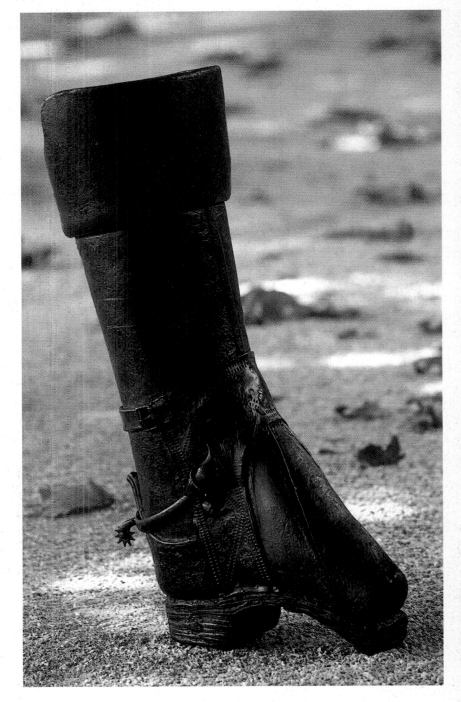

271. Burne-Jones. *Cinderella*, 1863. Watercolour and gouache on paper applied to canvas. Museum of Fine Arts, Boston.

272. Postilion's boot also called, "seven league boot". Weight: 4.5 kg. France, end of the 17th century. The seven leagues represent the distance covered by postilions between two posts. International Shoe Museum, Romans.

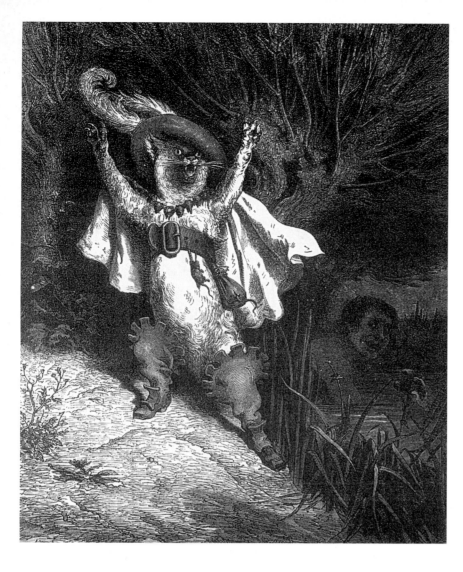

Petit Poucet
(Little Thumb)

One of Perrault's most popular fairytales, Little Thumb was widely published with many different variations and omissions beginning in the 18th century. The author's text gives a precise itinerary for a pair of seven-league boots, the indispensable accessory to a giant ogre's magic power, which Little Thumb will acquire through exceptional ingenuity.

The ogre's house is the starting point for the itinerary of the boots. When he learns that his seven daughters have ruined him, the ogre tells his wife, "Quick, give me my seven-league boots so I can catch them."

This is how Little Thumb and his brother discover the power of the ogre's seven-league boots: "They saw that the giant was going from one mountain to the next and that he crossed rivers as easily as if they were tiny streams."

The ogre's magic boots correspond to the winged feet of Hermes, the Greek messenger of the gods who could instantaneously cross the sky. While the ogre sleeps, the audacious Little Thumb takes off his boots and takes hold of their power.

"Little Thumb drew near to the giant, gently pulled off his boots, and immediately put them on. The boots were extremely wide and long, but since they were magical, they could expand or shrink according to the leg they clothed; so it happened that they fit his feet and legs as if they had been made for him."

Dressed in these magical boots, he returned to the giant's house to seize his gold, telling the giant's wife: "It is such a pressing matter he wanted me to take these seven-league boots and carry on post haste…"

Little Thumb returned to his father's home with all the giant's riches. But Perrault leaves the end of the story up in the air: "Many people disagree with this last detail… They attest that when Little Thumb put the giant's boots on he went to court where he knew that an army two hundred leagues away was desperately needed, as was new from the front. He sought the King, they say, to whom he offered to bring news of the army before the end of the day. The King promised Little Thumb a large sum of money if he was successful. Little Thumb returned that very evening with the news and this first run brought him attention and he had all the work he needed. The King paid him handsomely to carry his orders to the army and countless women would pay any price for news of their lovers, and this was his greatest profit. Some wives gave him letters to carry to their husbands, but they paid him so little and it was such a small thing that he dared not reveal what he earned from that side of the business. After working as a courier and having amassed a fortune he returned to his father's house where he was received with unimaginable joy."

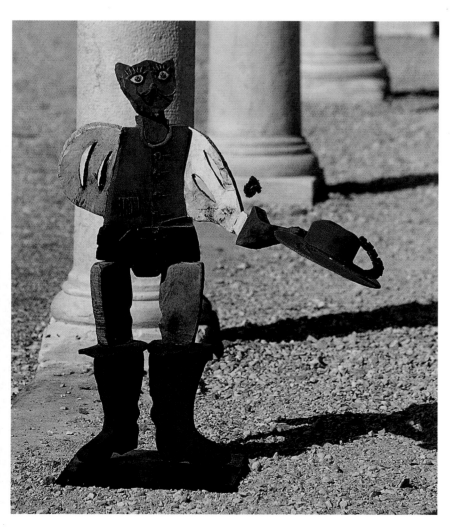

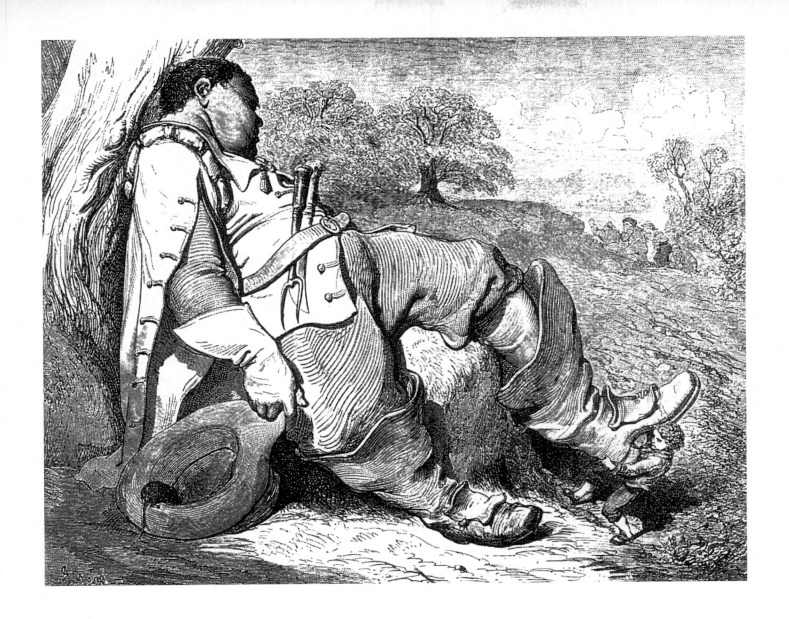

Coachmen's boots, also called "seven-league boots" in the 17th century are connected with Little Thumb and his role as the King's courier. In the last paragraph, ignored in the versions adapted for children, beautiful 17th-century women imitate their ancient Roman counterparts by entrusting amorous letters to Little Thumb.

Ovid's *The Art of Love* sanctioned the role of confidants carrying gallant messages in their sandals for their mistresses, and Perrault allows himself the same privilege with the seven-league boots. Charles Perrault pictures the power of the seven-league boots making Little Thumb the King's best courier and saves the child and his family from poverty.

Much later, Marcel Aymé based his tales of the Perched Cat on these stories. By placing the seven-league boots in a Parisian setting in Montmartre where dream and reality are combined he gives the story a contemporary, urban twist.

In these three fairytales, Perrault makes the shoe an emblematic accessory in the search for happiness, glory, power, and fortune.

273. *Puss in Boots*, tales by Perrault, engraving by Gustave Doré. 19th century.

274. Henri Terres. *Puss in Boots*. 1995. International Shoe Museum, Romans.

275. *Tom Thumb*, tales by Perrault, engraving by Gustave Doré. 19th century.

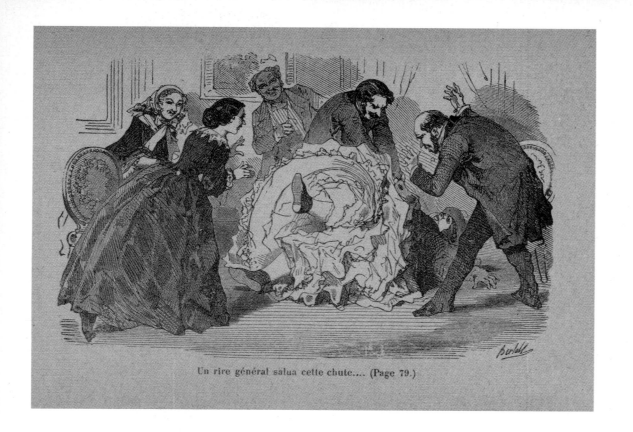

Un rire général salua cette chute.... (Page 79.)

The Countess of Ségur, *Good Little Girls*
"The Shoe of Madame Fichini"

The Countess of Ségur, born Sophie Rostopchine, was a children's book writer of Russian decent. Her trilogy of Sophie, *Les petites filles modèles* (Good Little Girls), followed by *Les malheurs de Sophie* (Sophie's Troubles) and *Vacances* (Vacations) are crown jewels among children's book collections and have a Second Empire ambiance.

The 1857 publication of *Petites filles modèles* (Good Little Girls) details the showy elegance of an upstart named Madame Finchini right down to the shoes when she arrives at Madame de Fleurville's country house: "'Here I am Dear Ladies,' she said stepping out of the car and revealing her big foot dressed in lilac satin shoes that matched her dress and had lace ornaments" (Ch. IX, p.76, Hachette).

A lilac faille ankle boot preserved in the Galliera Museum in Paris resembles this description as does Bertall's illustration reproduced in the 1857 edition, showing Madame Fichini's spectacular fall with her leg in the air and her foot in the shoe.

276. *The Little Girl Models: Fall of Madame Fichini*, illustration by Bertall,
former publishing house of Hachette booksellers.

277. Pair of lilac bottines by Camille Di Mauro. Around 1860. Galliera Museum,
Fashion Museum, Paris. Photo by Lifermann, PMVP.

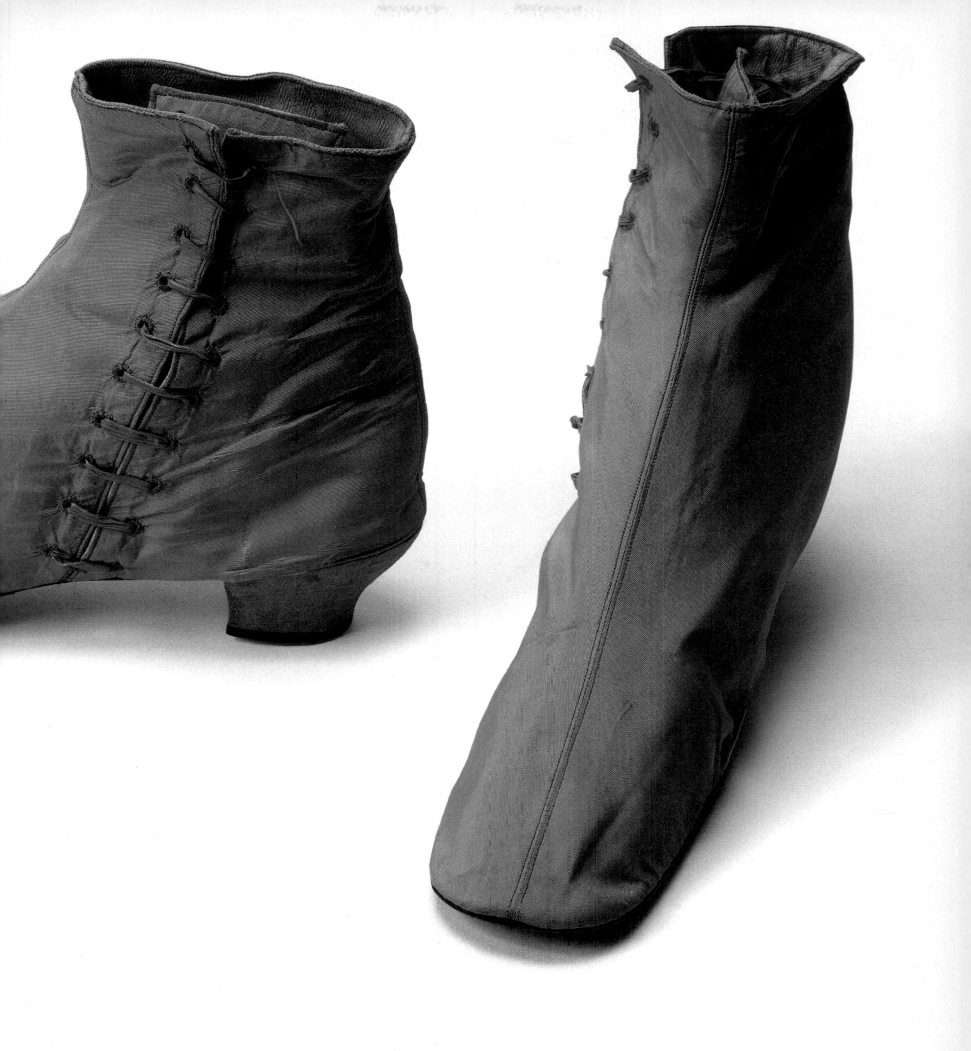

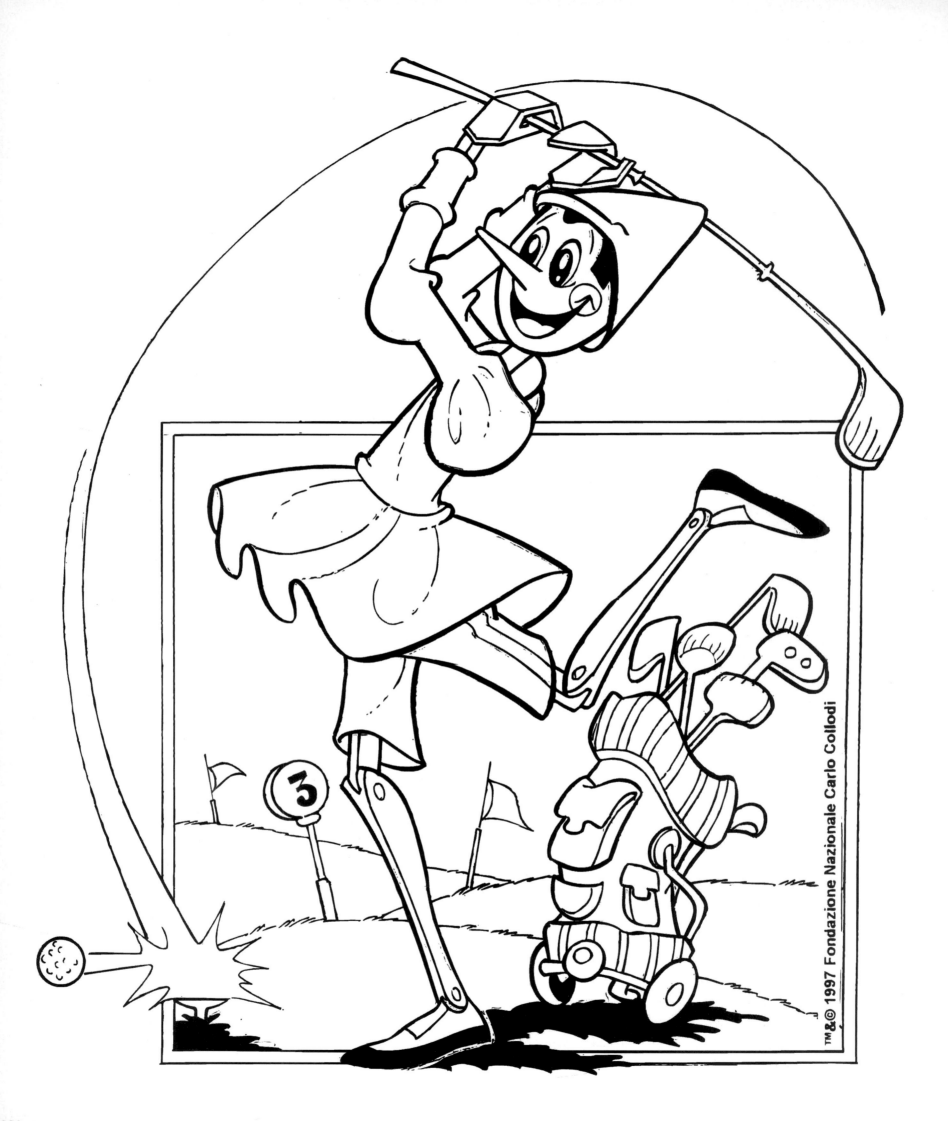

Carlo Collodi: *The Adventures of Pinocchio*
"Feet and Shoes"

Carlo Collodi's adventures of Pinocchio were first published in serial form. The book was immensely successful when it finally appeared in 1883. From the wooden puppet made by Gepetto to his metamorphosis into a real little boy with the help of a blue-haired fairy, the author uses the word for foot fifty-four times; the verb to walk fifteen times; the verb to run thirteen times; the verb to jump five times; the verb to leap four times; the verb to climb once; and a word for shoe six times. The vocabulary allows Pinocchio to make remarkable use of his feet. Pinocchio, a woodenheaded vagabond without a brain who is always in trouble due to his lies and has a nose that grows if he fails to tell the truth, also shows an exceptional capacity for exercise through mountains and valleys by means of his nimble feet handmade by his father Gepetto. Studying how Pinocchio employed his feet in different circumstances reveals the puppet's psychology: insolent feet, careless feet, defensive feet, and even angry feet.

Pinocchio's insolence starts the moment he is made: "The legs and feet still had to be made. When Gepetto finished them he received a kick in the nose" (*The Adventures of Pinocchio*, Gallimard p.12). There was more monkey business from the puppet when he tries out his new feet after his father had guided his first steps, teaching him to walk: "Then he lifted the puppet under its arms and sat it down on the floor in the room to make it walk. Pinocchio's legs were heavy and he did not know how to use them, so Gepetto took his hand and guided him, teaching him how to put one foot in front of the other. When his legs had loosened up, Pinocchio started to walk on his own and began running all over the room; suddenly he opened the door, leapt into the street, and fled. Poor Gepetto ran after the puppet, but was unable to catch up with him, because this naughty Pinocchio leapt like a hare and his wooden feet striking the pavement made as much noise as twenty peasants in wooden clogs" (Gallimard, p.12). But his carelessness has consequences as he sleeps: "He returned home soaked to the core, dead tired, and hungry; and as he was too weak to stand, he sat down hanging his dripping wet feet over the brazier full of still flaming embers. He feel asleep in this manner and while he was sleeping, his feet, which were made of wood, caught fire and little by little burned to ashes, which fell to the floor" (Gallimard, p.22).

During a fight with his friends, it is his feet that all called into action to defend him:

"Although he was alone, Pinocchio defended himself heroically. He used his hard wooden feet so well that he kept his enemies at a respectable distance at all times. When his feet were in striking distance they always left a memorable bruise" (*The Adventures of Pinocchio*, p. 92, Gallimard).

In this particular situation, Pinocchio hurls verbal abuse upon a large, moralizing crab who sounds "like a trombone with a cold" when it tries to break up the fight:

"'Shut-up boring old crab! You'd be better off taking two lichen tablets to cure your sore throat'" (*The Adventures of Pinocchio*, p. 92, Gallimard).

Finally, Pinocchio's feet get angry when he returns to the fairy and the chambermaid; a large slug is slow to answer the door and takes hours to go down four flights of stairs. The puppet loses all patience: "'Ah, hello?' cried Pinocchio, becoming overwhelmed with rage. 'And if the top part of the door gives way I'll keep banging it with my feet.' With that he stepped back and gave the door a tremendous kick. The blow was so strong that his foot halfway entered the wood and when the puppet wanted to pull his foot out, all his efforts were in vain: his foot remained stuck in the wood, like a well-driven nail. Imagine the poor Pinocchio! He had to spend the whole night with one foot on the ground and the other foot in the air." (*The Adventures of Pinocchio*, pages 102-103, Gallimard).

When the blue-haired fairy finds Pinocchio half-dead in her house, a victim of the collusion of two crooked assassins (the cat and the fox), she calls three doctors to the puppet's bedside for a consultation: a crow, an owl, and a cricket. The house call is in response to the fairy's request: "'Please tell me if this unhappy puppet is dead or alive!'... To this request, the crow approached first, took Pinocchio's pulse, then felt his nose, then his little toe; when he had palpated all that he made the following solemn pronouncement: 'In my opinion, the puppet is dead in every sense of the word, but if by some misfortune he was not dead, we would then be certain that he is alive'" (*The Adventures of Pinocchio*, p.54, Gallimard).

In Pinocchio's case, an examination of his little toe helps the practitioner make a diagnosis. As for shoes, they are mentioned six times surrounding Pinocchio, once relating to Medor (the fairy's poodle) and once in relation to the team of donkeys about to leave for the Country of Toys. After the episode of the burned feet, Gepetto remakes new feet for the puppet who resolves to go to school:

— "I'm going to start school immediately."
— "That's good my boy."
— "But I will need a few clothes to go to school."

Gepetto was so poor he did not even have one penny in his pocket, so he made Pinocchio a little outfit out of flowered paper, a pair of shoes from tree bark and a little hat out of soft bread. All the same, Pinocchio plays truant from school finding the attraction of a marionette theater irresistible. Since he lacks the four sous needed for admission, he offers to sell his shoes to a little boy, who declines the offer:

— "You don't want to buy my shoes?"
— "They're only good for lighting the fire" (Gallimard, p.30).

Medor, the blue-haired fairy's poodle, could stand on his rear legs like a man. Carlo Collodi created charming, elegant and amusing clothing for the dogs, immersing us in fantasy and wonder: "The poodle was dressed like a livery coachman for a gala. On his head was a tri-corned hat trimmed in gold braid, atop a white wig, whose curls fell below the shoulders; he wore a long, chocolate-coloured vest with diamond buttons and two large pockets for storing the bones that his mistress gave him for lunch, crimson velvet pants, silk stockings, little slippers, and behind, he carried a blue satin umbrella that he removed from a sort of scabbard when it started to rain" (*The Adventures of Pinocchio*, p.54, Gallimard). The author's inspiration here is the 18th-century fashion for pants, silk stockings, and flat shoes. Pinocchio discovers the fox and the cat and leaves with them to plant four gold pieces in the Field of Wonders located on the outskirts of city called the "City of Simple Simons": "'We're here,' said the fox to the puppet. 'Now get down and dig a little hole with your hands and put your gold pieces in it.' Pinocchio obeyed. He dug the hole from a little earth, deposited the four remaining gold crowns and then covered the hole. 'And now,' said the fox, 'Go over to that canal over there and fill a pail with water to give your planting a drink.'" "Pinocchio went to the canal, and since he didn't have a pail with him, he took one of his old shoes, filled it with water, and watered the spot where he had covered the hole" (Gallimard, p.62). The improvised watering can, employed here to show Pinocchio's naiveté, is used a second time: "He got near the field and stopped to look and see if by chance he had missed a tree with branches filled with gold pieces; but he saw nothing... He went to the canal and once again filled his shoe with water and went to water the ground over his gold pieces again" (Gallimard, p.64). The story of Pinocchio's departure for the Country of Toys in a donkey-drawn vehicle creates a stunning scene with the spectacle of a team of twenty-four little donkeys each with four hooves dressed in ankle boots; this amounts to a total of forty-eight pairs, for a grand total of ninety-six ankle boots! "Then the wagon arrived without the slightest sound because its wheels were wrapped in hemp fibers and rags." "Twelve pairs of donkeys, all the same size, but with different coats drew it. Some were gray, others white or with salt and pepper markings, while others still were adorned with large yellow and blue stripes. But the most singular thing was this: the twelve pairs, in other words, eighty donkeys, instead of being shod like any other animal or beast of burden had their feet in white calfskin ankle boots like humans wore" (Gallimard, p.109).

These ankle boots were symbols of the former state of the little boys who had metamorphosed into donkeys because of their laziness. But Pinocchio's good heart helps him overcome his naughty faults. The idle and lazy puppet turns himself into a worker. With his savings he decides to buy shoes: "One morning he said to his father, 'I'm going to the market nearby to buy myself a jacket, a little beret, and a pair of shoes'" (Gallimard, p.140). Pinocchio finally stops being a puppet and becomes a little boy. The fairy appears to him in a dream and forgives him for all his naughtiness and praises his good behavior: "At that moment, the dream ended. Pinocchio sat up and his eyes were wide open just like that. Now imagine his astonishment when he realized that he was no longer a wooden puppet, but that he had become a little boy like all the others. He glanced about and instead of the thatched cottage's straw walls he saw a beautiful little room that was furnished and decorated with an almost elegant simplicity. Leaping from his bed, he found beautiful new clothes and a beret laid out for him, as well as a pair of leather ankle boots that fit him like a glove" (Gallimard, p.141). Henceforth liberated from the slavery of laziness, Pinocchio acquires dignity. He is no longer one of the barefooted; his ankle boots were the obvious symbol of his condition.

Marcel Aymé, *Les contes du Chat Perché*
(Tales of the Perched Cat)
High Heels Oh!

Marcel Aymé transports his readers to the French countryside to tell the story of Delphine and Marinette in the lucid, spontaneous, and fresh style of the *Contes du Chat Perché* (Tales of the Perched Cat). The two little girls are leading a tame life focused on school and the farm, when their cousin Flora comes to visit, looking like a silly goose in high heels. From then on the girls are totally preoccupied with style and frilly ornaments: "One day Delphine and Marinette told their parents that they didn't want to wear clogs anymore. This is what had happened. Their older cousin Flora, who was almost fourteen and who lived in a big city, came to spend a week on the farm. As she had just one month earlier received her diploma, her mother and father had bought her a wristwatch, a silver ring, and a pair of high-heeled shoes … Therefore, the day after Flora left, the little girls placed their hands on their hips to give themselves confidence and Delphine said to the parents: 'Clogs are not really that practical if you think about it. First of all, they make one's feet hurt and what happens too is that water gets inside, whereas with shoes there is less risk, especially if the heel is a little bit high, and shoes are much prettier…'

The parents took a deep breath and after looking at their frowning daughters for a moment responded with a terrible voice. The little girls dared not speak anymore to their parents about hair, dresses or shoes. But when they were alone, going back and forth to school, or out in the pastures guarding the cows, or in the woods picking strawberries, they put rocks in their clogs so as to have a higher heel, turned their dress inside out to give the impression of having changed and put their hair up with a string."

This 1939 text still remains extremely topical through a subtle partnering of past and future. With an apparent ease full of subtlety, the writer's gift for observation translates the psychology of many young girls anxious to step into adulthood; high-heeled shoes, symbol of feminine seduction, summon them. Simultaneously, using the power of affective memory as a true magic mirror, the author takes adults back to the world of their own childhood.

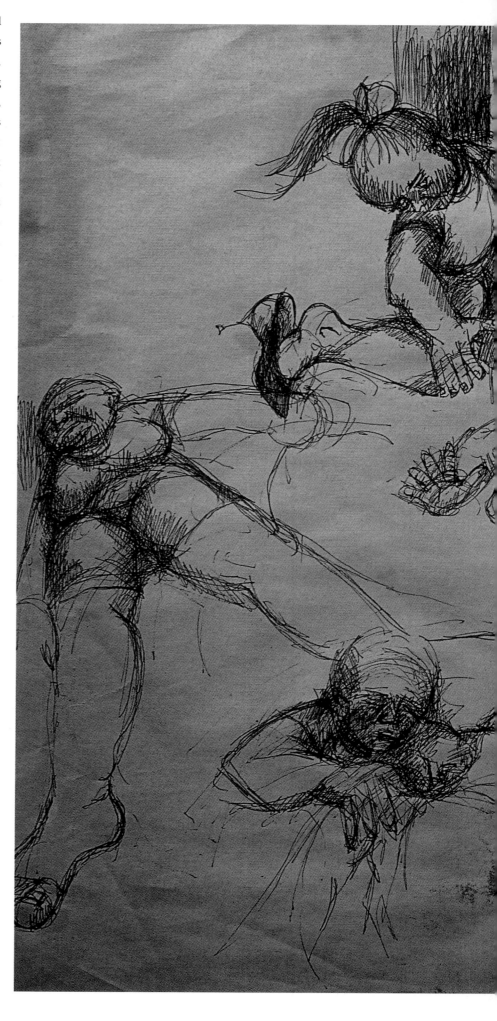

Previous page:

278. Drawing of Pinocchio. Carlo Collodi National Foundation.

279. Christina Tarares. "High Heels Oh!"

232

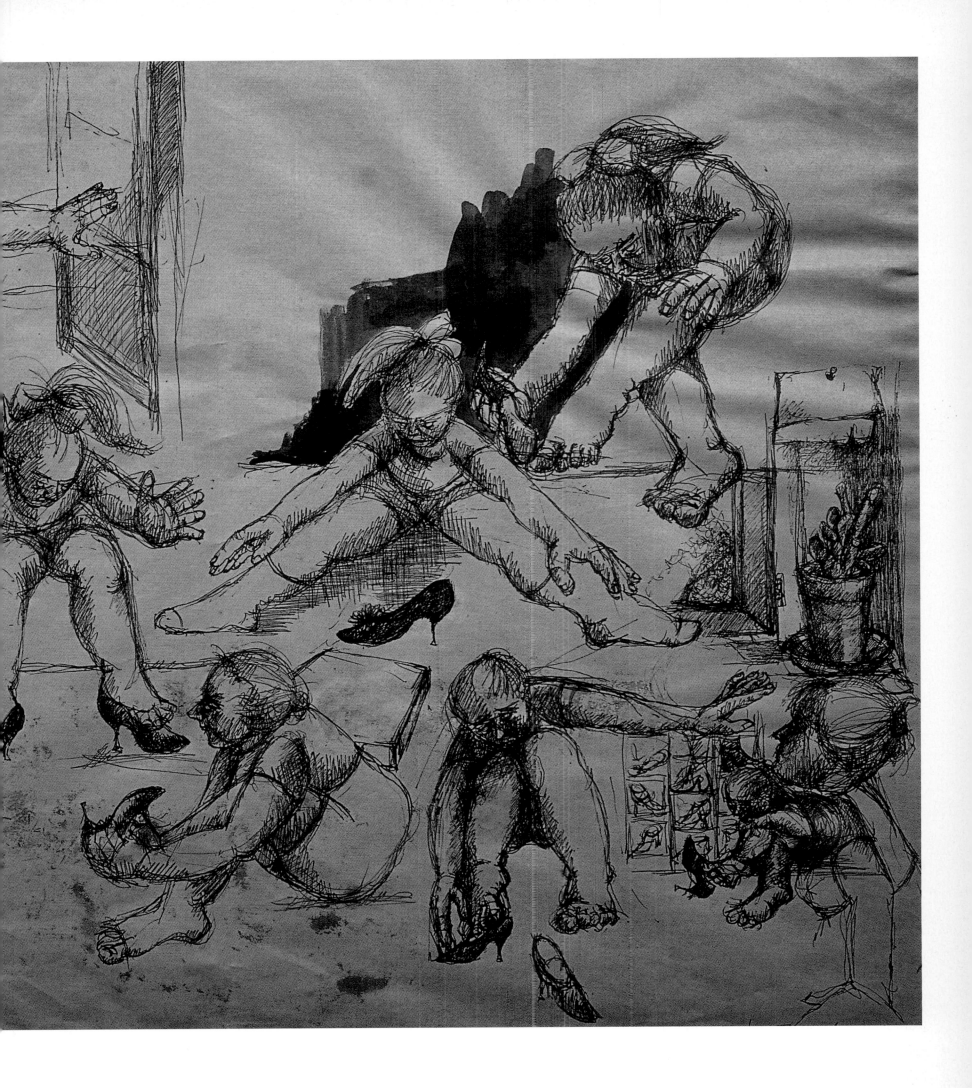

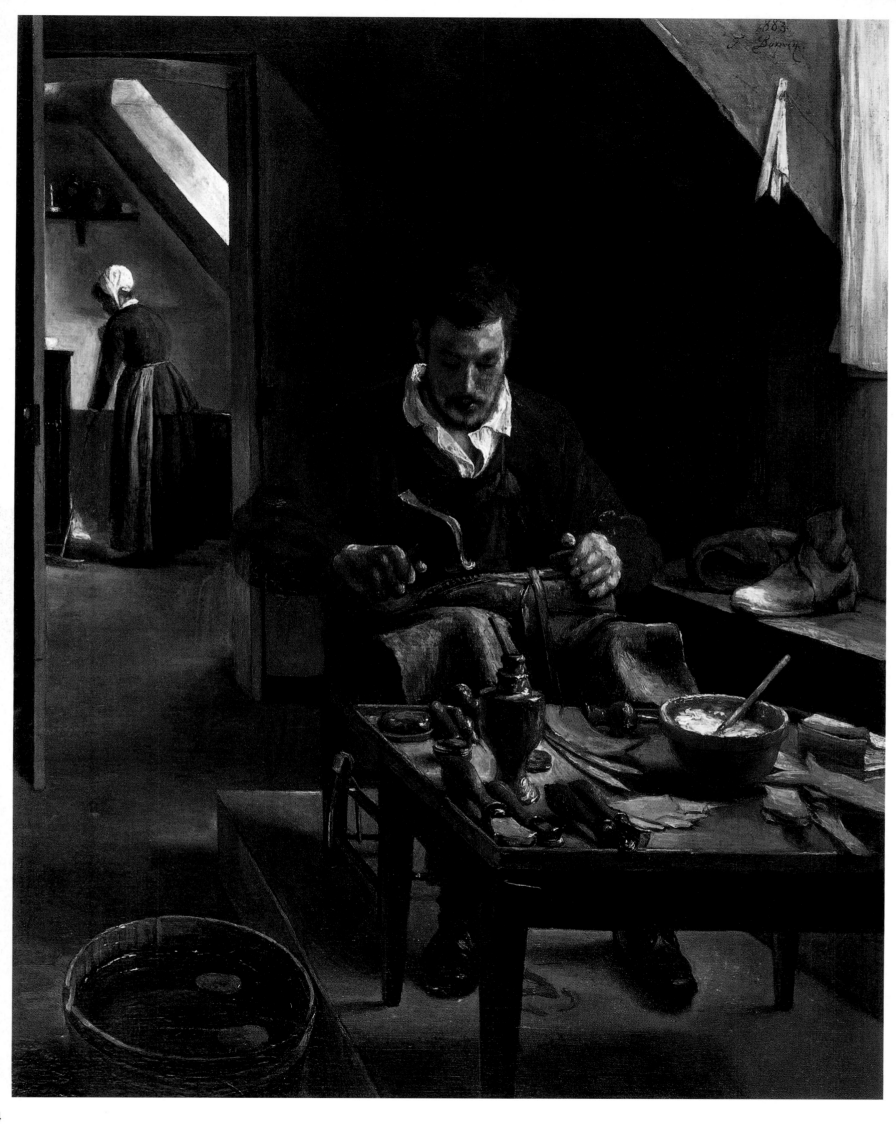

234

The Shoe and Art

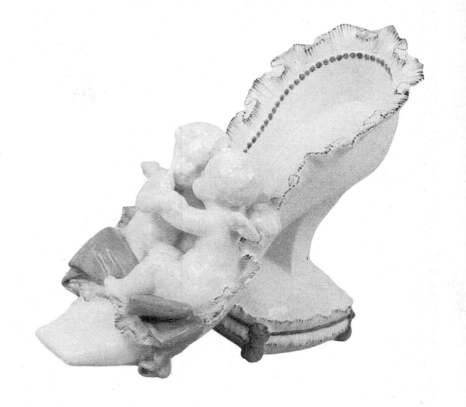

Conceived for walking, the shoe is an essential everyday object, but its aesthetic qualities can elevate it to the status of art. As art objects, shoes say a lot about their creator's personality, but above all they express the ideas and manual skill of the shoemaker, whether famous or anonymous. Shoes are also inexhaustible sources of iconography that have nourished the imagination of artists throughout the world, throughout time, in drawing and sculpture and in the decorative and plastic arts. This part of the book is therefore primarily visual, devoted to the contemplation of selected works from the countless examples of shoes transformed by artistic inspiration.

In 1832, Delacroix travelled to North Africa, a major episode in his career that transformed his vision, his technique, and his aesthetic. Maurice Serullaz, in his book on Delacroix, lists the various items the artist brought back, as indicated by the notes in Delacroix's travel journal:

"Five pair of slippers; eleven pairs of slippers with double soles; two small pairs; one small women's pair; common woman's slipper; man's slipper without quarter; four pairs of boots" (Maurice Serullaz, Delacroix, Ch. VII, "Living Antiquity", Light and its Coloured Reflections, p.173).

Delacroix shared his shoe observations in a letter he wrote to Félix Grullemardet as he approached Tangiers on January 24, 1832:

"After a lengthy crossing of thirteen long days, dear friend, I am damp facing the African river and with a view of this town, the first in the Moroccan empire with which we communicate. This morning I had the pleasure of watching a boatload of Moroccans come aside our corvette to bring over our consul whom we had contacted. These people exhibit a mélange of fascinating costumes: several were a little like the Barbary coast outfits one sees in Paris, except the men have bare legs and feet: only the lords wear slippers" (Maurice Serullaz, Delacroix, Ch. VIII, "Living Antiquity" Light and its Reflections, p.145).

Delacroix hardly considered shoes a superfluous accessory. According to what he wrote to George Sand in 1838, he felt quite the contrary:

"I had to run to both ends of Paris all day… I will try to come see you tonight and put on your shoes; I love the slippers, stockings, and legs (in the Arab fashion). Send word if I cannot see you and kindest regards."

As Maurice Serullaz points out: "And he signed with a visual pun he rarely used: Eugène 2, the musical note la, and a cross," which sounded out his name when spoken in French: deux, la, croix. (Maurice Serullaz, Delacroix, Ch. X, Les bibliothèques du Palais-Bourbon et du Palais du Luxembourg 1838-1848, p.203).

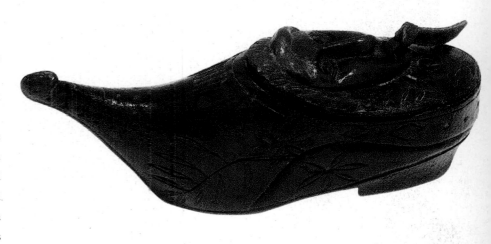

280. François Bonvin. *Shoemaker's Workshop*, 19th century. Beres Gallery Collection.

281. Court shoe in Dresden china, 19th century, International Shoe Museum, Romans.

282. Clog-shaped snuffbox. Rural Museum of Popular Arts, Laduz.

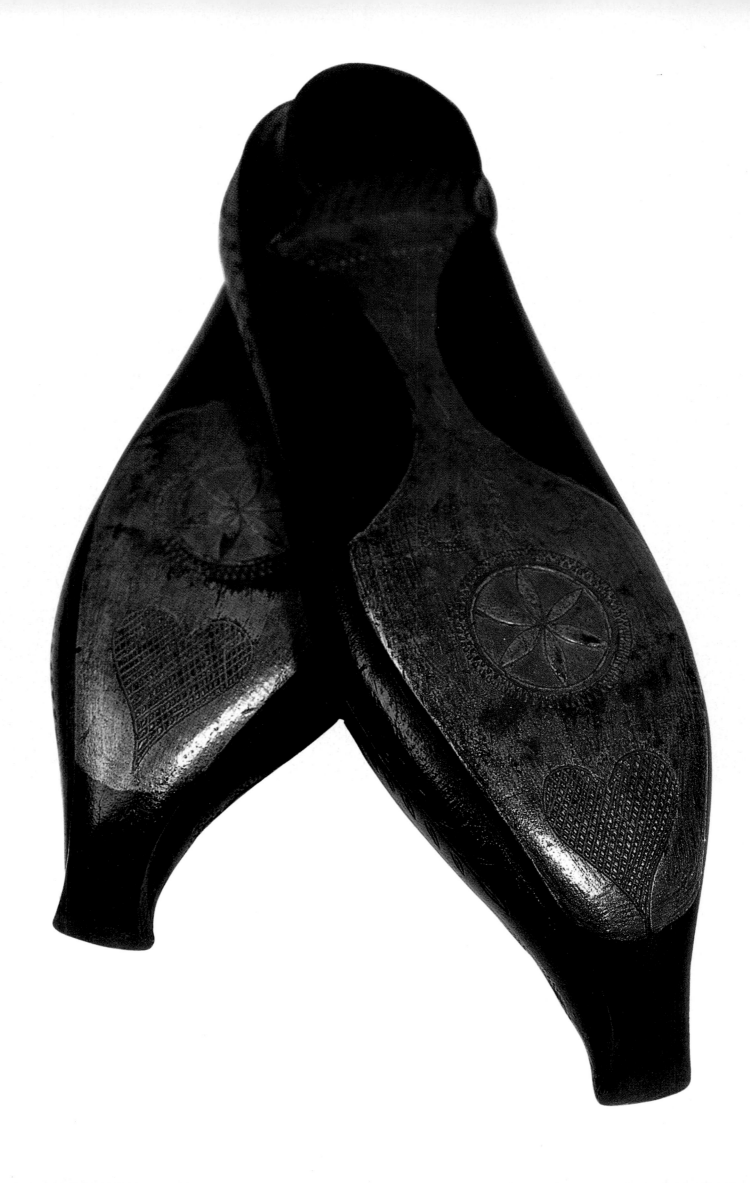

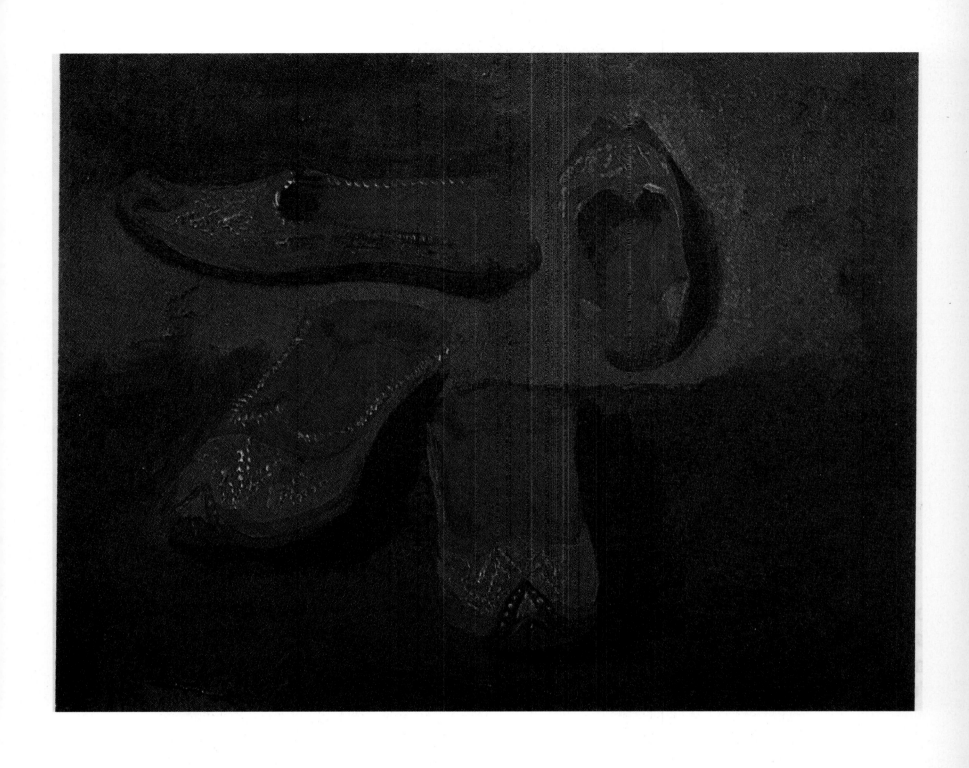

283. Marriage clogs. 19th century. Rural Museum of Popular Arts, Laduz.

284. Eugène Delacroix. *Babouches*, 1832. Louvre Museum, Paris.

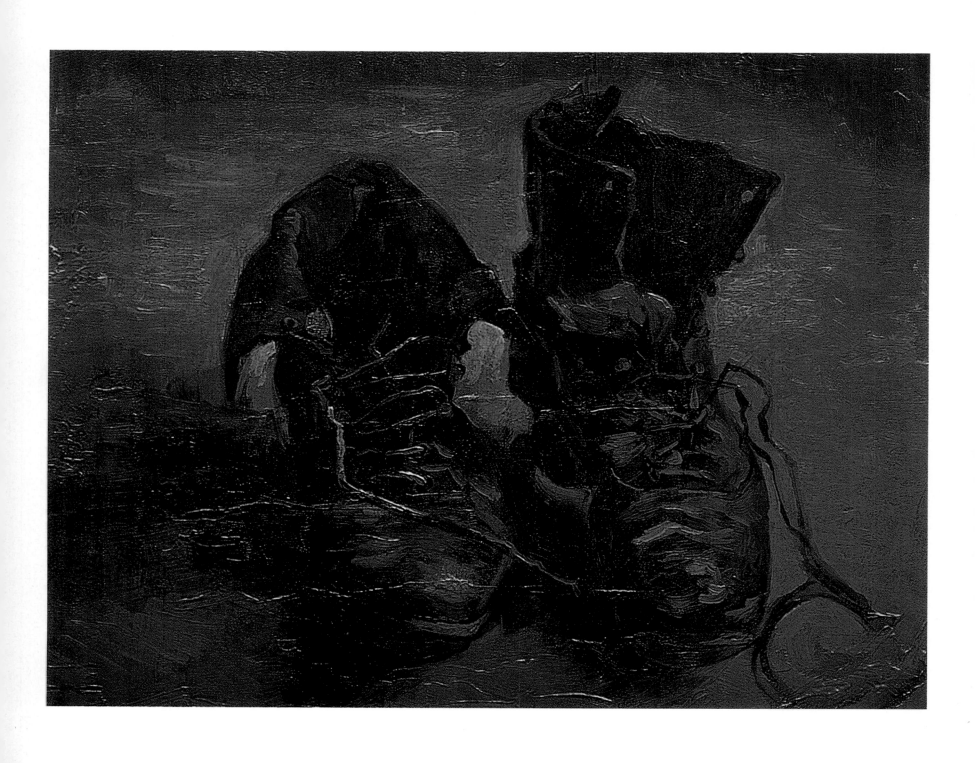

285. Vincent van Gogh. *A Pair of Shoes*, Paris, autumn 1886.

Rijksmuseum Vincent van Gogh, Amsterdam.

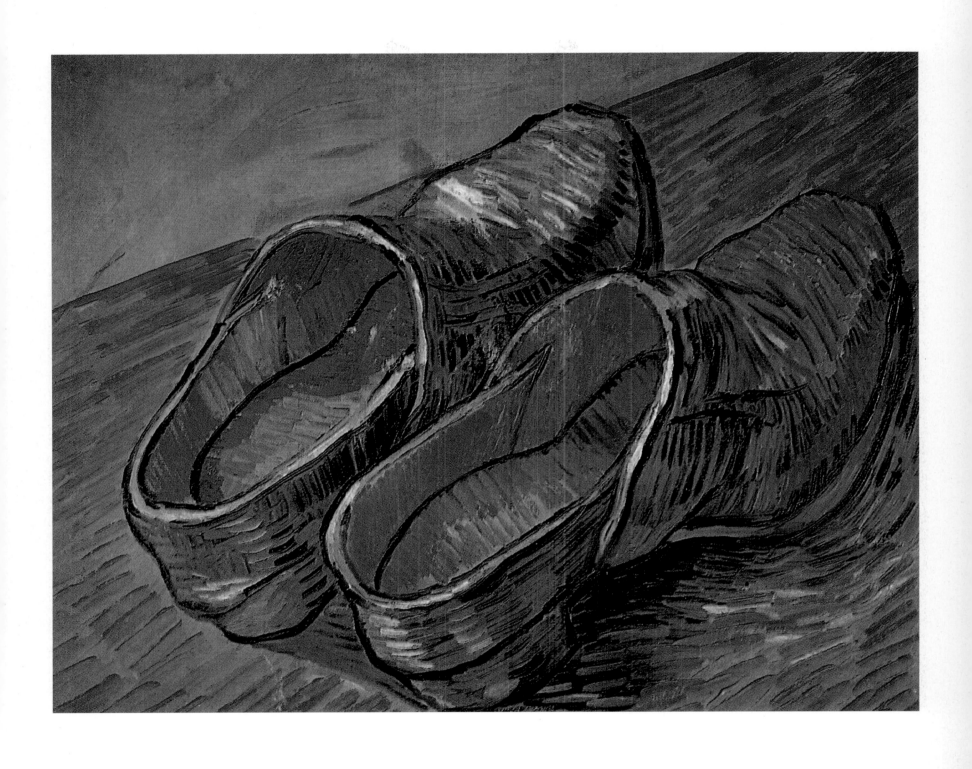

286. Vincent van Gogh. *A Pair of Leather Clogs*, 1888.

Rijksmuseum Vincent van Gogh, Amsterdam.

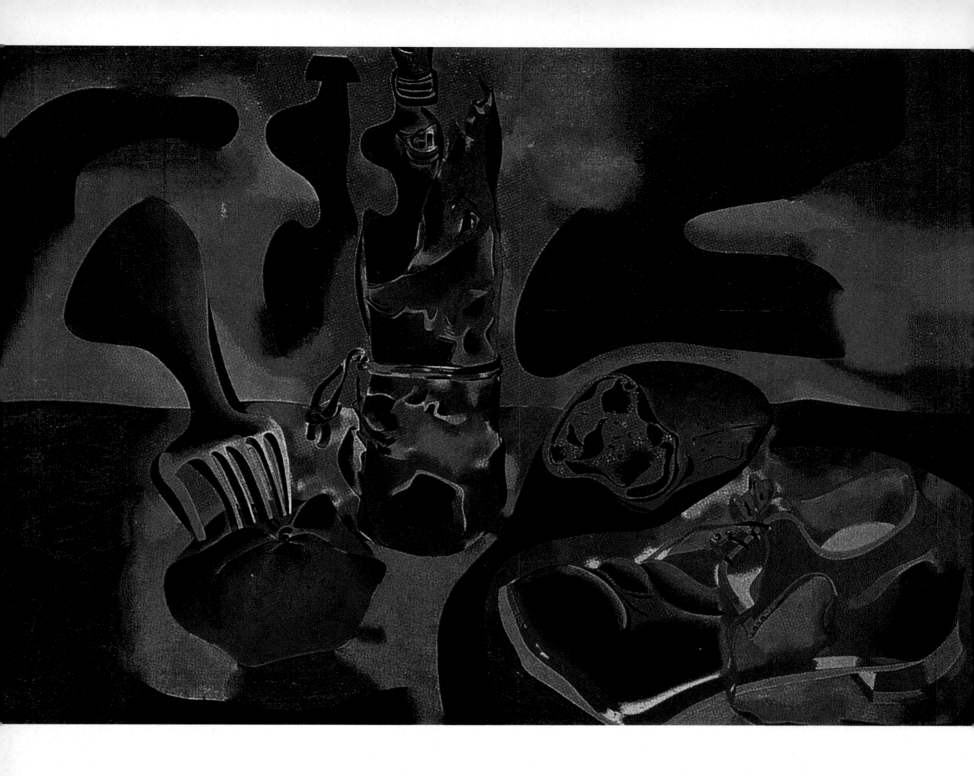

287. Miró. *Still Life with Old Shoe*, 1937.

288. Arroyo. *Spanish Caballero*, 1970. Borgogna Art Gallery, Milan.

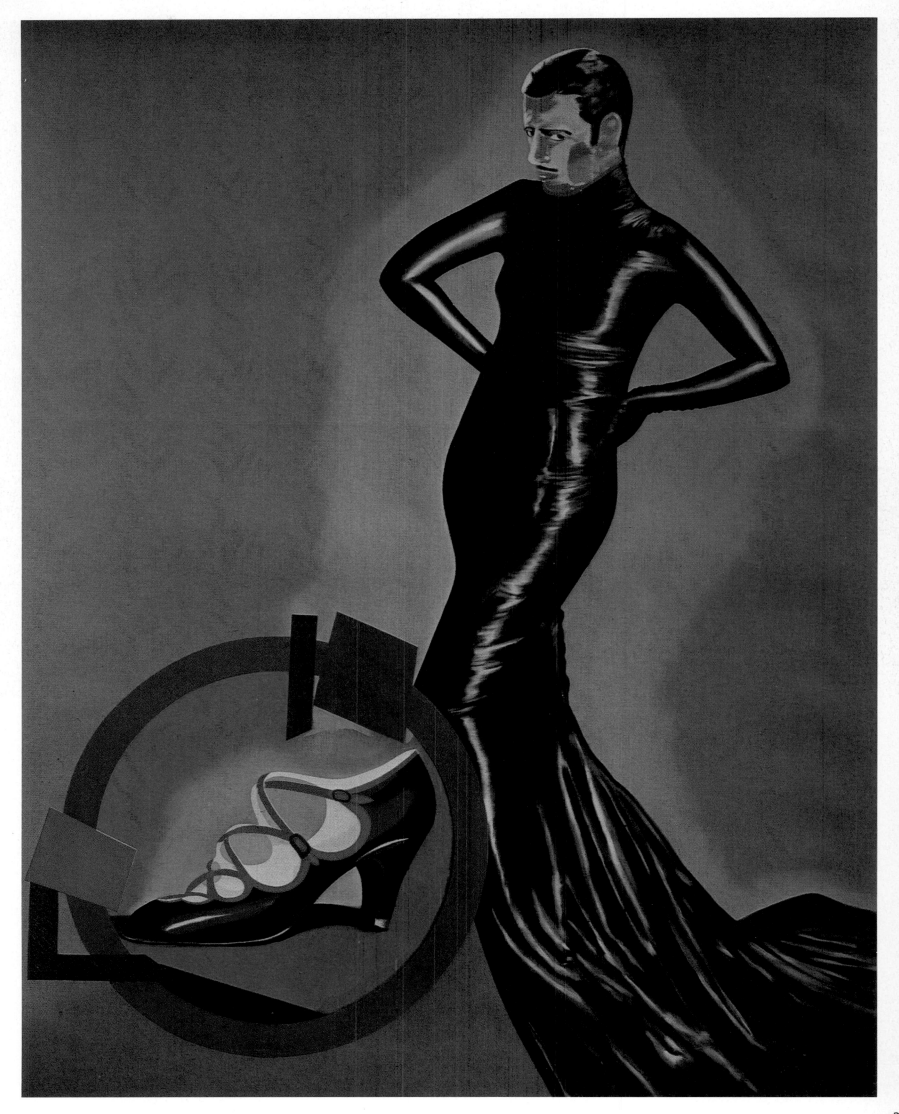

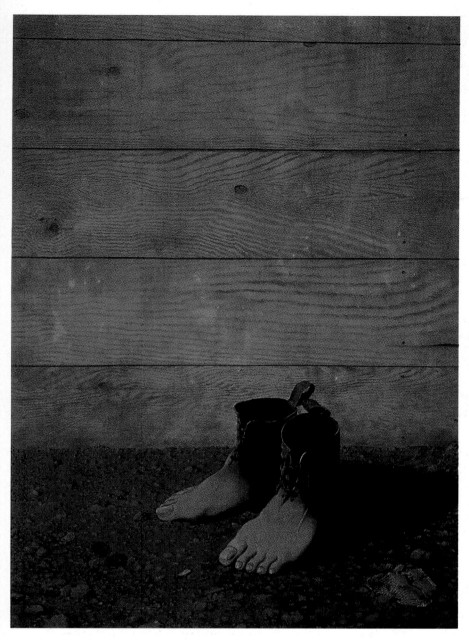 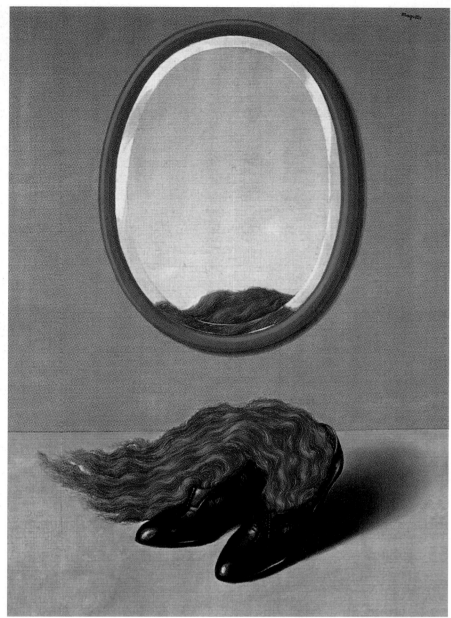

289. Magritte. *The Red Model III*, 1937.

Boijmans-Van Beuningen Museum, Rotterdam.

290. Magritte. *Love disarmed*, 1935. Private collection.

291. Magritte. *Philosophy in the Boudoir*, 1947.

Private collection, Washington.

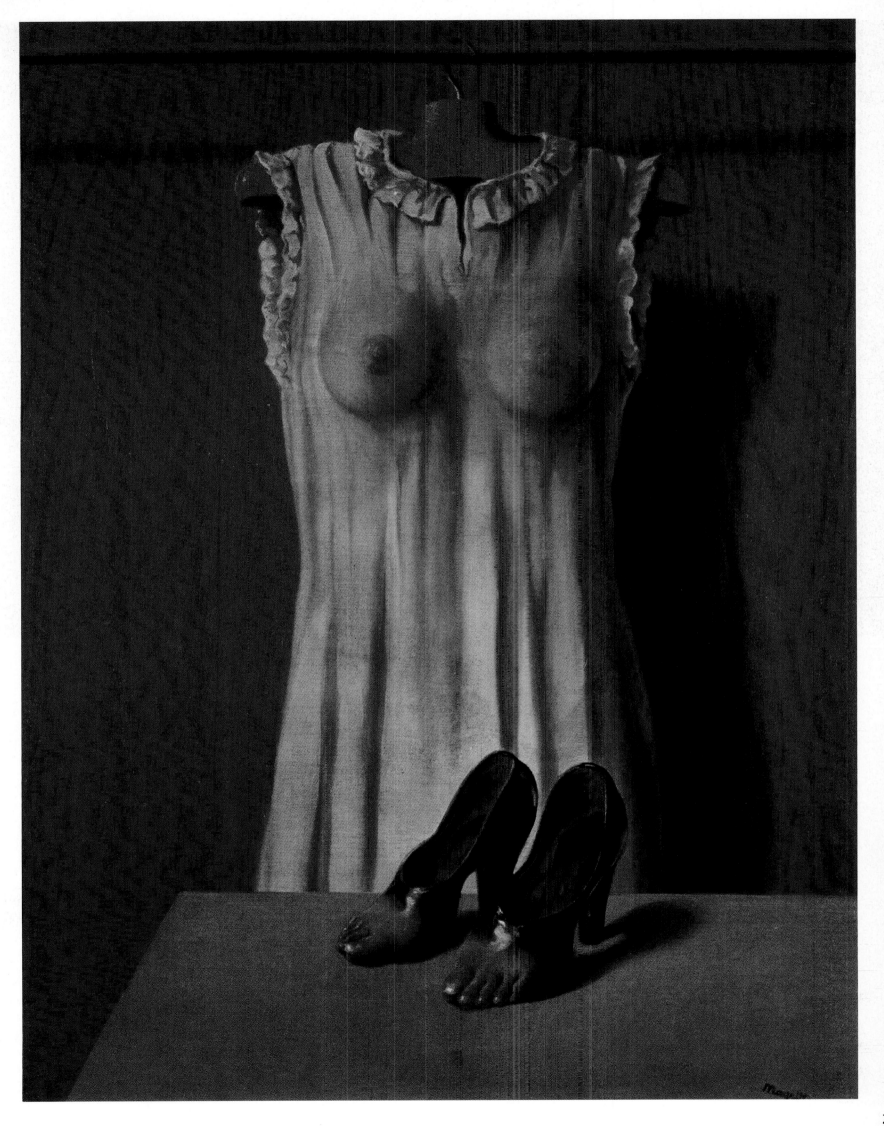

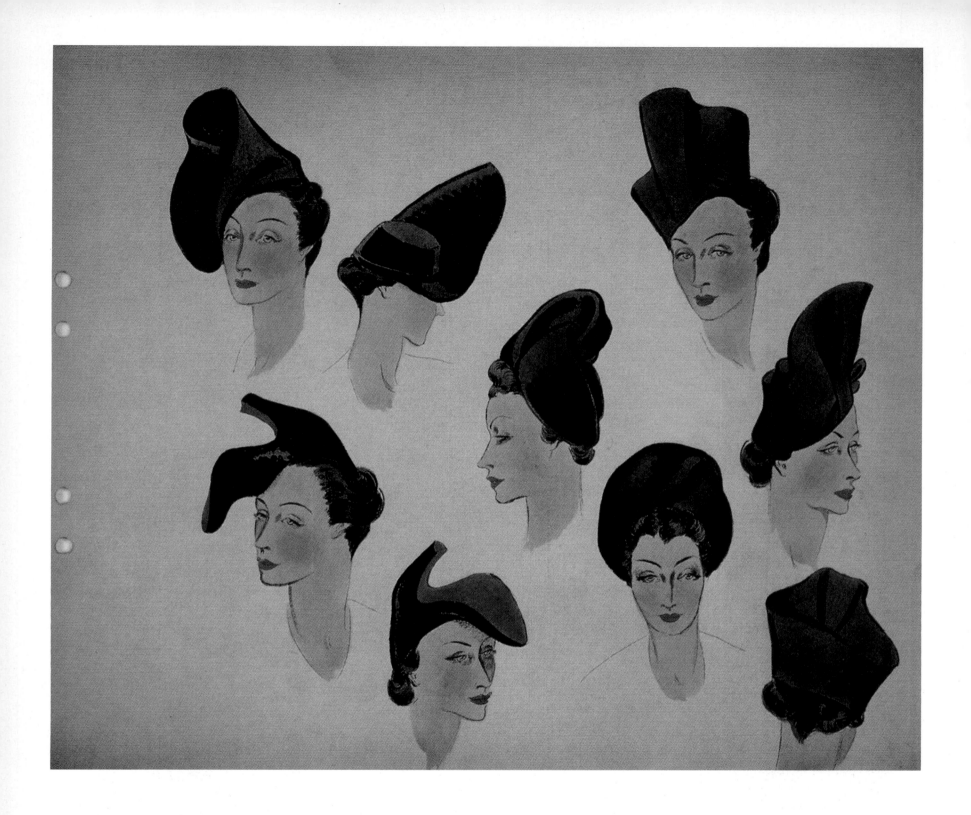

292. Schiaparelli Studio, drawing, winter 1937: shoe-shaped hats.

French Association of Costume Arts.

293. Dalí. *Cannibalism of Objects. Head of a Woman with Shoe*, 1937.

Private collection.

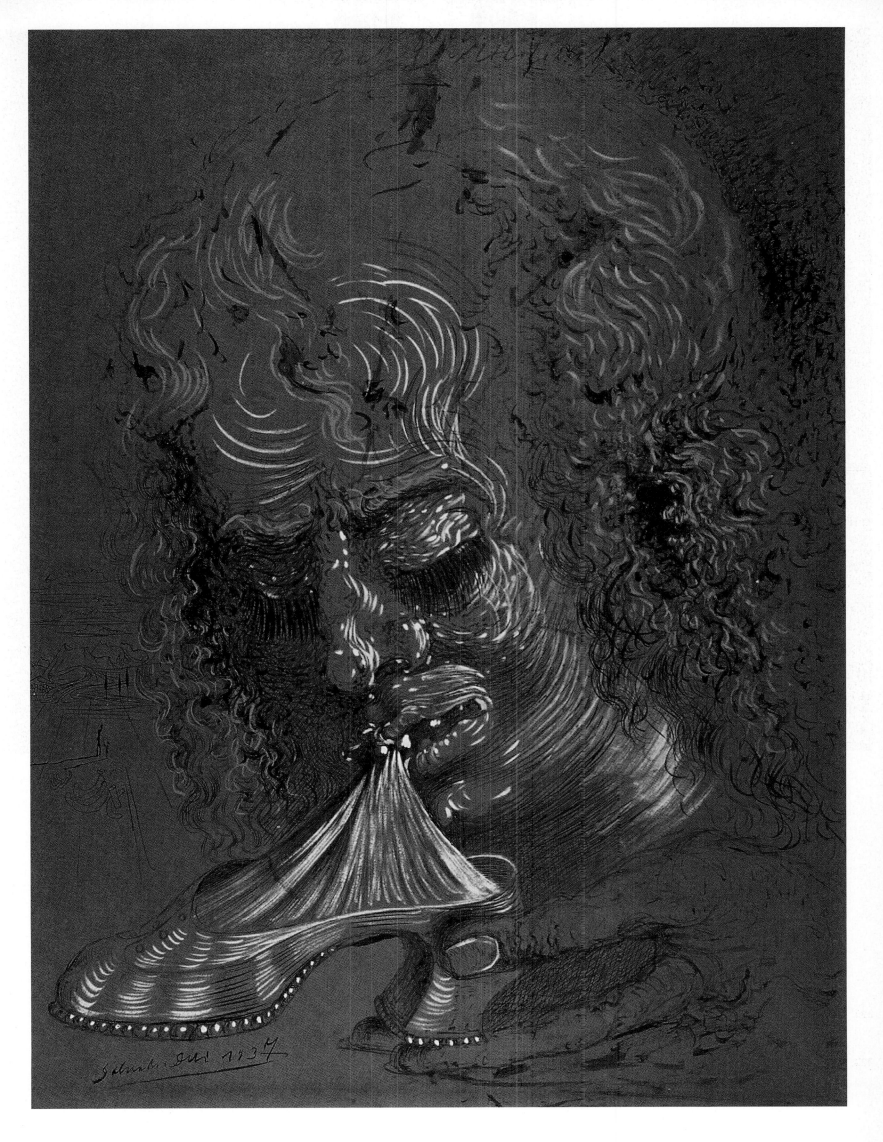

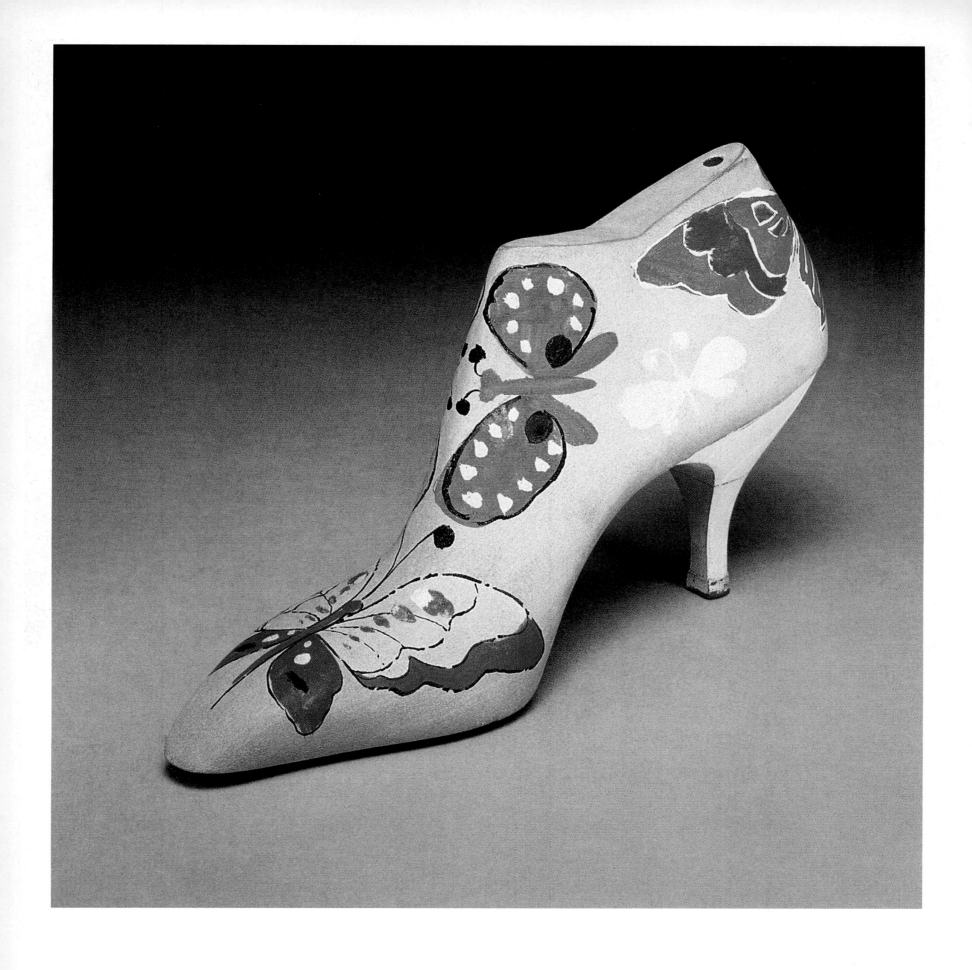

294. Warhol. *Shoe*, 1950-1953. Collection of José Mugrabi.

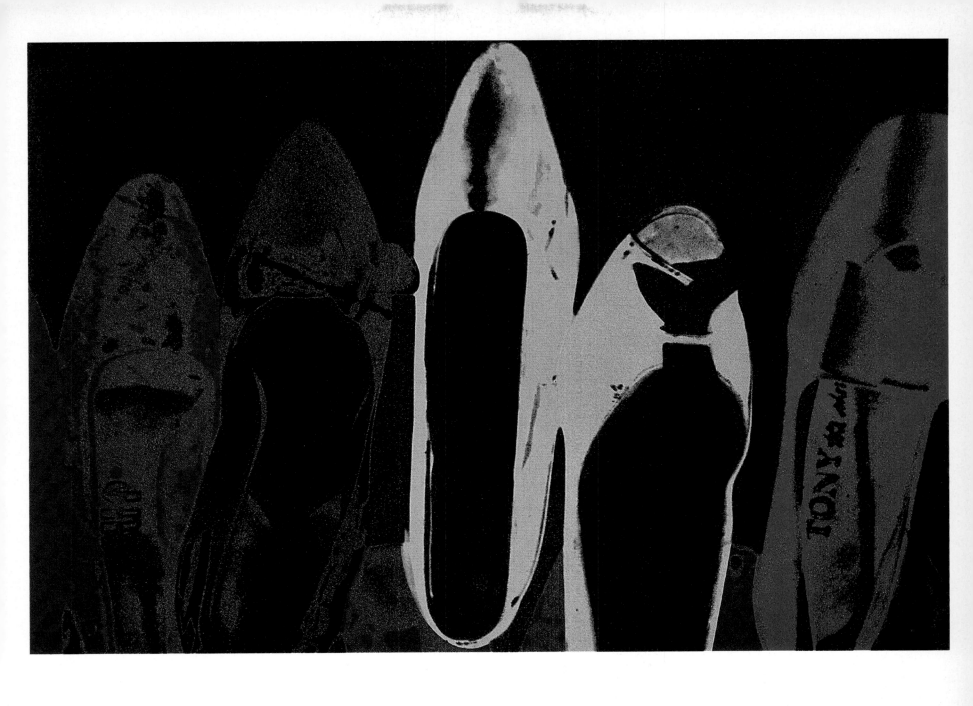

295. Warhol. *Tony Shoes*, 1980. Collection of José Mugrabi.

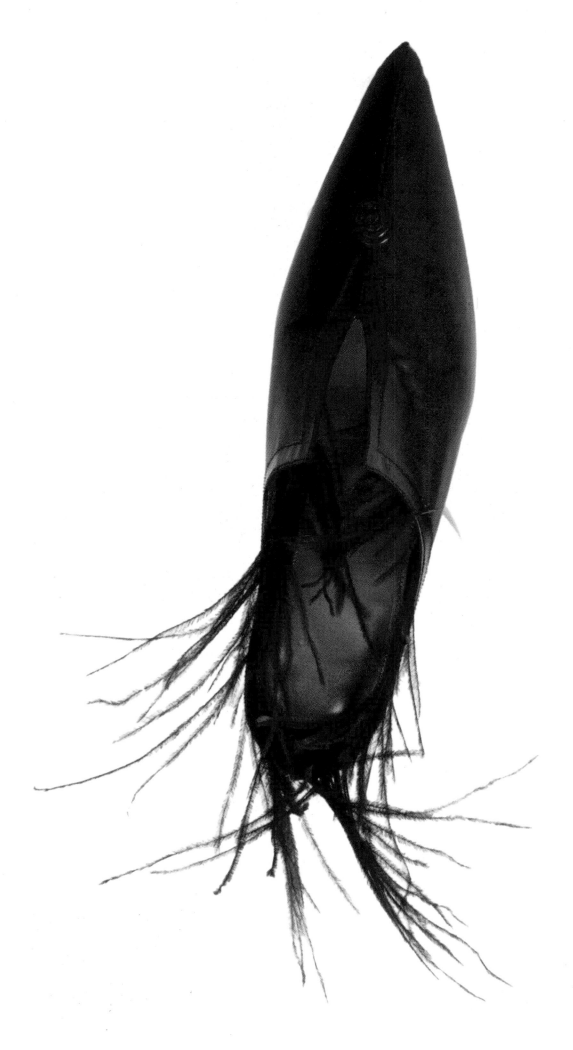

296-297. Shoes of Zita Attalaï. Ledermuseum, Offenbach.

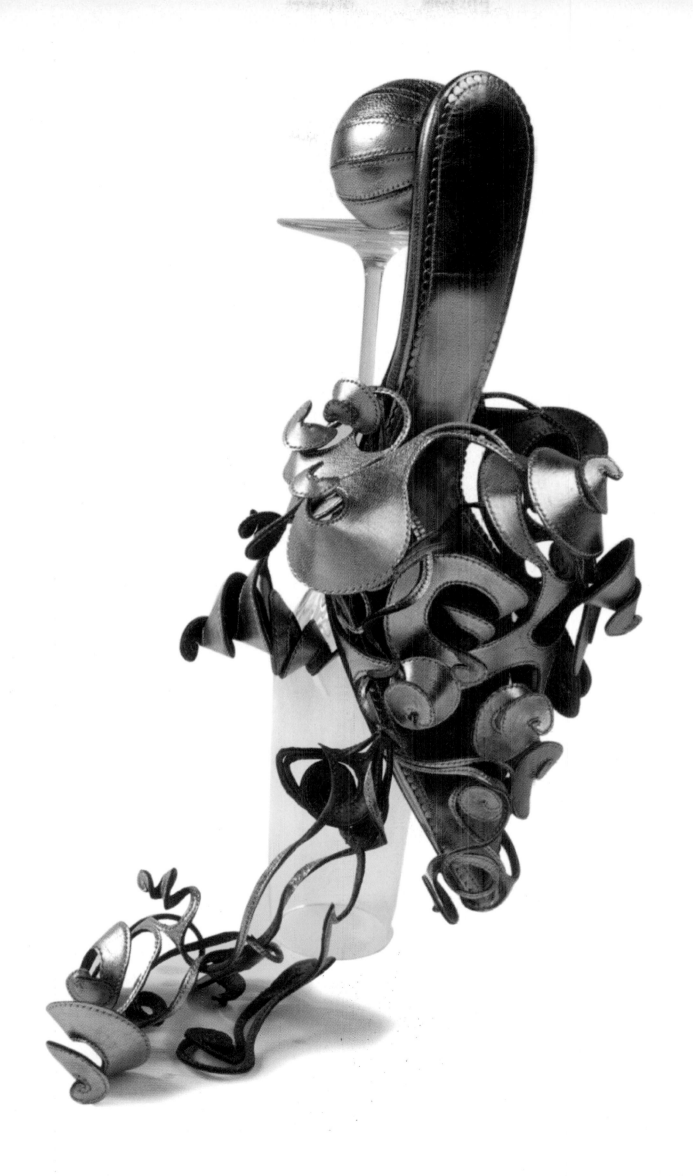

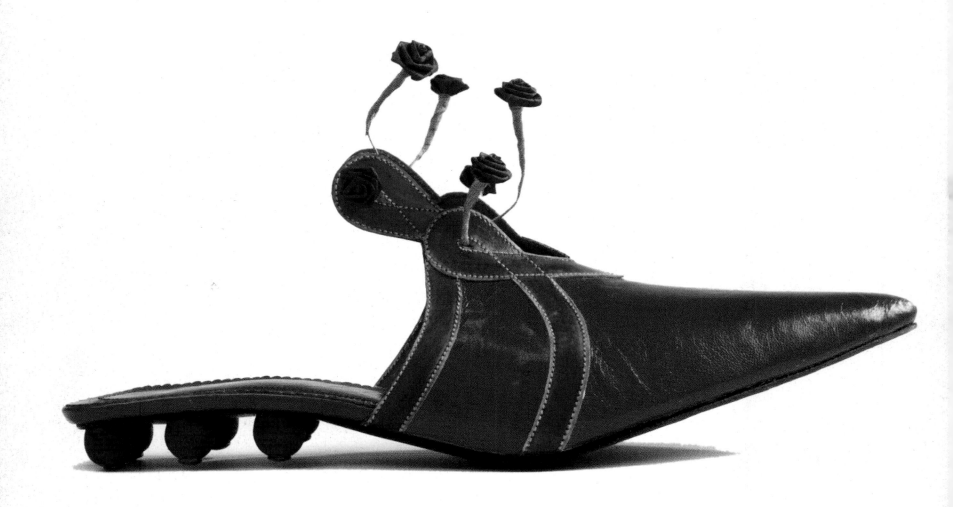

298. Shoe of Zita Attalaï. Ledermuseum, Offenbach.

299. Ex-voto executed by Berluti.

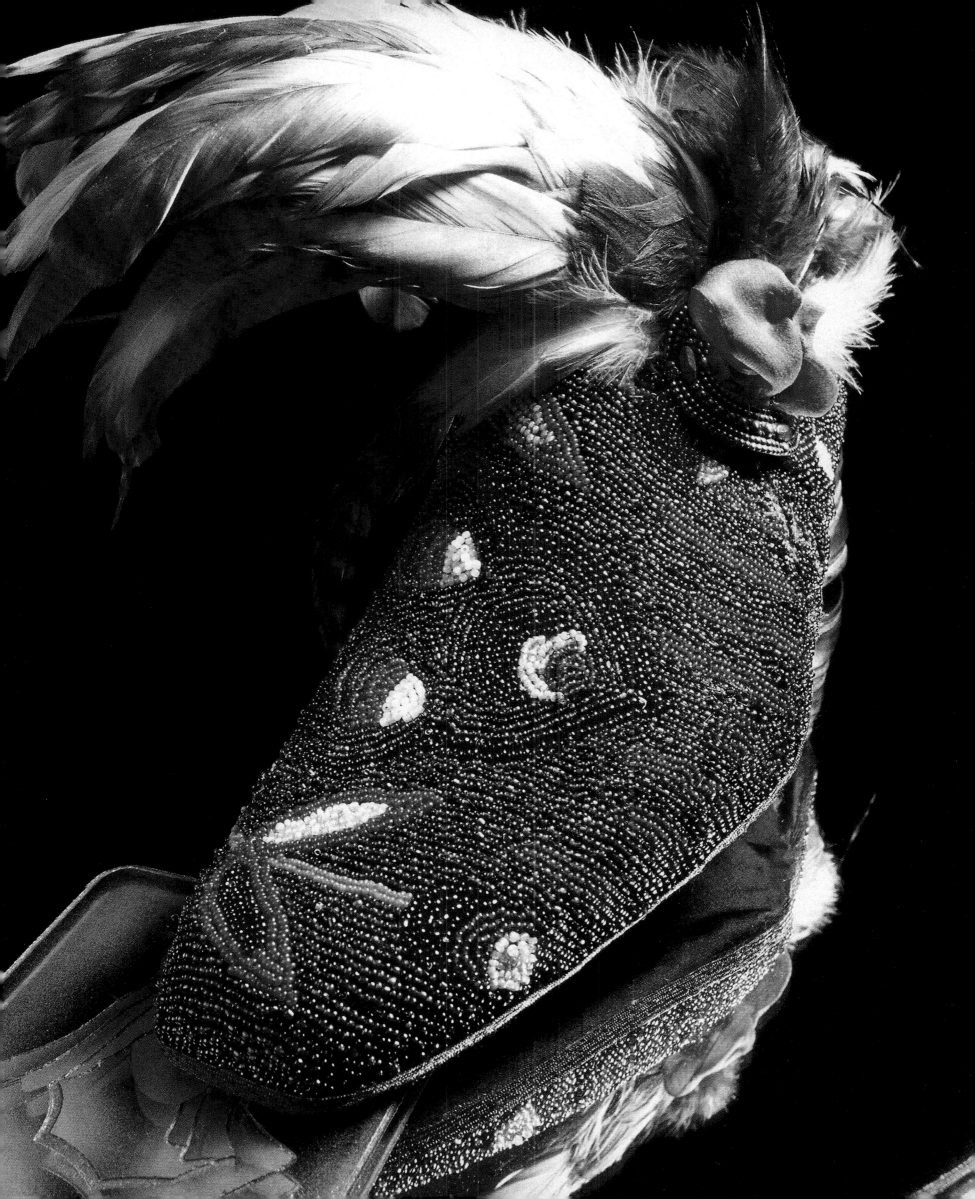

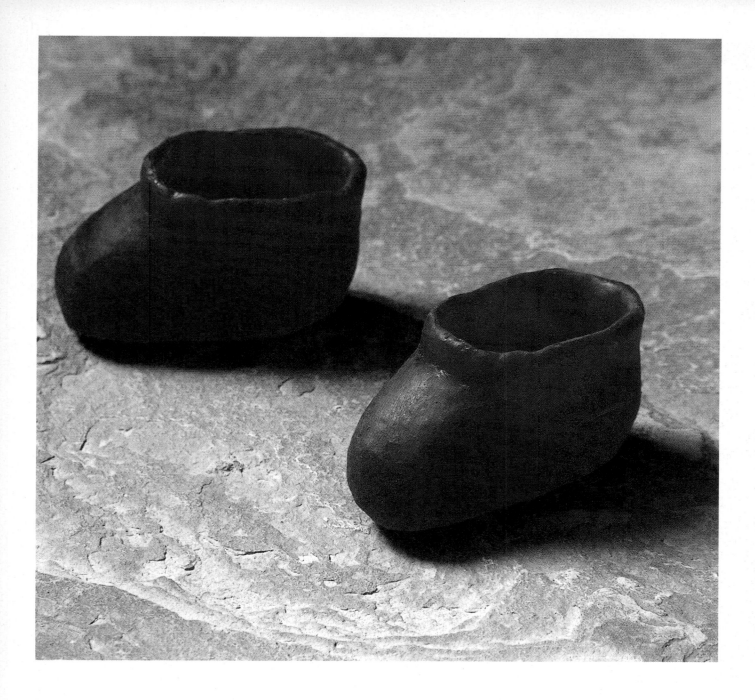

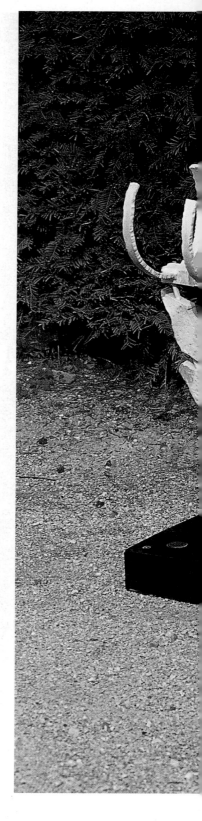

Henri Terres

Henri Terres was born in Oran in 1948 and devoted himself to drawing and lithography under the influence of surrealism before exhibiting his first sculptures in 1990. Primarily metal works (iron, steel, and bronze), these sculptures were decidedly figurative. At first the artist assembled his pieces by welding recycled materials that he had re-cut and polished. An important final stage involving polychrome resulted in truly painted sculptures. When recycled materials seemed to offer him a limited and repetitious formal vocabulary, Terres abandoned their use in 1992, turning instead to thick slabs of sheet metal. The two themes most frequently depicted are the human face and bestiaries.

300. Glass bottillons by Christine Crozat. Paris 1997-1998.
International Shoe Museum, Romans.

301. Henri Terres. "Paleontology" or "pump's skeleton." 1995.
International Shoe Museum, Romans. Photo by Joël Garnier.

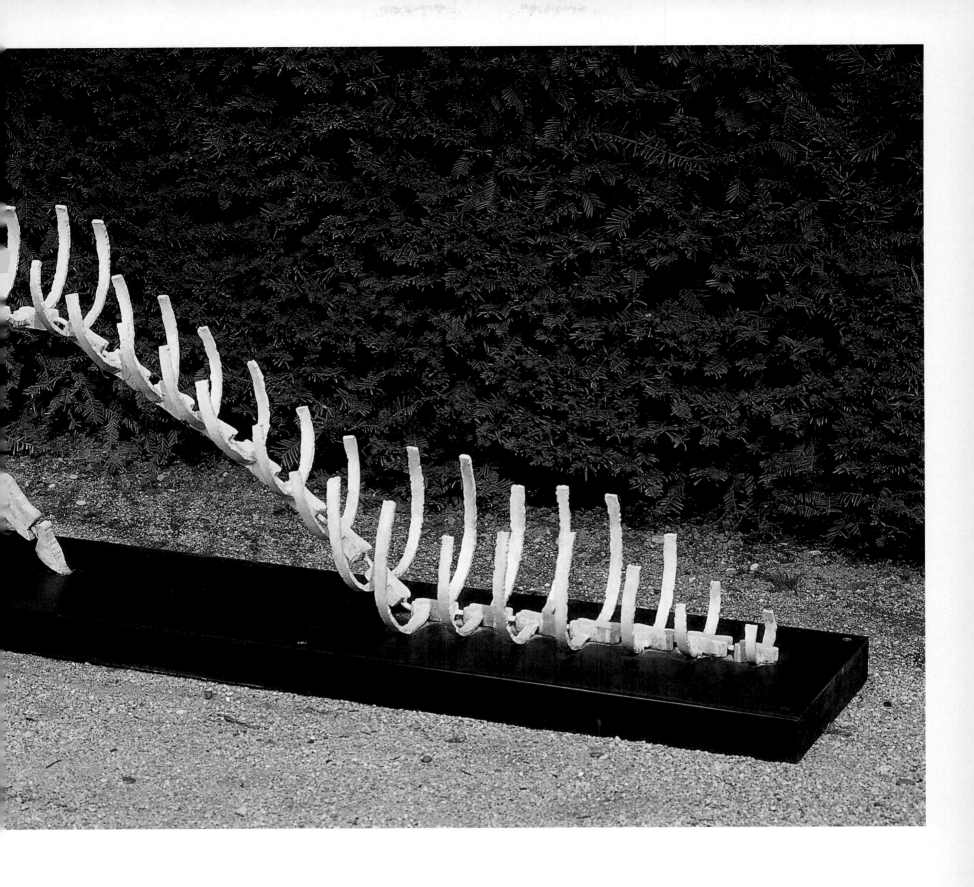

In 1995, Terres exhibited a sculpture series at the International Shoe Museum, Romans. Humorously entitled "Fancy Shoes," the theme was the seven deadly sins. The exhibition consisted of bas-reliefs made from a mixture of crushed stone and resin, which had been patinated with polychrome or painted with acrylics before receiving a final polish. Frames, formed during the first stage of the work and painted along with the bas-relief, were an integral part of each sculpture.

That year Terres also participated in a group exhibition called "Roger Vivier and his world," at Galerie Enrico Navarra in Paris. This exhibit brought together the work of a number of artists, including César.

The Berluti firm retains over three thousand wood forms crafted for famous and anonymous clients.

Today, Olga is restoring and adorning them with fabric and embroidery chosen to match the personality of each client represented. The shoe forms have been transformed into votive offerings by her inspired hand. Art objects in their own right, they tremble with life.

For twenty years a costume designer for the film industry (another facet of her great talent) Olga Berluti, finds her inspiration to immortalize the uniqueness of these individuals constantly renewed.

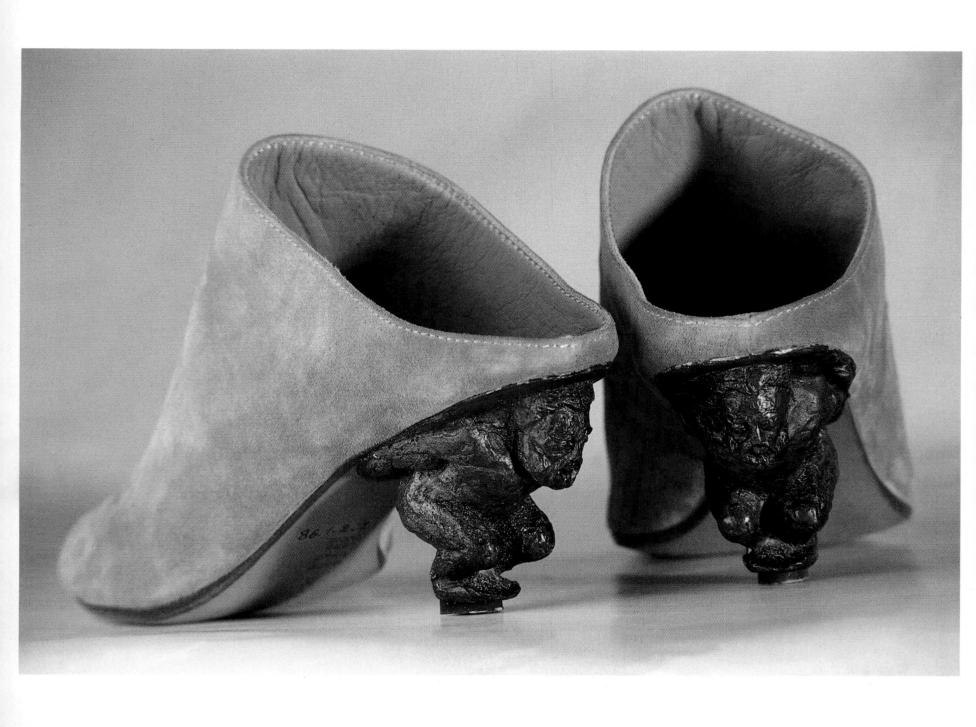

302. Mules in suede by Anne-Marie Beretta. Metal heel shaped as a crouched Titan.

International Shoe Museum, Romans.

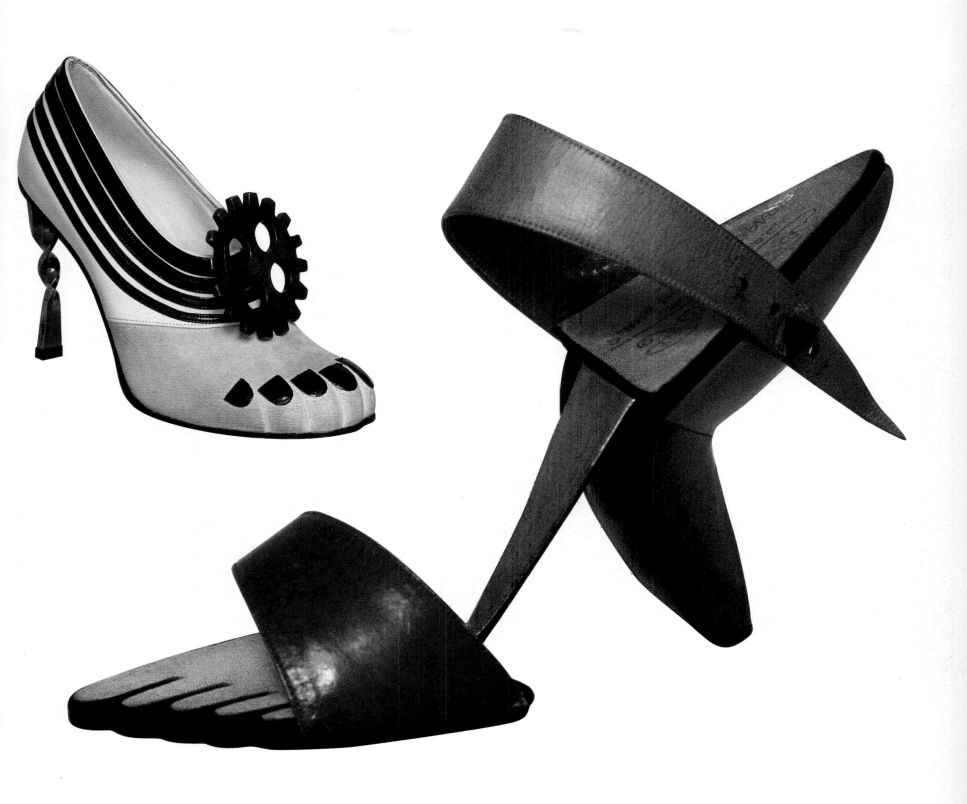

303. Shoe in white velvet calfskin and calfskin glazed black from Perugia, emphasized relief of fingers, metal wheel, twisted metal heel, style created after a painting by Fernand Léger. Around 1955. International Shoe Museum, Romans.

304. Perugia style after a painting by Picasso. Sandal in red and blue kidskin, forepart in the shape of fingers, metal arch, geometric heel. Around 1955. International Shoe Museum, Romans.

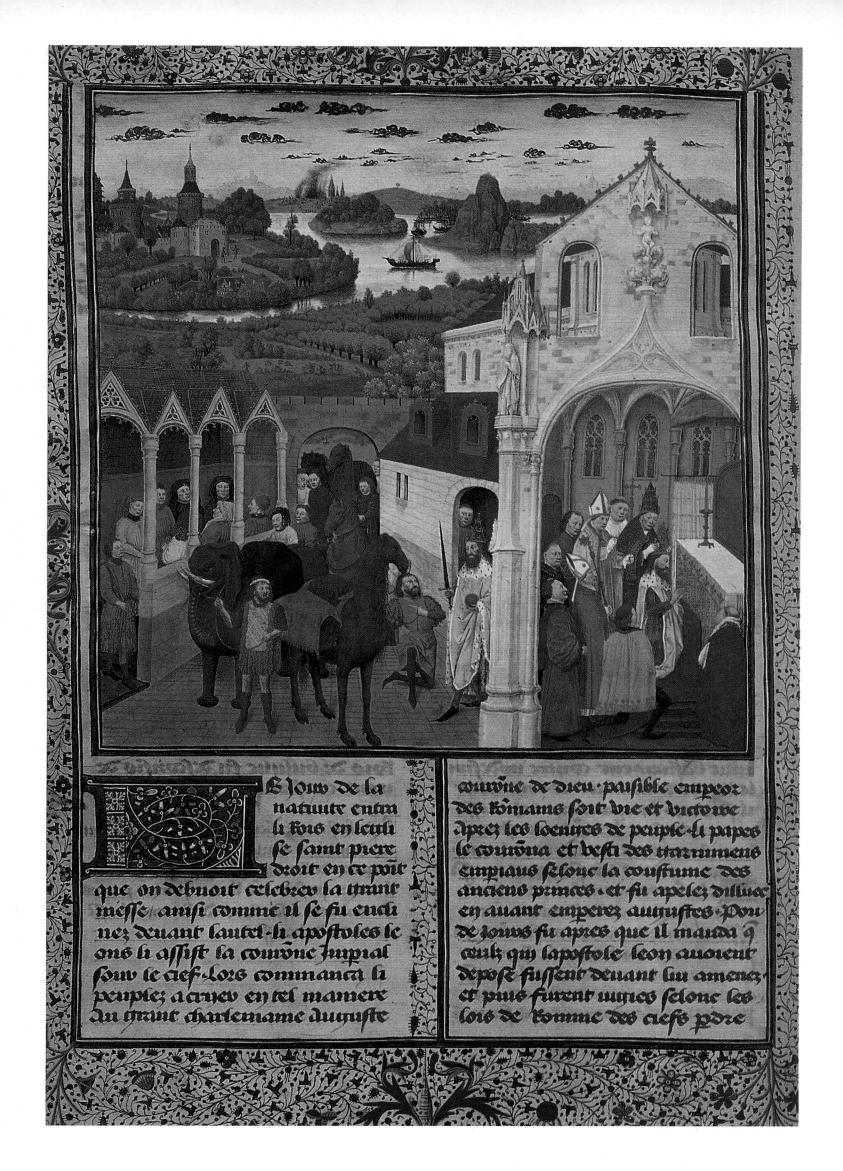

ES Jour de la
natiuite entra
li Rois en leu li
se sainr piere
droit en ce poir
que on debuoit celebrer la trainr
messe. ainsi comme il se fu encli
nez deuant lautel li apostoles se
ons li assist la courone imprial
souz le cief. lors commanca li
peuplez a crier en tel maniere
au trainr charlemaine auguste

courone de dieu pausible empeor
des romains soit vie et victoire
apres les loenges de peuple li papes
le couröna et vesti des haranimens
empiaus selonc la coustume des
ancieno princes et su apelez dilluec
en auant emperez auguistes Poi
de jours fu apres que il manda q
ceulz qui lapostole leon auoient
depose fussent deuant lui amenez
et puis furent iugies selonc les
lois de romme des ciefs pare

Appendix

The story of Rhodopis

A beautiful courtesan named Rhodopis was bathing in the Nile when an eagle swooped down and carried off in its beak a sandal that she had left nearby. Flying towards Memphis, the bird dropped its prey on the knees of the Pharaoh, who was busy dispensing justice. Pleasantly intrigued by the sandal's delicacy and elegance, the Pharaoh ordered a search be immediately undertaken throughout Egypt to locate its owner. He eventually found her and made her his wife. This ancient legend, told in the first-century of our era by Strabo predates the famous fairytale of Cinderella written by Charles Perrault in the seventeenth century.

Empress Foot

Any young woman could compete for the title Empress of the Byzantine Court. Candidates were judged on their beauty, charm, intelligence, and smallness of foot. In a tradition that endured until the 11th century, a pair of winged crimson shoes embroidered with pearls were handed over to the lucky woman "with great solemnity" by a court princess.

The Outlawed Poulaine

1 – The order of Charles V prohibiting the king's secretaries and notaries from wearing the shoes.

2 – Letters patent of Charles V (1368)

The letters patent prohibited "any person of any status or position whatsoever from the future wear of the shoe known as the poulaine, at the risk of paying a fine of ten florins, because this ostentation goes against good manners and disrespects God and Church with its worldly vanity and foolish presumption." In France, the Cardinal Curson prohibited a Université de Paris professor from wearing these scandalous shoes in 1215.

3 – Papal bulls (Urban V)

The papal bulls contained severe admonitions to priests and monks about the insolent luxury displayed in their costume and in particular their shoes. Pope Urban V was especially critical of their wearing the poulaine.

4 – The Council of Lavaur

The Council prohibited clerics from wearing long-tipped boots and prohibited their servants from wearing poulaines.

Bertrade with the Big Feet

Bertrade, mother of Charlemagne (742-814), had one foot that was much larger than the other, hence her nickname, "Big-foot Berthe."

Charlemagne's foot measured thirty-two centimeters, four millimeters and corresponded to a size 48 shoe, which was also General de Gaulle's size. By imperial order Charlemagne's foot become an official unit of measure, remaining in use until the metric system was adopted in 1795.

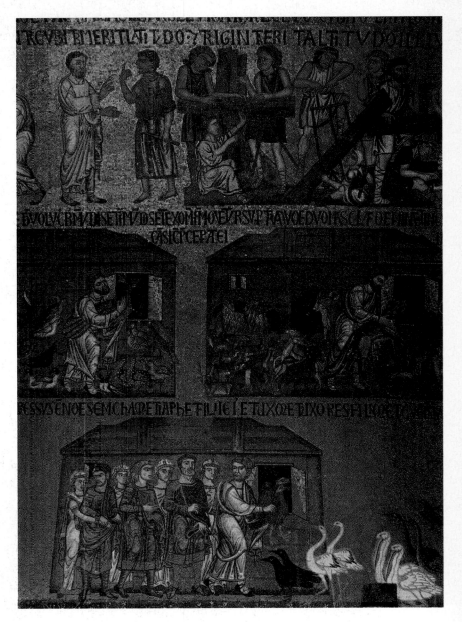

305. Coronation of Charlemagne. *The Grand Chronicles of France*, mid 15th-century. The Hermitage Museum, Saint Petersburg.

306. Story of Noah's Arc, detail, from a mosaic from the 13th century. Saint Mark Basilica, Venice.

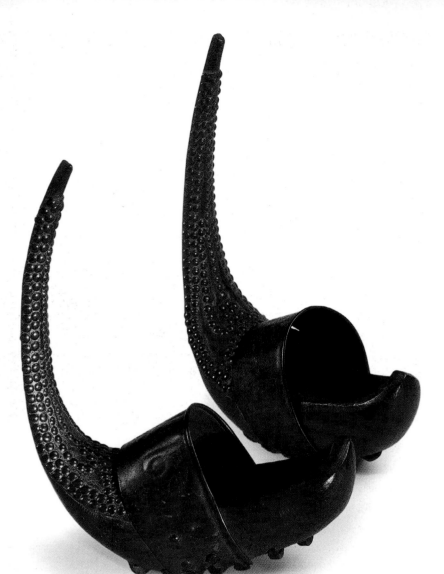

The Legend of Bethmale's Boots
(from the Saint Girons area, county Foix in Ariège)

The Bethmale Valley in Ariège was a center of Christian resistance during the Moorish invasion in the 12th century. It was at that time that Boedbit, the Moorish leader, became enamored with Esclarelys, who was engaged to a young man named Dannaert. Dannaert rallied opponents to fight the invaders and they took up position in the mountains; one of them was captured by the enemy, strung up by his feet, and beaten senseless with a boot. Meanwhile, the carefree and superficial Esclarelys, whose name meant étoile de lis, a reference to the Lily, had given into temptation and run off with her seducer, and was happily whiling away the hours cheating on her fiancé, and to a certain degree, collaborating with her country's enemies. A little later, Dannaert and his comrades captured the Moorish camp, taking the Moors prisoner and placing them in chains. Dannaert then ordered all the unmarried girls to be lined up for his review, and when he inspected them he was wearing strange boots with long, pointed tips held up vertically and from which dangled two pieces of skewered flesh. These were the hearts of the two lovers Boedbit and Esclarely, removed from their bodies by the scorned fiancé. He had just tossed their remains to wild mountain lions in a fit of vengeance.

Ever since then, engaged couples in the Bethmale valley have made similar boots for themselves and their betroved decorated with brass tacks arranged in the shape of a heart: it is said the deeper the love, the more finely sharpened the nail. The ancestral tradition of this engagement gift reminds the future couple of the value of engagement, commitment, and faithfulness in marriage.

307. Clogs from the Bethmale Valley, Ariège.

Wood, nail decoration in heart shape. Ariège, 18th century.

Guillen Collection.

308. Clogs typical of the Bethmale Valley, Ariège.

Gift from fiancé to the young woman; the higher the toe, the bigger the love.

Rural Museum of Popular Arts, Laduz, Yonne.

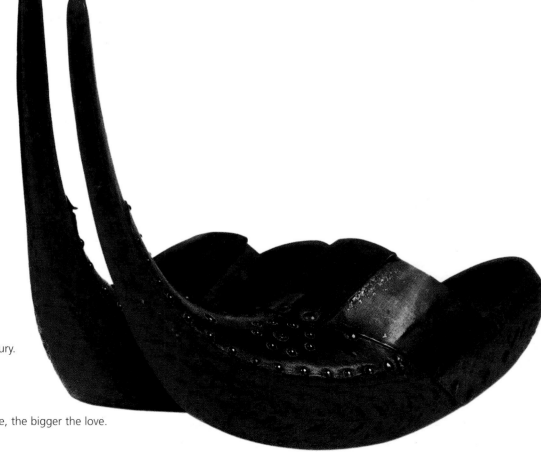

Shoemaker Brothers after Saint Crispin
In the footsteps of Saint Crispin and Saint Crispinian

Three men from three very different worlds came together in 1645 against the backdrop of 17th-century Paris to found the brotherhood of the shoemakers after the example of Saint Crispin and Saint Crispinian.

The three men were:

– Henri Buch. Born in 1598 to a poor family in Arlon, Belgian Luxembourg, he learned the shoemaker's trade training in his uncle's workshop.

– Gaston de Renty. Born in 1611 in Bessy Bocage, Normandy. Surrounded by luxury, this wealthy gentleman (godson of Gaston d'Orléans, Louis XIII's brother) led a life of abstinence in the spirit of the Gospel's Beatitudes.

– Jean-Antoine le Vachet. Born in 1601 to a bourgeois family in Romans-sur-Isère, a town in Dauphiné where tanners and mégissiers (tanners who used a special alum-based preparation) enjoyed great prosperity, this highly educated priest conducted his ministry in Paris, following the example of Vincent de Paul, with whom he was a close friend.

The workshop, which was located on the rue de la Tixanderie, at the crossroads between the rue de Rivoli and the rue Lobau, was close to the sumptuous town houses then coming under construction, and resembled a devoted secular brotherhood within the world of 17th-century Paris labour. The three founders shared a common objective: to eradicate the deep-rooted causes of extreme poverty. To achieve this goal, the volunteers embraced the social problems of their time, dividing the job among them as follows.

The one nicknamed "le bon Henri" or "Wise One," due to his knowledge of the trade, became the superior and was in charge of the workshop. Gaston de Renty, the community's patron, thought it insufficient to provide for the immediate needs of the poor and the marginalized in hospitals and in prisons; instead, he became a proponent of reintegration by promoting the value of work, an innovative concept at the time. Jean-Antoine le Vachet, the advisor and spiritual guide was part-contemplative, part-apostle, and he too lent his support to these artisan models of personal and communal piety. At the outset they numbered seven; later, an alliance with married laity and former community members would help spread the movement to Toulouse, Lyon, and other countries.

Dressed modestly (the costume of the era's labourers consisted of a smock and an apron), the Frères Cordonniers took no vows and lived uncloistered. They worked six days a week from five to eight following a fixed daily schedule that began with the day's offering, prayers being read aloud, and a meditation. After that they headed for the workshop thinking of Jesus working with Joseph. One of them would take turns going to mass on behalf of the whole community. At mealtime, in accordance with convent regulations, the reading was read aloud. Short breaks allowed them to converse before they picked up their hammers and awls amidst the smell of new leather, dye, and polish. These humble artisans dedicated their work to God and worked under his watchful eye, which was enough to make them happy. And their behavior at work confirmed it: they sang canticles while beating the leather, producing quality shoes and maintaining their good reputation at the same time.

The priest, the artisan, and the gentleman directed their combined efforts towards the neediest cases, attending to the poor, the sick, and the imprisoned. They made themselves poor among the most impoverished. The Thirty Years War and the Fronde had resulted in soaring destitution: from 1648 to 1651 there were over one hundred thousand beggars and vagrants in the capital and its outskirts. Many confined in the general hospital of Paris were considered a volatile force to be feared. And the 17th-century prison environment was hellish for both guilty and innocent.

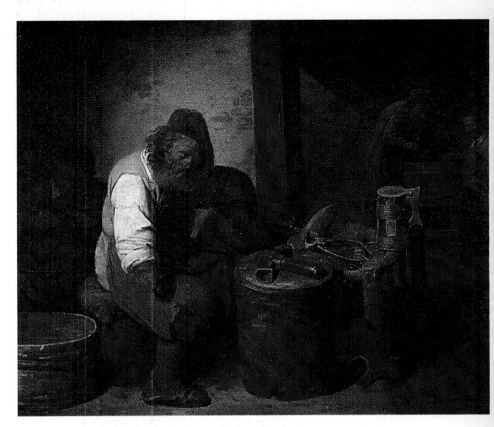

Prison cells unfit for human habitation held men eaten away by vermin, their feet wearing nothing but heavy chains for shoes. Father Vachet made every effort to obtain the just release of many. The active ministry of the Frères Cordonniers in the face of so much adversity enabled some caught in the flood of despair to rebuild their lives by apprenticing to the trade. In the interest of hospitality and sharing, the community obtained work for handicapped and homeless people reduced to indigence.

The Frères Cordonniers knew that goodness never attracted attention. Today we owe our knowledge of their exemplary conduct to Eugénie Debouté and his remarkable book, Without hearth or home: The story of Jean-Antoine le Vachet, a spiritual leader during the Fonde.

The Origin of the Godillot Shoe

Born in Besançon in 1816, Alexis Godillot became an army supplier in 1854 and developed the equipment necessary to manufacture shoes by machine. He owned factories in Saint-Ouen, Bordeaux, and Nantes, as well as in Paris on the rue Rochechouart. Godillot shoes weighed three kilos, so they did not make things any easier for the soldiers, who covered twenty-five to thirty kilometers a day. Sold commercially for seven francs, the army paid eight francs twenty-five for them. After making his fortune and being decorated by the Legion of Honor, Godillot retired to Hyères where the Palm-lined avenue running from the train station is named after him.

309. David Ryckart. *Cobbler and his Companions in his Workshop*, 1864.
Museum der bildenden Künste, Leipzig.

Shoemakers and Shoe Repairmen
A Brief History

In all likelihood, shoemaking has existed ever since prehistoric man thought of protecting his feet with the aid of primitively cut and assembled animal skins. But the ancient Egyptians were probably the first to ply the trade, as attested by a reconstructed fresco from the XVIII dynasty (1567-1320 BC) depicting a sandal maker at work in the collection of the Metropolitan Museum, New York.

Shoemaking flourished in Greece, supporting entire villages, such as Sicyon, where very expensive shoes were made. A painted Greek vase dating to 500 BC now in the Ashmolean Museum, Oxford, is decorated with the image of a shoe repairman in his workshop. In ancient Rome, emperor Numa Pompilius (715-672) divided citizens into nine colleges; shoemakers, called sutores in Latin, were ranked fifth. Roman shoemakers therefore were not slaves, but citizens and they worked in shops. A bas-relief from Ostia dating to the 2nd century BC in the National Museum of Rome depicts a shoemaker at work.

Although many images in painting, pottery, and sculpture portray shoemaking in Antiquity, the etymology of the French word cordonnier (shoemaker) only dates back to the Middle Ages. Originating in the 11th-century adoption of cordouannier (it would become cordonnier in the 15th century), cordonnier signified a person who worked leather from Cordoue (Cordoba), as well as the artisans authorized to use this leather to make shoes, which were generally reserved for the aristocracy. Shoes made by savetiers (shoe repairmen) were less refined. In the Middle Ages, shoes reached exorbitant prices. This explains why shoes appear in medieval wills and notary deeds, and were part of the general bequest a feudal lord made to his vassal and donations made to monasteries.

Beginning in the 12th century, shoemaking expanded in France and provided work to no less than four corps of tradesmen, each with its own specialty and bylaws. These were the cordouaniers (shoemakers), sueurs (leather sweaters), savetonniers (shoemakers who worked with basane, a tanned lamb's skin they prepared themselves), and the savetiers (shoe repairmen).

The cordouaniers, who alone knew the secret of making cordouan, produced expensive shoes and had the right to affix their mark. The sueurs applied the final treatments to the leather and sewed the soles previously cut by the shoemakers. The savetonniers or basaniers made soft shoes in small sizes and were prohibited from using any type of leather except basane, a tanned lamb's skin that they prepared themselves. As for the savetiers, they contented themselves with mending old shoes, by replacing or repairing the soles and the uppers. The general public gave them colorful nicknames, such as: carreleurs de souliers (shoe masons), orfèvres en cuir (shoe smiths), courvoisiers, and bobelineurs.

During the 10th and 11th centuries, these artisans formed guilds, which were labour organizations that brought together merchants, artisans, and artists. Prevalent in northwestern Europe up to the 13th century, the guilds transformed themselves into corporations at the end of the 11th century, whence they enacted their own rules and monitored compliance in the following areas: pricing; quality control, production control, work time, and the acceptance of apprentices, later called compagnons. After apprenticing with a master, the apprentice had to make a "tour" meant to expand and improve his knowledge by working alongside other masters. This education lasted from six to nine years but came to be limited to eighteen months beginning in the 17th century. After this training period, the young man executed a masterpiece to prove his craft before a jury of examiners. Upon passing the examination, the apprentice obtained the title of master and the right to membership in the corporation.

King Charles the Wise established the brotherhood of shoemakers in the Cathedral of Paris in 1379. The shoemakers took Saint Crispin and Saint Crispinian as their saints. The corporation loosed its regulations in the 17th and 18th centuries, which explains how a shoemaker was able to have his shop in the same town where he apprenticed. Eventually, the profession was divided into groups according to categories of shoes, with each group restricted to producing the type of shoes they had been designated to make. Thus there were men's shoemakers, women's and children's shoemakers, boot makers, shoemakers who only worked in lambskin, and finally, the shoe repairmen, also known as cobblers.

A special craftsman called le talonnier made wooden heels. Form makers (formiers) made the shoemaker's forms and shoetrees, but had neither standing nor oath. Working without a master, many were themselves poor master shoemakers. Nevertheless, the jurors of the shoemaker community tried in vain to gain control over them. Out of all these groups, it was the cobbler, whose lifestyle was immortalized by Jean de la Fontaine in his famous fable, The Cobbler and the Financier. Prints from the 17th century depict the blatant distinction between shoemakers and their customers when they illustrate scenes of shoe shops. It is usually a cavernous space where masters and journeymen measure the feet of a customer whose elegance indicates his class. In reality, the sale took place in the street: the shoe shop, backed up against a house, could only contain two people. As for the didactic plates in the Encyclopedia of Diderot and d'Alembert featuring tools of the shoemaker's trade accompanied by explanatory notes, they give us a valuable introduction to the art of fabrication in the 18th century. In the years before the French Revolution, shoemakers managed thriving shops. The writer Sébastien Mercier records that, "in their black outfit and powdered wig, they look like Clerks of the Court." In the 19th century the profession became organized, leading to the formation of la société des Compagnons Cordonniers Bottiers du Devoir du Tour de France (the Workers' Association of the Shoemaker and Boot maker Companions of Duty). The Tour de France sponsored by the Compagnons du Devoir was an itinerate work-study program that enabled an apprentice to successively acquire mastery of his trade in a number of French towns called villes du devoir, or towns of service.

In 1829, Thimonier invented the sewing machine, which gradually established itself in the workshops and transformed traditional shoemaking. In today's shops, shoemakers continue to uphold the cobbler's tradition by repairing shoes and boots, and making custom shoes like the shoemakers of old.

The shoe shop: Its appearance remained unchanged for a long time. The center of the room held a workbench upon which various tools lay about. These tools fall into three main categories: Pattern-cutting tools and other cutting tools: punch, compass with points, cutter's knife, triangular file for sharpening the leather knife, sharpening stone, and a type of mechanic's file for forming or adjusting patterns. Tools used for assembling and execution: awl, working cutter, lasting pincers, joiner's pincers, nails, steel tack claw, nail hammer, peen hammer, hand protector, rand cutter, rasp, and stirrup. Tools used for finishing: a tool for polishing and smoothing soles, various leather polishing tools, and wooden mallets.

A glass globe enclosing a candle or oil lamp provided the workshop's dim lighting and was called a boule de cordonnier or shoemaker's globe. Under the table was a bucket of water used to soak the leather called the baquet de la science. The shoemaker and the shoe repairman usually worked seated on a stool. The shop always seemed to have a birdcage called the cage aux serins or canary cage. Tradition required a shoe repairman to have a pot of basil or an orange tree called the oranger du savetier to mask the smell of old shoes. An artisan could refer to himself as cordonnier en vieux et en neuf, or maker of shoes old and new, indicating that he made new shoes and repaired shoes already worn.

The paintings in the International Shoe Museum, Romans, apart from their pictorial interest, enable us to visualize the world of shoe fabrication from the 17th to the end of the 19th century. Above all, they teach us about the permanence of the specific tools used to create shoes over the centuries, tools that visitors can still recognize in contemporary workshops.

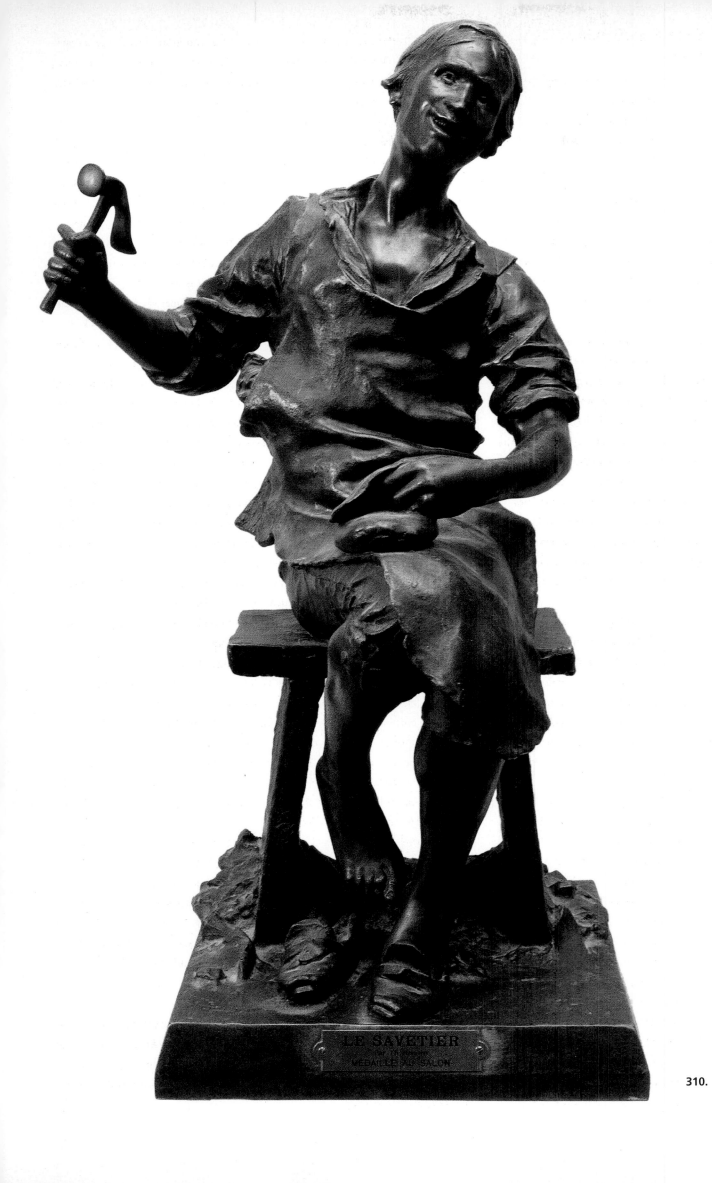

310. *The Cobbler*, bronze by Théodore Rivière. 19th-century, Romans.

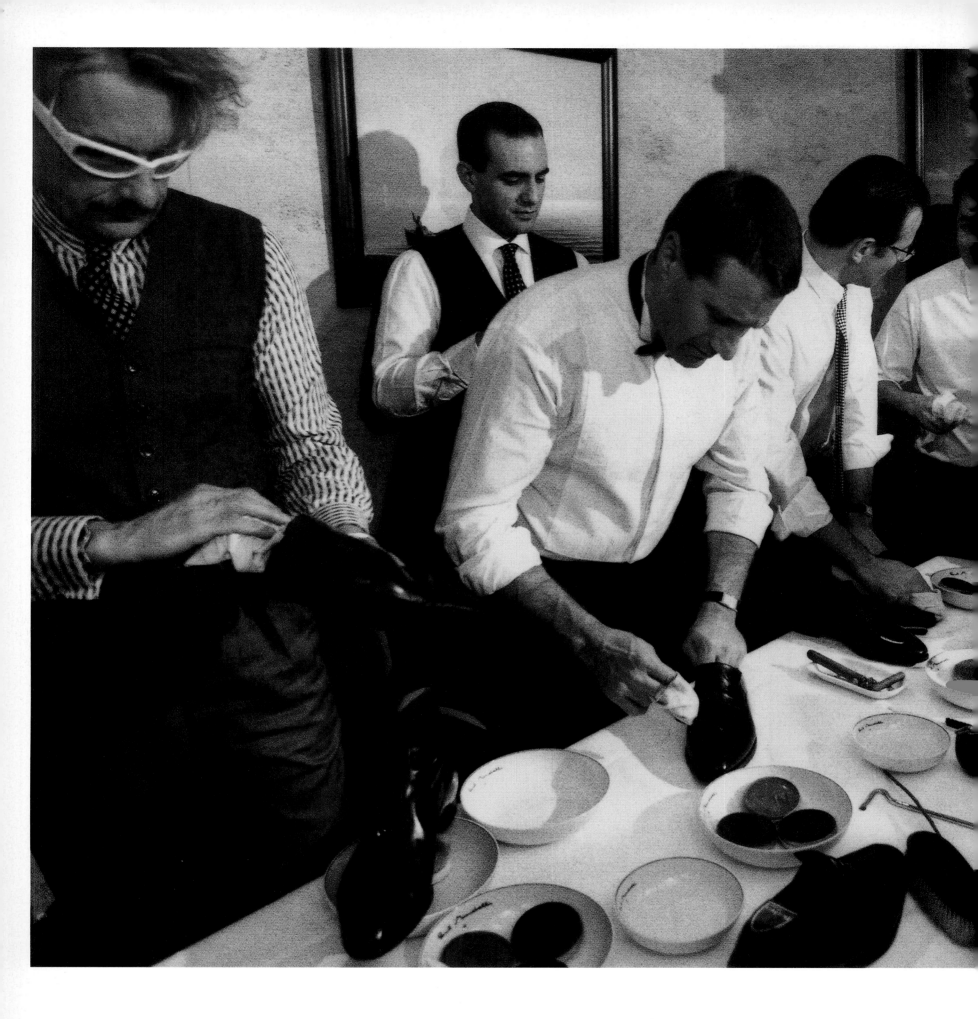

311. Members of the Swann Club during a polishing session at Paul Mincelli in 1996.

Page 264:

312. Louis Vuitton open checked pump. Paris, 1998.

International Shoe Museum, Romans.

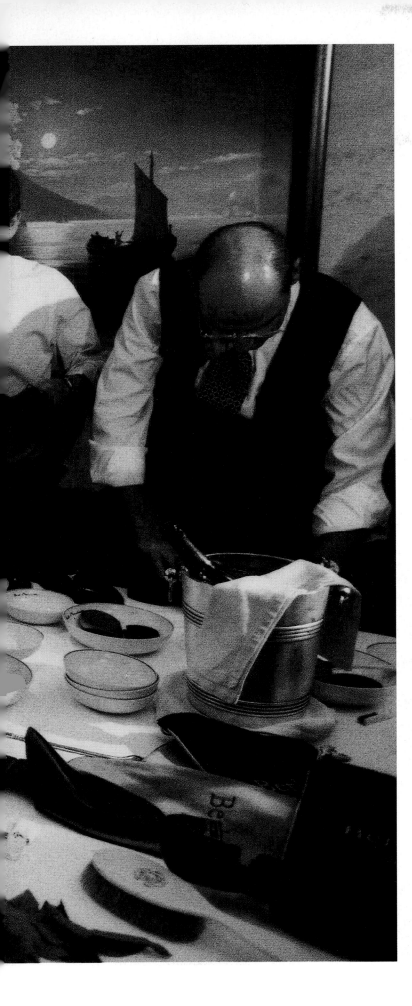

The Swann Club
Olga Berluti's Lessons in Polishing

The very special art of polishing shoes by moonlight invented by Olga Berluti sheds some light on her research into the art of polishing. Aficionados of beautiful shoes, during stops outside rue Marbeuf, would listen to Olga impart her knowledge in such romantic terms that they were swept away to another world. These meetings, at once professional, friendly, and animated, gave birth to the Swann club, in memory of the refined atmosphere in the works of Marcel Proust.

The one hundred members admitted to this circle of privileged aesthetes met once a year for a light-hearted lesson in polishing that was orchestrated by Olga's magic.

Always under moonlight, the faithful removed their shoes and placed them on a table. The table was covered with a white damask tablecloth whose brilliance was enhanced by the light from candelabras illuminating the ceremony's main event. Fingers were swaddled in squares of Venetian linen, immersed in wax, to massage the leathers. Then came buffing, at first using water but followed by champagne.

The entire Swann Club never came together at one time. Some lived far away, but eagerly made the trip. The location of the get togethers would change. Boredom was unheard of at these unique evenings, which provided a blissful moment of escape.

René Caty

Among the most famous names in fashion, Adolphe Carraz's shoe factory for expensive women's shoes opened in 1909 and employed thirty-two workers. Around 1931, through a family alliance, the firm became the company known as "Carraz et Caty." In 1948, it brought a new article to the market called the "ballerina," which quickly became a smashing success, peaking at the end of the 1950s.

The Continuity of Myths
Cinderella in China

Well before Charles Perrault and after Strabo, the 9th-century Chinese text relates an Asian version of the Cinderella myth. There once was a powerful man with two wives, each of whom had a daughter. One daughter was named Sheh-Hsien. When her parents died, Sheh-Hsien continued to live with her stepmother, who used to send her to draw water. One day Sheh-Hsien withdrew a fish with red fins and gold eyes. She carried the fish to a pond where everyday the fish would come when she called.

Taking advantage of Sheh-Hsien's absence, the stepmother killed the fish, ate it, and hid the fishbone under a manure heap. The young girl cried when she could no longer find her fish. Then a figure descended from the sky and told her to remove the fishbone from the manure heap and place it in her room where it would allow her to obtain her heart's desire. In this way, Sheh-Hsien obtained gold, pearls, and food.

Now her half-sister and her stepmother had gone to the village celebration leaving Sheh-Hsien to watch the house. While they were gone, she put on a blue dress and gold shoes and went to the celebration herself where her appearance left everyone speechless. In her haste to get back to the house before her stepmother and half-sister, she lost one of her gold shoes. The powerful king of a neighboring island purchased the shoe. In vain he tried it on all the young girls in his kingdom. In the end, he found the other shoe at Sheh-Hsien's house and married her.

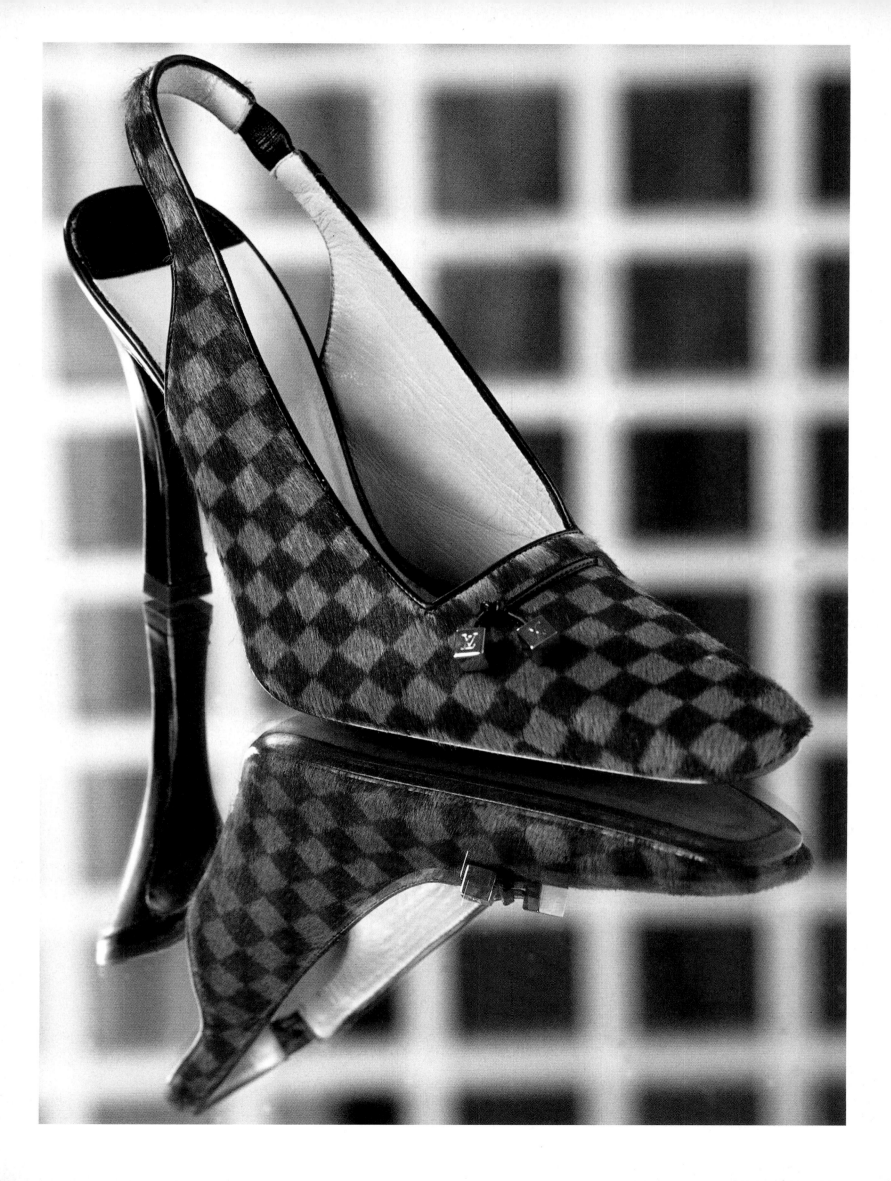

Glossary

Babouche

The babouche, "slipper of colored leather with neither quarter nor heal" (Littré), is probably of Iranian origin as proved by the Persian word PAPOUTCH (from *pa*, "foot" and *pouchiden*, "to cover").

Blake

Lyman Reed Blake (1835-1883), American technician who, in 1858, invented a machine to sew right through the insole to the sole using a chain stitch. His patents were acquired and subsequently perfected by Gordon Mackay.

Boot

Shoe covering the foot and the leg at the same time and rising to various heights.

Ankle boot

Woman's shoe very fashionable in winter since 1940. Strictly speaking, it is a short boot with a fur-lined interior, the fur-lining peeking out and serving as decoration.

Bottine

Small boot, of which the upper rises above the ankle to cover the calf at various heights, closed by lacing or buttoning. During the Middle Ages, bottines were called boots without soles that were slipped over the shoe like gaiters or houseaux.

In the 19th century, from the end of the Restoration, women wore bottines, whether of fine leather or fabric with or without heal, in following the mode. One found laced bottines and bottines with buttons, for which came the invention of the buttonhook.

At the beginning of the 20th century, women wore very elegant bottines with a high upper rising to the calf. The vogue of bottines began to disappear after the war of 1914-1918.

Buckle

Generally metallic accessory, with or without a tongue, which serves to fasten the shoe.

Ornamental buckle: buckle strictly for decoration.

During the 17th century, shoe buckles were most often made of precious metals. In 1670 and 1680, buckles replaced bows on top of shoes. They were decorated with an entourage of real or fake pearls and diamonds. For mourning, buckles were bronzed and without precious stones. Buckles, kept in jewelry cases, adapted to different shoes. Small and rectangular, they became round and oval in the 18th century, following the fashion. Their dimensions increased at the end of the reign of Louis XV and appeared square under Louis XVI. The buckles of men's shoes covered the foot under Louis XVI.

Floral toe

Toe adorned with perforations of different sizes. The origin of this name goes back to the beginning of the 20th century for the motif represented was most often of flowers.

Polishing brush

Horsehide brush used for shining shoes.

Shankpiece

Elongated piece of leather, wood, steel or plastic placed in the shank to give firmness to the arch of the shoe and support the arch of the foot.

Campagus

Ancient shoe worn in Rome. The campagus takes the shape of a bottine leaving the foot uncovered. Trimmed with fur, often decorated with pearls and precious stones, it is the shoe of generals. When crimson in color, it is reserved exclusively for emperors.

Shoehorn

Strip of metal, horn or plastic used to aid the foot in entering the shoe. According to the *Historical Dictionary of Arts, Trades and Professions Exercised in Paris since the 13th Century*, by Alfred Franklin, in the 16th century, a leather strap or a horn is used. A royal account of 1570 contained the following two notes: "for having cut a quarter of morocco leather hide, to make shoehorns to put in the wardrobe…", "for three horn shoehorns to serve the pageboys…"

Trévoux's dictionary (1704-1771) reproduced this passage almost word for word and added: "In the past one made it of horn and even of iron."

In a word, the Academy, in its 1778 edition, pointed to this proverb: It is inside without shoehorn, which means: "It succeeded with no trouble and more easily than one believed."

Slipper

Light and supple shoe suited to various uses: house slippers, ballet slippers, fencing slippers, bootees.

Interior, removable part of a ski boot or walking shoe assuring the tight and supple contact between the foot and the outer shell of the shoe.

Chopine

Woman's shoe worn in Venice in the 16th century, also called "stilted mule" or "cow's foot". These strange shoes, held to the foot by ribbons, demonstrate pedestals of an excessive height reaching up to fifty-two centimeters.

Chiquet

Small, not very high heel generally on flat, women's shoes.

Vamp

Top of a shoe, from the instep to the toe.

Espadrille

Cloth shoe with a braided rope sole worn throughout Spain and the Midi of France.

Stivali

In the 14th century, one called a stivali a light summer shoe. They were tall boots of supple hide or cloth, dyed in red or black and worn by both sexes.

Last-maker

Technician who creates or develops the lasts.
Manufacturer of lasts in industrial series.

Goodyear

Name of the patent (from the patronymic of the inventor) originally naming the method known as the Goodyear Welt.

In 1862, a patent is awarded to Auguste Detouy for a machine for sewing the leather sole by means of a curved needle. Charles Goodyear Junior (son of Charles Goodyear, American inventor of the process of the vulcanization of rubber) improves the method and registers a patent for a machine to sew the welt in 1869.
Louis Rama, in the *Technical Dictionary of Leather* gives the following technical definitions:
1 - hand-sewn welt:
type of manufacture in which the welt and the upper are hand-sewn on the wall of a plated insole.
2 - machine-sewn welt:
type of manufacture producing mechanically all of the operations of hand-sewing the welt on the wall of a plated insole.

Lacing

The most elegant horizontal lacing is typical of the oxford while lacing in the form of a cross is often used for derbies.

Ladrine

In the time of Louis XIII, when the wearing of boots was broad, this one rose to mid-leg and fell back like a funnel on the calf. It was called a ladrine or lazarine. The boot was decorated with useless spurs even worn to the ball and for which one made leather wheels to avoid tearing dresses.

Tongue

Until the end of the 15th century, shoes have tongues on the instep, usually tied by a string and which are called liripipes.

On an oxford or derby, instep's protective flap situated under the lacing.

On a loafer or moccasin without laces, part of the upper being an extension of the vamp that covers and hides the tightening elastic.

Mule

Light house shoe without quarter leaving the heel exposed.

Eyelet

Hollowed out, metal piece used to reinforce a perforation. Sometimes one places it in the lacing holes.

Throat

In shoe manufacture, the throat of a shoe is the extension of the vamp on the instep.

Buckle attachment strap

Short tie, sewn to a piece of the upper and folded in such a way as to form a part receiving a buckle

Pieds noirs (French settlers in North Africa)

It is not by chance that the descendants of North African settlers themselves (ah yes!) created this nickname for themselves that, supposedly, should have been given to them by the Arabs: Pieds noirs. So called for their solid shoes of "civilized" material as compared to the precarious babouches of the unworthy.

Pigage or Pigache

Shoe of the 12th century, with a pointed and hooked toe, sometimes decorated with a little bell and whose style goes back to antiquity.

Platform sole

Thick mid-sole, whose edge can be coated or decorated, inserted between the upper and the sole itself.

Size

Interior dimension of a shoe expressed in points and taking into account the length of the foot and its lengthening in a walk. Shoe size is expressed in points:
English point, sometimes also called wrongly American point: $1/3$ of an inch or 8.466 mm. French point or Paris point: $2/3$ of a centimeter or 6.666 mm.

Drawing bridge shoe (pont-levis)

Before Henri IV, men's shoes were heelless. At the end of the 16th century and the beginning of the 17th century, they were made heeled, leaving an empty space beneath the sole, which causes these shoes to be called drawbridge shoes (pont-levis).

Quarter

One of the two pieces symmetrically arranged that form the back of the upper and continue to the instep or thereabouts to close the shoe.

Rose

Under Louis XIII, to decorate men's and women's shoes, bows and ribbons are placed on the instep hiding the tie or buckle. Thus are formed shoe roses, often very big, gathered or goffered, resembling dahlias. Under Louis XIV, this mode is replaced by buckles.

Sable

Extremely fine method of weaving beads used in the 18th century for shoes and small objects: buckles, ornaments, etc...

Saint Crispin and saint Crispinian

Patron saints of shoe repairers, 1660. In *La Vie Parisienne*, operetta by Jacques Offenbach: "By saint Crispin, we arrive, and the way so as to dine put us in good spirits, by Saint Crispin…" (Final chorus Act II)

Sandal

Worn since Egyptian, Greek and Roman antiquity, this simplified shoe is made up of a sole and straps or strips of various widths and assembled in a variety of ways, between which the foot remains visible. Several religious orders still keep with the use of sandals.

Clog

Derived from the ancient soccus, shoes made of a wooden sole attached to the foot with straps.

Worn from the Middle Ages under leather soled chausses and shoes, they stay in use until the 17th century under town boots.

Soccus

Kind of slipper or shoe without any lacing entirely enclosing the foot. Worn in Greece by both sexes, in Rome it is reserved to women and comic actors, as opposed to the tragic cothurnus.

Solea

Roman sandal of the simplest form made up of a wooden sole with a string passing over the top of the foot.

Solleret

The solleret, formerly called pédieu, was, in the suit of armor, the part that imprisoned and protected the foot. First, it was a sort of steel gutter only protecting the instep and leaving the rest of the foot under the mail. This piece was then divided into several articulated lames forming a series of arches or a scorpion tail pointed toe in the 14th century and poulaines in the 15th century. Under Charles VIII, the solleret was spoon-billed, bear's footed until François I, then duckbilled. It disappeared under Charles IX.

Shoe

Covering for the foot but stopping at the instep.

Upper

As opposed to the sole, the superior part of the shoe, designed to dress and protect the top of the foot.

Boot hook

1- Hook that one passes through the bootstrap to help slip it on.
2- Sort of small plank having a notch in which one wedges one's shod foot to help remove one's boot.

Stirrup strap

Leather strap that fixes the foot in the process of manufacture or repair to the knees.

Welt

Small strip of leather sewn the length of the edge of a shoe's vamp to strengthen the sole.

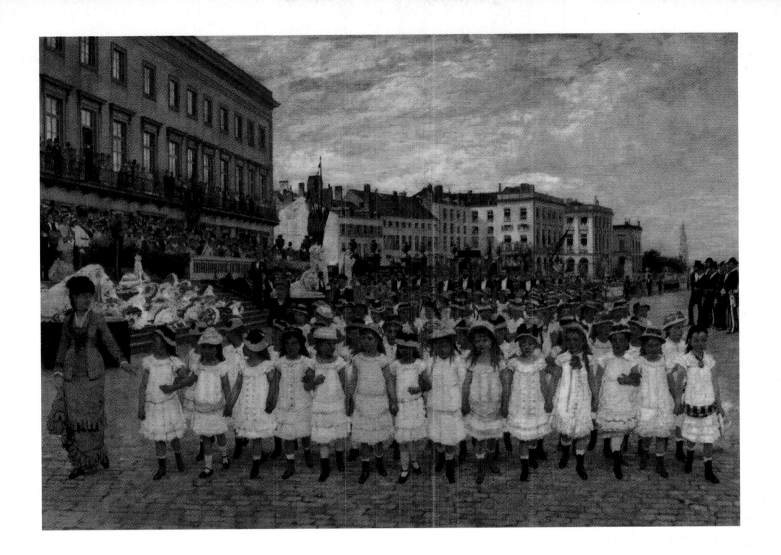

Bibliography

Marie-Josèphe Bossan, *Livre guide du musée international de la chaussure de Romans édité par l'association des amis du musée de Romans*, 1992.

François Boucher, *Histoire du costume*, Paris, 1965.

Eugénie Debouté, *Sans feu ni lieu un maître spirituel au temps de la Fronde – Jean-Antoine le Vachet*, Châtillon 1994

Yvonne Deslandres, *Le Talon et la mode*, 1980.

Catherine Férey – Simone Blazy, *Des objets qui racontent l'histoire*, Saint-Symphorien-sur-Coise, December 2000.

Paul and Jacqueline Galmiche, *La Saga du pied*. Erti, Paris 1983.

Victor Guillen, "La légende des sabots de Bethmale", in *Chausser*, Spezialausgabe.

Paul Lacroix, *Histoire des cordonniers*, Paris, 1852.

D. Pfister, "Les chaussures Coptes", in *Revue de l'Institut de Calcéologie n° 3*, 1986.

William Rossi, *Érotisme du pied et de la chaussure*, Cameron Sait Amand Montrond, 1978.

Jean-Paul Roux, *La Chaussure*, Paris, 1980.

Marie-Louise Teneze, "Cycle de Cendrillon", in *Bulletin n° 1 de l'Institut de Calcéologie*, 1982.

Marie-Louise Teneze, "Le Chat botté", in *Bulletin n° 2 de l'Institut de Calcéologie*, 1984.

Marie-Louise Teneze, "Le Petit Poucet", in *Bulletin n° 3 de l'Institut de Calcéologie*, 1986.

Jean-Marc Thévenet, *Rêves de Pompes, Pompes de Rêves*, Paris 1988.

Gabriel Robert Thibault, "L'exaltation d'un mythe: Rétif de La Bretonne et le soulier couleur rose." *in Bulletin n° 4 de l'Institut de Calcéologie*, 1990.

Loszlo Vass and Magda Molnar, *La chaussure pour homme faite main*, Germany, 1999.

Correspondance de Pasteur, gesammelt und mit Anmerkungen versehen von Pasteur Vallery-Radot, Flammarion, 1951.

Le Musée, la Chapelle funéraire, Institut Pasteur.

Dictionnaire de la Mode au XXe siècle, Paris 1994.

La Mode et l'enfant, 1780-2000, Musée Galliera, Musée de la Mode de la ville de Paris, April 2001.

Le Soulier de Marie-Antoinette, Caen – Musée des beaux-arts, Caen 1989.

XVIIᵉ siècle, Lagarde and Michard, Bordas.

XIXᵉ siècle, Lagarde and Michard, Bordas.

XXᵉ siècle, Lagarde and Michard, Leonard Danel Loos (Nord), 1962.

Grammaire des styles
– *Le costume de la Restauration à la Belle époque.*
– *Le costume de 1914 aux années folles.*
– *4000 ans d'histoire de la chaussure*, Château de Blois, 1984.

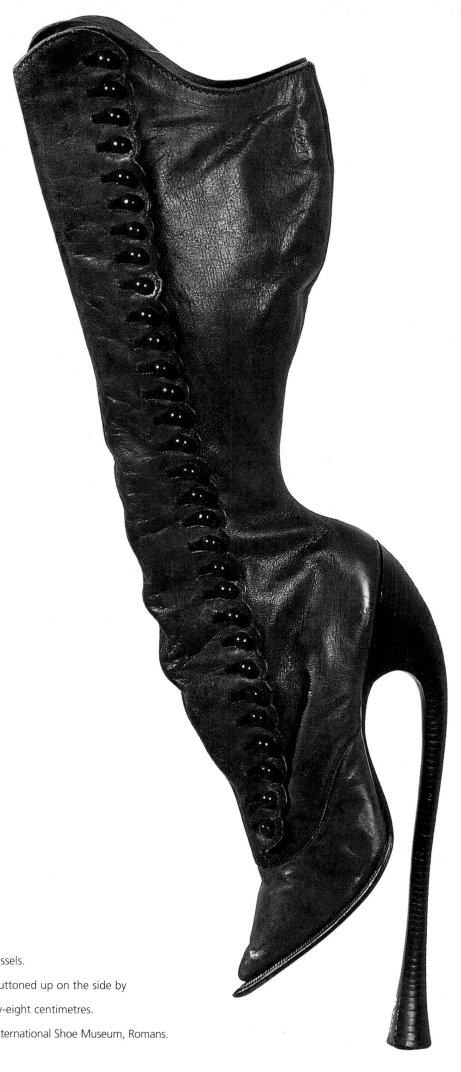

Page 267:

313. Jan Verhas. *The Review of Schools*, 1878.

Royal Museums of Fine Arts of Belgium, Brussels.

314. Fetishist boots, unsuitable for the market, buttoned up on the side by

thirty-two fastenings. Height of heel: twenty-eight centimetres.

Vienna, Austria, c. 1900. Guillen Collection. International Shoe Museum, Romans.

Photograph: Joel Garnier.

Table of Contents

Note of Thanks

Association des amis du musée de Romans, Véronique Auroux, Association Charles Trenet, Mouna Ayoub, Muriel Barbier (Musée Galliera), Laure Bassal, Guy Blazy (Conservateur en chef du Musée des Tissus et des Arts Décoratifs de Lyon), Simone Blazy, (Conservateur en chef du Musée Gadagne, Lyon), Docteur Jean Bénichou, Galerie Berès, Paris, Olga Berluti, Henri Bertholet (Maire de Romans), Georgy Bidegain, Paul Bocuse, Bon Marché Rive Gauche, Olivier Bouissou (Délégué général de la Fédération française de la chaussure, Commissaire général du MIDEC et de Mod'Amont), Docteur Simon Braun, Pierre Brissot, Stéphanie Busuttil, Marie-Noëlle de Cagny (Bureau de style, chaussure maroquinerie cuir, Paris), Jean-Claude Carrière, Professeur Jean-Paul Carret, Pierre Caty, Charles Jourdan, Centre historique de la résistance en Drôme et de la Déportation, Centre Technique du Cuir, Lyon, Professeur Guy Chouinard, Robert Clergerie, Le Conseil National du Cuir, Patrick Cox, Astrid Sarkis Der Balian, Kegetzique Sarkis Der Balian, Sophie Descamps (Conservateur au département des antiquités grecques et romaines, Musée du Louvre), Henri Ducret, Thierry Dufresne, Jean-Pierre Dupré, Pierre Durand, Françoise Durand, Fabienne Falluel (Conservateur au Musée Galliera, Paris), La Fédération française de la chaussure, Ferragamo, Marc Folachier, Elisabeth Foucart (Conservateur en chef au département des peintures, Musée du Louvre), Jacques Foucart (Conservateur général au département des peintures, Musée du Louvre), Jean-Paul Foulhoux, Ginko, Pascal Giroud, Dominique Goberthier, Bernard Gouttenoire, François Gravier, Cécile Guinard (Musée de Romans), Nicole Hechberg (chargée du Centre de documentation du musée de Romans), Claude James, Véronique Jeammet (Conservateur au département des antiquités grecques et romaines, Musée du Louvre), Claudette Joannis (Conservateur en chef du Patrimoine, Adjoint au Directeur du Musée de Malmaison et Bois-Préau), Roland Jourdan, Daly Jourdan-Barry, Isabelle Julia (Conservateur à l'Inspection Générale des Musées), Stéphane Kélian, Geneviève Lacambe (Conservateur général du Patrimoine), Christiane Laffont (Adjointe chargée de l'urbanisme, du patrimoine et des arts plastiques), Françoise Laigle (journaliste), Karl Lagerfeld, Lydie Laupies, André Laurencin (Conservateur honoraire du Musée Denon), Bénédicte Leblan, Christian Lebon, Sylvie Lefranc (Fondatrice et ancienne Directrice du Bureau de style chaussure maroquinerie cuir, Paris), Éric Le Marec, Jeannie Longo, Françoise Maison (Conservateur en chef chargé des collections du Second Empire, Château de Compiègne), Christiane Marandet (Conservateur général honoraire du patrimoine), Suzanne Marest (Styliste conseil au Bureau de style chaussure maroquinerie cuir, Paris), Laurence Massaro, Raymond Massaro, Docteur Jacques Mazade, André Meunier, Docteur Jean-Jacques Morel, Comte et Comtesse Moussine-Pouchkine, Musée d'art et d'histoire, Genève, Musée Bally, Schoenenwerd (Suisse), Musée de l'Homme, Paris, Rosita Nenno (Conservateur Musée Allemand du Cuir et de la Chaussure, Offenbach), Catherine Perrochet (Musée de Romans), Anne Rondet, Annick Perrot (Conservateur du Musée Pasteur), Andrea Pfister, Patrick Pichavant, Pascal Pitou, Hervé Racine, Stefania Ricci (Conservateur du Musée Salvatore Ferragamo), Huguette Rouit, Joël Roux, Jean-Paul Roux (Directeur de recherche honoraire au CNRS, Professeur titulaire honoraire de la chaire des Arts Islamiques à l'École du Louvre), Le Service Communication de la Ville de Romans, Brigitte et Jean Schoumann, Alexandre Siranossian (Directeur de l'École nationale de musique et de danse), Docteur Tan Sivy, Jean Tchilinguirian, Henri Terres, Françoise Tétart-Vittu (Chargée du Cabinet des arts graphiques au Musée Galliera, Paris), Olivier Thinus, Tod's, Pierre Troisgros, Gérard Turpin, Gérard Benoît-Vivier.